# Freud and the Scene of Trauma

# Freud and the Scene of Trauma

*John Fletcher*

FORDHAM UNIVERSITY PRESS

NEW YORK 2013

Fordham University Press has no responsibility for the persistence or accuracy of URLs for external or third-party Internet
websites referred to in this publication and does not guarantee
that any content on such websites is, or will remain, accurate or
appropriate.

Fordham University Press also publishes its books in a variety of
electronic formats. Some content that appears in print may not
be available in electronic books.

Library of Congress Cataloging-in-Publication Data

Fletcher, John, 1948 January 2- author.
    Freud and the scene of trauma / John Fletcher. — First edition.
        p. ; cm.
    Includes bibliographical references and index.
    ISBN 978-0-8232-5459-0 (cloth : alk. paper) —
    ISBN 978-0-8232-5460-6 (pbk. : alk. paper)
    I. Title.
    [DNLM: 1. Freud, Sigmund, 1856–1939.   2. Freudian
Theory—history.   3. Hysteria—psychology.   4. Medicine in
Art.   5. Medicine in Literature.   6. Stress Disorders,
Traumatic—psychology. WM 460.5.F9]
    RC532
    616.85'24—dc23

                                                        2013024365

Printed in the United States of America

15  14  13      5  4  3  2  1

First edition

*In Memoriam*
*Jean Laplanche (1924–2012)*

CONTENTS

FIGURES

# ACKNOWLEDGMENTS

To Iain Bruce for four decades of love and companionship, generosity and *cordon bleu* cooking, without whom this book might not have had a consistent referencing system, an index, or any illustrations.

To Nicholas Ray, a fellow 'Laplanchean,' and collaborator, for his helpful comments on an early draft, his intellectual comradeship, resourcefulness, and staying power in hard times.

To Judith Butler and Peter Fonagy, who very kindly read various drafts and versions of this book, my gratitude for their support and encouragement.

To generations of students, both undergraduate and postgraduate, who took courses with me on Literature and Psychoanalysis, Freud's Metapsychology, Psychoanalysis and Cultural production or wrote dissertations and theses in the field, many of whom were enthusiastic, some of whom claimed it changed their lives, and some of whom swore never to do it again.

The project for this book first emerged, backwards and unexpected, out of a research term funded by the old Arts and Humanities Research Board to enable the writing of a theoretical introduction to a collection of my essays but which turned into something else. They wanted immediate product, upfront, and were not best pleased. Ten years later, here it is. Thinking and writing take time.

Thanks to the University of Warwick for two periods of research leave to work on and complete this project.

A previous version of Chapter 5 appeared as "The Scenography of Trauma: A 'Copernican' Reading of Sophocles' *Oedipus the King*," *Textual Practice* 21, no. 1 (2007): 17–41.

A previous version of Chapter 12 appeared as "Freud, Hoffmann and the Deathwork," *Angelaki* 7, no. 2 (August 2002): 125–41.

This book is a study of the central role of trauma in Freud's thought. It argues that it is Freud's mapping of trauma *as a scene*, the elaboration of a *scenography* of trauma, that is central to both his clinical interpretation of his patients' symptoms and his construction of successive theoretical models and concepts to explain the power of such scenes in his patients' lives. This attention to the scenic *form* of trauma, and its power in the determination of neurotic symptoms, presides over Freud's break from the neurological model of trauma he inherited from Charcot. It also helps explain the affinity that Freud and many since him have felt between psychoanalysis and literature (and artistic production more generally) and the privileged role of literature at certain moments in the development of his thought.

A number of alternative theoretical models are to be found in Freud's work: traumatic seduction, screen memory, inherited primal fantasy (*Urphantasie*), the individually constructed originary fantasy (*ursprüngliche Phantasie*). All involve the analysis of sequences of scenes layered one upon the other in the manner of a textual palimpsest, with claims to either material or psychical reality. The notion of a 'primal scene,' a central term for this study (which argues that it has been misconstrued by later generations of psychoanalysts), designates the site of a trauma that deposits an alien and disturbing element in the suffering subject. These signifying traces of the seductive or traumatizing other person resist assimilation and binding into the ego's narcissistic structures and personal archives; they function as an internal foreign body and so give rise to deferred or belated aftereffects. Trauma, involving the breaching of psychical boundaries by an excessive excitation and leading to an unmasterable repetition, characterizes both Freud's first encounter with sexuality under the sign of seduction and with the death drive under the various forms of the compulsion to repeat, from the negative clinical transference to shell shock and war trauma.

The book begins with the figure of Charcot and the role of key psychological elements in his predominantly neurological model of trauma and traumatic hysteria. It was Freud's encounter with Charcot and his treatment of hysteria, in Paris in 1885–86, that turned him from a career that had been based on laboratory dissection, the anatomy of the central nervous system in the lower animals (eels and crayfish) to a concern with hysteria as a psychological condition based on traumatic shock and the operation of unconscious ideas, although he continued throughout the1890s to do highly regarded neurological work on infantile brain diseases. Freud was to break from Charcot to develop a properly psychological theory of hysteria (and, by extension, all psychopathology) based on the operation of traumatic memories and their affects. The problem, both clinical and theoretical, that confronted Freud was the status of the 'scenes' that his patients reproduced, either through recall and association or through acting out. His model of traumatic causality gains in complexity in the texts of 1895–97, especially through the elaboration of a traumatic temporality with the concept of *Nachträglichkeit* (deferred action/afterwardsness). At the same time it is progressively narrowed to a sexual etiology of seduction/abuse in childhood, Freud's notorious 'seduction theory.' Along with the problems of his clinical practice, the development of a concept of fantasy internal to the model of traumatic seduction precipitates the crisis or turning point of September 1897, in which Freud privately rejects his seduction theory in a letter to Wilhelm Fliess. Freud falls silent in public, but in his correspondence with Fliess and his self-analysis he oscillates between the model of traumatic memory and its repudiation in a turn to an emergent model of infantile sexuality. Here he proposes as a 'universal event' an emotional configuration that is not until 1910 labeled the 'Oedipus complex,' but which in the crisis months of late 1897 is outlined through a brief commentary on Sophocles's *Oedipus the King* and Shakespeare's *Hamlet*. This turn to tragedy as a model of male subjectivity is more fully elaborated in *The Interpretation of Dreams* (1900). It crystallizes a shift in focus from symptom to subjectivity, from the narrower field of psychopathology to a concern with psychical structure and a developmental model of sexuality as such in the *Three Essays* of 1905.

This book also examines a second crisis or turning point, that of 1919–20. Here the turn to literature (E. T. A. Hoffmann and the associated aesthetic question of the uncanny) accompanies the return of trauma under the rubric of the compulsion to repeat and the death drive. At both moments of theoretical crisis and change (1897 and 1919) Freud turns to literary texts that exemplify a repeated pattern of traumatic scenes and that dramatize precisely a traumatic scenography. He then submits his chosen texts to an 'oedipal' reading that marginalizes or excludes the 'daemonic' repetition that characterizes them. The book argues that Freud's engagement with literature at key moments of theoretical impasse and crisis, as well as his long study of Leonardo da Vinci, constitutes thought experiments in the imaginary space of literature and painting. When the chosen works of Sophocles, Shakespeare, Hoffmann, and da Vinci are read in the light of the tension verging on conflict in Freud's thought, between what Jean Laplanche has called a 'Copernican' or other-centered model of trauma and a 'Ptolemaic' or self-centered model of development, the insights of his rejected 'traumatology' return to challenge and disturb his dominant developmentalist framework. It will be argued that the texts to which Freud is drawn both invite and resist his oedipal readings, while themselves bearing imaginative witness to the foundational relation to the traumatic or seductive other, even as Freud's readings refocus them on the impulses of the centered, single individual.

Where conventional accounts often see the repudiation of the theory of traumatic seduction as the maturing, if not the foundation, of psychoanalysis as such, this book develops the thesis of Jean Laplanche that in this shift from a traumatic to a developmental model, along with the undoubted gains embodied in the theory of infantile sexuality, there were crucial losses, specifically, the recognition of the role of the adult other and the traumatic encounter with adult sexuality that is entailed in the ordinary nurture and formation of the infantile subject. It also argues that Freud's attention to the power of scenes—scenes of memory, scenes of fantasy—persists, both in his general psychology of dreaming and his major case studies. Along with this persistent Freudian 'scenography' is the recurrent surfacing, at different moments of his thought, of key elements of the officially abandoned model of trauma.

The conceptual focus for the book arose out of an engagement with the work of Jean Laplanche, beginning with the classic essay coauthored with J.-B. Pontalis on fantasies of origin, "Fantasy and the Origins of Sexuality," around which an important Anglophone anthology was built, *Formations of Fantasy*, edited by Victor Burgin, James Donald, and Cora Kaplan (London: Methuen, 1986). Its immediate context is my long-term project of translating and presenting Laplanche's work to an Anglophone public: *Jean Laplanche: Seduction, Translation and the Drives*, coedited with Martin Stanton (London: ICA, 1992); Jean Laplanche, *Essays on Otherness*, edited with an introduction by John Fletcher (London: Routledge, 1999); a special issue of *New Formations* 48, "Jean Laplanche and the Theory of Seduction," which translates and presents the work of Laplanche and his co-thinkers, published in 2003; and, most recently, *Freud and the Sexual: Essays 2000–2006* (New York: IP Books, 2011). My overview of Laplanche's revision of Freudian metapsychology that situates him in relation to Freud, "Seduction and the Vicissitudes of Translation: The Work of Jean Laplanche," appeared in *Psychoanalytic Quarterly* 76, no. 1 (2007): 1241–91.

Laplanche's work, as will be obvious to any reader, is therefore a recurrent reference point, and its insights into the logic of trauma, its topography, temporal dimensions, and fundamental relation to the other are an incitement to the book's tracing of the evolution, disappearances, and serial returns of the traumatic in Freud's work. My enthusiasm for a Freudian scenography, however, is not something that the late Laplanche would probably have shared.

# Freud and the Scene of Trauma

*Freud's Scenographies*

"Everything goes back to the reproduction of scenes."[1]

On January 24, 1897, at the high point of his commitment to the theory of infantile seduction as the cause of the major forms of psychopathology, Freud wrote to Wilhelm Fliess, his intimate friend and long-term correspondent:

> The early period before the age of 1½ years is becoming ever more significant. . . . Thus I was able to trace back, with certainty, a hysteria that developed in the context of a periodic mild depression to a seduction, which occurred for the first time at 11 months and [I could] hear again the words that were exchanged between two adults at that time! It is as though it comes from a phonograph. (Masson 1985a, 226)

It is an extraordinary claim, but not for its postulation of traumatic aftereffects resulting from very early sexual abuse (nothing surprising there), nor even for its confidence in obtaining such detailed information about a long past event (Fliess is not told if it was obtained from the patient only, or whether it was corroborated by another source as some of Freud's inferences and his analysands' memories often were). Freud's claim is extraordinary because of its *form*. This goes beyond the postulation of a causal event

1. Letter of May 2, 1897. *The Complete Letters of Sigmund Freud to Wilhelm Fliess 1887–1904*, trans. and ed. Jeffrey Moussaieff Masson (Cambridge, Mass.: Harvard University Press, 1985), 239. Henceforth, Masson (1985a).

impacting on the organism in the form of visible damage, as in traditional medical models of physical trauma (the literal meaning of the word is a wound or break in the organism's skin surface or boundaries). It also differs from neurological models of trauma, where shocks to the nervous system produced a range of belated contractures, paralyses, and anesthesias (the prototypical incident here was the railway accident). In these models of trauma the explanation involves a relatively direct cause-and-effect relation, even if as in Charcot's model of traumatic hysteria the symptoms appeared belatedly after a time lapse or an incubation period. What we have here, however, are not so much the aftereffects of a causal event in the past as the activity in the present of a *scene* played out with all the immediacy of a present event. In the instance Freud cites here, it takes the form of an adult dialogue that could not have been understood let alone remembered, in any ordinary sense of the word, by an infant of eleven months. Nevertheless, Freud claims, a dialogue is reproduced with such vividness "as though it comes from a phonograph" (we are not told through the medium of what inscriptions, although he calls it a "case of epileptiform convulsions," thus indicating its presenting symptoms). This emphasis on the present effectivity of *scenes* is also apparent in Freud's turn of phrase in the following letter, "Imagine, *I obtained a scene* about the circumcision of a girl," and in the previous letter he writes of a patient, "Eckstein *has a scene* where the diabolus sticks needles into her fingers" (my emphasis, Masson 1985a, 227, 225).

Unlike the railway accident, what is involved is not just the shock of a physical impact and its accompanying affect of fright but the human and signifying effect of other persons, their interactions and intentions, however opaque or incomprehensible. In a letter four months later (April 6, 1897), Freud comments that what had previously escaped him about hysterical *fantasies* was that they often "go back to things that children overhear at an early age and understand only subsequently [*nachträglich* – JF]. The age at which they take in information of this kind is, strangely enough, from six to seven months on!" (234). Here it is the exciting but incomprehensible speech of adults that implants the traumatic seed of later hysteria.

Where the emphasis in the previous scene is on hearing and exchanged words, other scenes that Freud retells to Fliess, as in this from the letter of December 22, 1897, have the visual dimensions of a tableau:

The intrinsic authenticity of infantile trauma is borne out by the following little incident which the patient claims to have observed as a three-year-old child. She goes into a darkened room where her mother is carrying on and eavesdrops. She has good reasons for identifying with this mother. . . . The mother *now* stands in the room and shouts: "Rotten criminal, what do you want from me? I will have no part of that. Just whom do you think you have in front of you?" Then she tears the clothes from her body with one hand, while with the other she presses them against it, which creates a very peculiar impression. Then she stares at a certain spot in the room, her face contorted by rage, covers her genitals with one hand and pushes something away with the other. Then she raises both hands, claws at the air and bites it. Shouting and cursing, she bends over far backward, again covers her genitals with her hand, whereupon she falls over forward, so that her head almost touches the floor; finally, she quietly falls over backward onto the floor. Afterward she wrings her hands, sits down in a corner, and with her features distorted with pain she weeps.

For the child the most conspicuous phase is when the mother, standing up, is bent over forward. She sees that the mother keeps her toes strongly turned *inward*! (Masson 1985a, 288–89)[2]

Freud's reason for retelling this terrible scene is its confirmation of the "authenticity of infantile trauma," of the perverse and often violent scenes that featured in so many of his analyses. At least three moments are linked together here: the enigmatic tableau that the mother enacts and on which the small child uncomprehendingly stumbles; the shadowy 'primal scene' behind the frozen moment of the mother's tableau; and its persistence and retelling, now, in the present moment of the analysis by the adult daughter. A fourth moment can also be postulated, that of Freud's retelling to Fliess, affirming once again the reality of infantile trauma, in the attempt to resolve his uncertainty about the status of these scenes as either 'real events' or 'fantasies.' However, there is more to the letter than a move in a theoretical

---

2. To bring out the sequence of the scene, I have cut the following, which makes clear the basis for her identification with her mother: "The father belongs to the category of *men who stab women*, for whom bloody injuries are an erotic need. When she was two years old, he brutally deflowered her and infected her with his gonorrhea, as a consequence of which she became ill and her life was endangered by the loss of blood and vaginitis" (Masson 1985a, 288).

debate, or, rather, the latter is in part driven by Freud's palpable need to pass this haunting scene on to someone else, to unburden himself and bear witness to its distress. He ends the letter with a quotation from Goethe's *Mignon*:

> A new motto: "What has been done to you, poor child?"
> Enough of my filthy stories.[3]

The scene in the darkened room remembered by the daughter is the mother's acting out of a tableau, which has an arrested or fixated quality. Something is being repeated that one feels has been repeated many times before, like a compulsive ritual. In her solitude the mother is, nevertheless, not alone, for she addresses and cries out against an absent presence. The small witness does not understand what is happening, but her attention is drawn to certain "conspicuous" details, such as her mother's "toes turned strongly *inward*," to a certain action of the hands, "which creates a very peculiar impression." The mother's postures and gestures are enigmatic signs whose meanings are not spoken but acted out, and which seem to belong elsewhere, to another scene, whose violence shadows the repetitive tableau in the darkened room, and where those puzzling signs would regain some of their lost meaning if not their origins. Freud comments on the foreclosure of meaning here by comparing it to the "Russian censorship" exercised over foreign newspapers at the frontier: "Words, whole clauses and sentences are blacked out so that the rest becomes unintelligible." By analogy, Freud argues that "a Russian censorship of that kind comes about in psychoses and produces the apparently meaningless *deliria*" (289).

Freud attempts to read this tableau and its foreclosed meanings, through both the uncomprehending gaze of the child and the retrospective narration of his now grown-up patient, with an attention and expectation attuned by his understanding of the hysterical attack derived from Charcot's model of traumatic hysteria, and elaborated by Breuer and himself in their *Studies on Hysteria*, published almost two years previously in 1895. In this early account the attack is the reproduction of a scene, which is assumed

---

3. I quote here from an alternative translation provided in Masson's earlier book, *The Assault on Truth: Freud's Suppression of the Seduction Theory* (Harmondsworth: Penguin Books, 1985), 117.

to be both the moment of the hysterical symptoms' first appearance and therefore their origin. In the course of the intervening two years Freud's developing account of hysteria had dislocated this direct causal connection in ways that we will consider later, but which still anchored it in a specifiable traumatic event of external origin (albeit of a very particular kind).

> Can one doubt that the father forces the mother to submit to anal intercourse? Can one not recognize in the mother's attack the separate phases of the assault: first the attempt to get at her from the front; then pressing her down from the back and penetrating between her legs, which forced her to turn her feet inward. Finally, how does the patient know that in attacks one usually enacts both persons (*self*-injury, *self*-murder), as occurred here in that the woman tears off her clothes with one hand, like the assailant, and with the other holds onto them, as she herself did at the time? (Masson 1985a, 289)

The apparent meaninglessness of the mother's distraught behavior, her speech to a hallucinated other person, makes sense for Freud as the reproduction of an earlier scene of sexual violence, of marital assault, which he reconstructs through its repetitions, the layers and relays of its transmission. What governs Freud's selection of the clinical material for retelling to Fliess is a concern with the "authenticity" of the traumatic tableau witnessed by the child, and its relation to its other scene. Freud reads the mother's postures as the signs of particular forms of adult sexual assault, first frontal and then finally from the rear, which would be unintelligible to the child. Even more telling for Freud are the mother's gestures, so striking and "peculiar" for the child, which exemplify a crucial fact about the processes of identification in play in a hysterical attack. "How does the patient know that in attacks one usually enacts both persons . . . as occurred here?" This feature of the clinical material is significant at this point for Freud because it appears to confirm the scene's authenticity, to bear witness to psychological processes that the child and later the analysand would have no knowledge of. Freud's wondering question implies: How could she reproduce such telling details unless she had actually witnessed such a scene, which itself bears traces, signs, of an even earlier scene? Consequently, he concludes both that his patient had witnessed as a child the scene she describes her mother performing, and that such a scene itself bears testimony through its form and significant details to an earlier scene of which the child is not aware but which can be inferred from the fixated, repetitive response of its adult victim. Freud's focus in the letter is not on the child's experience of abuse referred to in passing but to her witnessing of her mother's scene of hallucinatory repetition. Of course Freud is writing a compressed clinical anecdote in a private letter and not a publicly presented and elaborated case study, so we have no access to the daughter's own network of associations and emotions connected with the incident (one might have wondered whether her own experience of paternal abuse might not have been reactivated by or resonated within her experience of this strange maternal scene). What is so striking about the anecdote, and prefigures the argument of this book, is the structure of repetition in which a past moment is not so much the absent past cause of present effects but is acted out and appears to be immediately present and alive as a current event.

One of the surprising things about this second letter is its date, December 22, 1897. In the eleven months between it and the letter I began by quoting, Freud had written his famous repudiation of his seduction theory in the letter of September 21, 1897, giving Fliess four reasons why he no longer believed in the scenes of early child sexual abuse on which the chains of association and inference in his clinical cases seemed to converge (discussed in Chapter 4). Even more striking is that in a series of letters in October and November, Freud formulates the germ of the Oedipus complex (complete with references to Sophocles's *Oedipus* and Shakespeare's *Hamlet*), of infantile pregenital sexuality and of 'normal' (i.e., nontraumatic) repression, which were to replace the seduction theory and become the cornerstone of classical Freudian psychoanalysis. Yet here again in December, some three months after his letter of repudiation, we find Freud compelled by the structure of scenic repetition, by the relay from scene to scene, to reaffirm "the intrinsic authenticity of infantile trauma" *in the face of his own previous objections.*

As the letters to Fliess throughout the late 1890s testify, despite the famous repudiation and turning point of September 1897, Freud returns again and again to the hypothesis of an originary traumatic event and the uncovering of later scenes in which it appears to be encoded. As late as January 8, 1900 (at the time of the publication of *The Interpretation of Dreams*), Freud is writing: "In E's case, the second genuine scene is coming up after years of preparation; and it is one which may *perhaps* be confirmed objectively by asking his elder sister. Behind it a third long-suspected scene approaches" (395). We have the same palimpsestic structure of scene upon scene, and the same patience as of an archaeologist slowly uncovering sedi- mented layers and deposits (two sentences previously Freud had written: "In the evenings I read prehistory and the like, without any serious pur- pose"). Even *after* his so-called 'abandonment' of the seduction theory (an- nounced privately to Fliess in September 1897) had become public and official in 1906,[4] Freud still pursues and seeks to reconstruct originary or 'primal' scenes that operate with the force and structure of psychical trau- mas, in case studies such as that of the Rat Man (1909) and the Wolf Man (1918). Laplanche and Pontalis were the first to point to this persistence of key elements of the 'abandoned' theory in Freud's later work and to attempt a structural explanation of it, while Maria Torok and Nicholas Rand have traced the recurrent oscillation between fantasy and the external event in Freud's thought.[5]

The question of the abandonment of the so-called seduction theory is often described in terms of a simple turn or change of mind, from sexual seduction by an adult in childhood as a causal paradigm or etiology for psychopathology to oedipal wishes and fantasies directed at the parents. Unfortunately Freud himself is largely responsible for this misleadingly simplified account. The further he moved away from his earlier theory, both in time and in thought, the more he was prone to give a misleadingly polarized retrospect on his now long abandoned 'error' and to present it in terms of a mutually exclusive opposition between fantasy and the real event. "On the History of the Psycho-Analytic Movement" (1914d) and *An Autobiographical Study* (1925d) in particular misrepresent both the complex- ity of the theory and the nature of the clinical materials on which it was

4. "My Views on the Part Played by Sexuality in the Aetiology of the Neuroses" (1906a), *SE* 7, 269–79.

5. Jean Laplanche and J-B. Pontalis, "Fantasy and the Origins of Sexuality" (1964), trans. in *International Journal of Psychoanalysis* 49 (1968), reprinted in Victor Burgin et al., eds., *Formations of Fantasy* (London: Methuen, 1986), and in Riccardo Steiner, ed., *Unconscious Phantasy* (London: Karnac Books, 2003); also see Nicholas Rand and Maria Torok, "The Concept of Psychical Reality and Its Traps," in *Questions for Freud* (Cam- bridge, Mass.: Harvard University Press, 1997, 24–44).

based. On either side of the so-called theoretical break or turn of September 1897, however, there is an array of closely related concepts, ranging from an increasingly complex model of trauma to the model of the screen memory, of primal fantasy (*Urphantasie*), of originary fantasy (*ursprünglich Phantasie*), and of transference, in which elements of memory and fantasy combine in different ways and repeat. In particular, in both trauma and the various forms of fantasy, what we find is the power of scenes, of a certain scenography, its capacity to conscript the individual and to replicate itself at different levels of the psychical apparatus, generating a force of repetition, a repetition-compulsion, that is to disrupt Freud's clinical practice and transform his metapsychology. It is to the development of this repertoire of concepts that we will now turn.

# Part I    The Power of Scenes

# Charcot's Hysteria: Trauma and the Hysterical Attack

Freud refers to the hallucinatory scene in the darkened room discussed in the Prologue as an 'attack,' and his theory of the hysterical attack, closely related to the notions of trauma and traumatic neurosis, derives from the work of the great French neurologist Jean-Martin Charcot (1825–93). Freud studied with Charcot for five months from October 1885 to February 1886 at La Salpêtrière in Paris, the vast women's hospital for nervous diseases with its five thousand resident 'incurables.' Freud's experience there under the influence of Charcot was a turning point for him. It initiated a shift from his medical training and laboratory experience within the field of neurology, with its concern with the anatomical structure of the brain and its relation to the central nervous system, to the problem of psychopathology, in particular, hysteria, the effects of trauma, and the practice of hypnotism. While Freud continued to make contributions to neurology for the next ten years or so and to gain a considerable reputation in the field, dealing in particular with the brain diseases of children, his passion was now for the study and clinical treatment of the psychoneuroses.

Charcot held the Chair in Neuropathology, established especially for him in recognition of his foundational role as "a unique organiser in the history of a new discipline ... the constructor of a medical speciality," and in acknowledgment of the importance of his work in consolidating neurology, the study of the nervous system and its diseases (neuropathology), as an autonomous medical field.[1] Charcot had won his reputation as a great identifier and classifier of nervous diseases, assigning each its typical clinical picture, based on its distinctive complex of symptoms, establishing the fully developed or extreme 'type' and then the various deviations from it. As Freud wrote,"with these types as a point of departure, the eye could travel over the long series of ill-defined cases—the *'formes frustes'*—which, branching off from one or other characteristic feature of the type, melt away into indistinctness."[2] In his admiring obituary of Charcot, two volumes of whose work he translated into German, Freud compared him, as a bringer of order to the chaos of symptoms and malfunctions, to Cuvier, the great classifier of species in the animal world, and even to the mythic figure of Adam, distinguishing and naming the creatures God brought before him in the Garden of Eden. Charcot's treatment of nervous diseases entailed the identification of characteristic combinations of symptoms and the demonstration of their basis in certain underlying pathological anatomical changes, distinguishing and describing multiple sclerosis, lateral sclerosis ('Charcot's disease'), and locomotor ataxy with its distinctive features ('Charcot's joints'), among others. From 1870 onward he turned his attention to hysteria. This coincided with, if it was not occasioned by, an administrative decision by the authorities at La Salpêtrière to split up the population of patients with the common symptom of convulsive fits (*'les convulsionaires'*) previously housed together. The mixed population of those with epilepsy and severe hysteria but not deemed insane was assigned to Charcot's 'service' and those considered insane to the care of an alienist (i.e. a psychiatrist).

1. Christopher Goetz, Michel Bonduelle, and Toby Gelfand, *Charcot: Constructing Neurology* (Oxford: Oxford University Press, 1995), viii; see also *Charcot the Clinician: The Tuesday Lessons*, trans. and ed. Christopher Goetz (New York: Raven Press, 1987).
2. Freud, "Charcot" (1893f), *SE* 3, 12.

In his inaugural lecture on taking up the new Chair in Neuropathology in 1881, Charcot outlined his 'anatomo-clinical method' as a correlation of the symptomatic disease pictures clinically encountered at the bedside with the lesions established by anatomy in the postmortem room. He also went on to argue, using the example of the new spinal pathology, that the progressive differentiation of the spinal cord into newly discovered regions, each with its circumscribed lesion, could reveal "the special functions belonging to the affected structures."[3] In other words, the field of physiological functioning and its failures, and the localization of functions in different parts of the brain and nervous system (a recent discovery of nineteenth-century anatomy), were annexed to the new field of neurology and subordinated to Charcot's method. To his initially triumphalist vision, hysteria and other neuroses "evidently having their seat in the nervous system" but "which leave in the dead body no material trace" posed a challenge. "These symptomatic combinations deprived of anatomical substratum" lack the appearance of "solidity" and "objectivity" and "come before us like so many Sphinx" (ibid., 12), Charcot declared.

In 1869, the year before taking over responsibility for La Salpêtrière's mixed population of epileptics and hysterics, Charcot had attended a meeting of the British Medical Association and heard a lecture by a leading London physician and expert on epilepsy, J. Russell Reynolds. Reynolds argued that "some of the most serious disorders of the nervous system, such as paralysis, spasm, pain, and otherwise altered sensation, may depend upon a morbid condition of emotion, of idea and emotion, or of idea alone," that they have the appearance of "complicated diseases of the brain or spinal cord," and that consequently in their case it is important to distinguish between the effects of "organic lesion" as distinct from those of "morbid ideation."[4] Reynolds, whose 1869 paper Charcot cited as seminal for his own work, belonged to a British tradition familiar to Charcot and beginning with Sir Benjamin Brodie's work in the 1830s on "local nervous affections" or "local hysterias," in which symptoms ranging from pains and swellings of

3. J. M. Charcot, *Clinical Lectures on Diseases of the Nervous System*, vol. III (London: The New Sydenham Society, 1889), reprinted and intro. Ruth Harris (London: Routledge, 1991), 11.
4. J. Russell Reynolds, "Remarks on Paralysis, and Other Disorders of Motion and Sensation, Dependent on Idea," *The British Medical Journal* 6 (November 1869): 483.

the joints to paralyses, nervous tremblings, loss of voice, back and neck pains, and urinary retention were found to have no organic basis.[5] In 1873 Sir James Paget published a series of lectures on what he called "nervous mimicry" or "neuromimesis," which he considered an objective disorder of 'the nervous centres' and not a question of either conscious simulation and deception, or the mental error of imagination. Imitated diseases are found in children and ignorant or slow-minded people, who know nothing of the diseases imitated.[6] Significantly, both Reynolds and Paget reject the assimilation of idea-based or imitated symptoms to hysteria. Paget is vehement: the term "hysteria" should be used, if at all, for patients with the classical hysterical symptoms of convulsions and suffocation "and those other signs of nervous disorder that are not imitations of other diseases." The characters of nervous mimicry "make a distinct group with another name . . . we may call them hyperaesthetic or hyperneurotic; anything but hysterical" (ibid., 173). While they were talking about the same range of symptoms, it is not clear that Paget conceived his involuntarily imitated diseases as ideogenic or idea-based in quite the same way Reynolds did, as he was concerned to protect their objective reality from any suggestion of the imaginary, by basing it in the "erroneous workings of sensitive and motor nerve-centres" (ibid., 183). Repudiating the idea that they might be understood as the effect of the mind over the body, Paget seems to want to postulate an involuntary and therefore objective production of the signs and symptoms of organic diseases by the organism, but without the organic lesions that would usually cause them. Nervous mimicry is distinct from mental disorder for "surely, any nervous centre may 'go mad' as well as any part of the brain" (ibid., 186).

Transferring his 'anatomo-clinical' method to the sphere of hysteria, Charcot, nevertheless, assimilated the range of ideogenic and imitated symptomologies to hysteria, despite the caveats of Paget and Reynolds. He proceeded to defend the genuineness and objectivity of hysterical phenomena even as he distinguished them from the organically based symptoms that

5. Mark Micale, "Charcot and *les névroses traumatiques*: Scientific and Historical Reflections," *Journal of the History of the Neurosciences* 4 (1995): esp. 103–5.
6. James Paget, "Nervous Mimicry," in *Clinical Lectures and Essays by Sir James Paget, Bart.*, ed. Howard Marsh (London: Longmans, Green and Co., 1875): 172–219.

they imitated and with which they were often confused. Citing Paget's term "neuromimesis" in his inaugural lecture, Charcot took the resemblance of hysterical symptoms to the hemianesthesia (one-sided loss of sensation) produced by cerebral lesions, or the paraplegia (paralysis) produced by spinal lesions, as a guide or clue to the enigma of hysteria. Instead of an organic, anatomical lesion, he posited what he called a functional or dynamic lesion as the immediate cause of hysterical symptoms; beyond the similarity of symptoms, the pathologist "perceives a similarity in the anatomical seat, and *mutatis mutandis*, localises the dynamic lesion from the data furnished by an examination of the corresponding organic one" (Charcot 1889, 14). Charcot read back from the imitated organic disease to its hysterical imitation and inferred the same location for the functional lesion as for the organic one. He continued to affirm his neurological project of explaining hysteria in terms of a localizable, albeit functional or dynamic, lesion, virtually up to his death in 1893, although he was never able to succeed in locating the lesions specific to hysterical symptoms and so enforce his ambitious claim, that the neuroses "do not form, in pathology, a class apart, governed by other physiological laws than the common ones" (ibid., 13).

However, in his last publication on hysteria in 1892, the year before his sudden death, in a long article for a British dictionary of psychological medicine, in response to the question, "What, then, is hysteria?," he wrote:

According to our notion it is less a disease in the ordinary sense of the word, than a peculiarly constituted mode of feeling and reaction. We do not know anything about its nature, nor about any lesions producing it; we know it only through its manifestations, and are therefore only able to characterise it by its symptoms, for the more hysteria is subjective, the more it is necessary to make it objective, in order to recognise it.[7]

This looks like a partial admission of his failure to draw hysteria within the law-like framework of neurology, at least as far as identifying an etiology specific to it. If the elusive lesion escaped Charcot, he had, nevertheless, he felt, submitted it to neurological law and order by having both enlarged

7. J. M. Charcot and Pierre Marie, 'HYSTERIA mainly HYSTERO-EPILEPSY,' in *A Dictionary of Psychological Medicine*, ed. D. Hack Tuke (London: J. & A. Churchill, 1892), 628.

and stabilized the hysteria diagnosis as a clinical picture and a symptomatic field, differentiating it from its neighboring nervous disorders, epilepsy and neurasthenia, as well as from the organically based and anatomically demonstrable diseases of the nervous system.

## La Grande Hystérie: The Hysterical Attack

In his influential nosography of the field of hysterical phenomena, Charcot divided it into two major forms, the convulsive and the nonconvulsive. Convulsions and the hysterical fit were part of the traditional description of hysteria going back to ancient Greek medical treatises. Charcot foregrounded this as central to the clinical picture, although he vigorously rejected the classical etiology (from *hystera*, meaning the womb) that located its cause in the wandering of the unsatisfied womb around the body, rising from the stomach or chest to the throat in the classical *globus hystericus*, or ball in the throat. In Charcot's account, hysteria was not a specifically female disease in the field of gynecology but a disease of both men and women in the field of neurology (although the uterine theory persisted among gynecologists, especially in Anglophone countries, right through the nineteenth century and into the early twentieth).[8] The description and spectacular clinical demonstrations of the ideal type of the hysterical attack in the lecture theaters of La Salpêtrière, often before an audience drawn from literary, artistic, and fashionable circles, and in its published photographic records, brought both high drama and notoriety to Charcot's study of hysteria.[9] Charcot called this *hysteria major* or *la grande hystérie*, having rejected the standard term 'hystero-epilepsy' for its misleading implication that this was basically epilepsy presenting in hysterical form, when what was at stake was in fact 'epileptiform hysteria,' a terminology that both he and

8. Mark S. Micale, "Hysteria Male/Hysteria Female: Reflections on Comparative Gender Construction in 19th Century France and Britain," in *Science and Sensibility: Gender and Scientific Inquiry, 1780–1945*, ed. Marina Benjamin (Oxford: Basil Blackwell, 1991), 223–26.
9. D. M. Bourneville and P. Regnard, *Iconographie Photographique de la Salpêtrière*, 3 vols. (Paris: Aux Bureaux du Progrès Médicale, DelaHaye & Cie., 1876–80).

Freud preferred.[10] 'Epileptiform convulsions' provided the presenting symptom or medium from which emerged the 'phonographic' reproductions that Freud heard in the case first cited at the beginning of the Prologue to this book, and this suggests that it belonged to the third phase of the *attitudes passionelles*, to be discussed later.

Charcot formulated a schematic outline of the full-scale hysterical attack, dividing it into a preliminary 'aura' followed by four main phases.[11] The aura consisted of anticipatory states of excitement, palpitations, constriction in the head with hammering in the temples and ringing in the ears, increases in body temperature, and a sense of suffocation from the notorious *globus hystericus* (ball in the throat) that rises from below and feels like a foreign body or obstruction. Very often the aura is characterized by an intense sensation starting from a single point, the hysterogenic point or zone, and spreading to the throat or head. In women this point is often in the ovarian region, although the zones may be located in other parts of the body, including the scalp, under the breast, and, in men, in the abdominal wall, testicles, and spermatic cord. Pressure brought to bear on these points can sometimes abort an attack or lower its intensity, although attacks can also be provoked by applying pressure on the same points.

The convulsive sequence or attack proper begins with the first epileptoid phase, which is characterized by agitation of the limbs, loss of consciousness, suspension of breathing and foaming at the mouth. The hands are pronated (bent inward), and the forearms and legs are rigidly contracted (the tonic subphase). This is followed by clonic spasms in which contractions and relaxations violently oscillate. Then stertorous and painful breathing begins again.

The second phase of *grands mouvements* or 'clownism,' involves contortions and acrobatic convulsions, such as the famous *arc de cercle*, in which the body, bent over backwards, rests on the feet and head and the trunk is raised

10. See Freud's appendix to his 1888 article "Hysteria" and his footnote to his translation of Charcot's *Tuesday Lessons* (1892–94), *SE* 1, 58, 142.
11. Charcot gave various descriptions of his schema of the *grande attaque*, sometimes with the final stage omitted. See the introductory lecture in his *Clinical Lectures on Diseases of the Nervous System*, vol.III: 13; Charcot and Marie, "HYSTERIA," in *Dictionary*, 629–31 (one of the most detailed descriptions in English); Freud, "Hysteria" (1888b), *SE* 1, 42–43.

up like a bridge. This gives way to 'salaam' movements in which the patient moves from lying back to sitting up, then to bending forward as if in salutation. Freud remarks that, "Hysterical movements are always performed with an elegance and co-ordination, which is in strong contrast to the clumsy coarseness of epileptic spasms" (1888b, 42).

It is, however, the third phase that was to become the significant one for Freud's reworking of Charcot's clinical picture into a psychoanalytic theory of hysteria. This is the phase of *attitudes passionelles*, in which "the psychical element begins to play the first part" and there appears the purposefulness that Charcot contrasts with the purposelessness of the purely convulsive second phase. It is characterized by what he calls "expressive mimicry" of a series of emotions—love, hatred, fear, fright, ecstasy—related to experiences that have played a part in the onset of the hysterical symptoms: "We sometimes see the patient recall a whole scene in his former life (some dispute, accident, etc.)" (Charcot and Marie 1892, 630). The mode of behavior is that of mimicry and enactment, involving screaming and the making of long speeches (Charcot's assistants referred to the imaginary addressees of these speeches as the patient's "Invisibles"[12]). Freud describes this phase as "distinguished by attitudes and gestures which belong to scenes of passionate movement, which the patient hallucinates and accompanies with corresponding words" (1888b, 43).

A final fourth phase of terminal delirium sometimes succeeds in which the patient repeats the themes and preoccupations of the third phase while gradually returning to normal. The four phases constitute the fully developed 'type.' The complete sequence of phases does not always appear in every attack, which may consist of one or two of the four phases, while some may be missing; or, the sequence may start over again halfway through with the first phase of epileptoid movements and continue on repetitively for hours, or in some cases days, in which hundreds of separate attacks might be recorded. It is as if a repeating mechanism has taken over the subject and plays itself out according to some internal balance of forces. In other cases the attack may be represented only in rudimentary or abbreviated form. Despite the varieties of combination of the different phases of the attack,

---

12. Daphne de Marneffe, "Looking and Listening: The Construction of Clinical Knowledge in Charcot and Freud," *Signs* 17, no. 1 (1991): 87.

Charcot confidently asserted that "it will always be easy for those who possess the formula to bring them under one fundamental type" (Charcot 1889, 13).[13]

This scenario of the *grande attaque* with the *attitudes passionelles* as its climax is one of the two key contributions that Charcot's clinical phenomenology of hysteria makes to Freud's later reconceptualization of what I am calling a *scenography* of hysteria, in a fully psychological rather than a neurological register. The second contribution is Charcot's theory of traumatic hysteria, which results from his use of hypnotism to make a connection between hysteria and the problematic of trauma and the traumatic neuroses. Just as he had included the ideogenic and imitated symptoms described by Reynolds and Paget under the heading of hysteria, so also he extended the hysteria diagnosis to include the post-traumatic nervous derangements caused by physical traumas, such as workplace accidents and the new high-speed means of travel (the notorious 'railway spine' and 'railway brain'[14]). Railway accidents, being the subject of much litigation and of claims for damages against the rail companies, were much studied and had become highly controversial in the last quarter of the nineteenth century. The rapid increases in paralyses and nervous symptoms that set in some time *after* the accident, and which lasted long after the healing of the often relatively minor physical lesions, were often considered examples of either simulation or a nebulous 'nervous shock' rather than any real anatomical damage. They also posed a challenge to the new science of neurology. They were conceived by German physicians such as Robert Thomsen

---

13. In the dismemberment of Charcot's model of hysteria that took place so rapidly after his death, the charge that the great hysterics such as Blanche Wittman were trained to perform the stages of the *grande attaque*, which could not be found outside the lecture rooms of La Salpêtrière, played a part, as it did in contemporaneous criticisms of Charcot. It is noteworthy, therefore, that modern physicians have reported striking parallels to Charcot's hysterical symptoms and attacks, for example, in patients from the poor white rural communities of the Appalachians. See E. M. R. Critchley and H. E. Cantor, "Charcot's Hysteria Renaissant," *British Medical Journal* 289 (July–December 1984): 1785–88. See also Mark Micale, "On the 'Disappearance' of Hysteria: A Study in the Clinical Deconstruction of a Diagnosis," *Isis* 84 (1993): 496–526.

14. Micale notes that "the single largest number of Charcot's *traumatisés* were either employees or passengers on trains who were caught in dramatic train wrecks." See Micale, "Charcot and *les névroses traumatiques*," 106.

and Hermann Oppenheim (whom Freud visited on his way back to Vienna from his period with Charcot in Paris) as examples of a distinct morbid entity in its own right, which they called 'traumatic neurosis.' They rejected Charcot's identification of these post-traumatic cases as 'hysterotraumatic,' that is, belonging to the ideogenic and imitated symptoms he had identified as nonconvulsive forms of hysteria (although many of his accident cases also displayed the classical pattern of the convulsive attack).[15] Charcot disputed the conventional location of the effective cause in the sheer physical impact of the trauma (and hence he rejected Thomsen and Oppenheim's hypothesis of undetectable microscopic lesions of the organs involved). Instead, Charcot attributed the cause to the emotional state of shock and fright in the accident victim taken by surprise. He designated this state as hypnoid by analogy with the state of somnambulism into which a hypnotized subject could be put.

Paralyses of the limbs with the same distinctive features as those of hysterical paralyses, which distinguish them from organic paralyses, could be produced by hypnotic suggestion, and Charcot demonstrated this in his clinical experiments with hypnosis in his public lectures. Here he induced a range of artificial symptoms from paralyses to contractures and anesthesias, and then removed them all through hypnotic suggestion. He also transferred preexisting hysterical symptoms, such as hemiplegias, from one side of the body to the other through hypnotic suggestion. For the young Freud trained in the strict materialist and 'somaticist' traditions of German physiology and anatomy, the experience was profoundly disorienting. "I found to my astonishment that here were occurrences plain before one's eyes, which it was quite impossible to doubt, but which were strange enough not to be believed unless they were experienced at first hand," Freud wrote in his report back to the University of Vienna on his experiences at La Salpêtrière (1956a [1886], 13).

Charcot argued that the same mechanism that produced the symptoms of common 'constitutional' hysteria, as embodied in the female *convulsionaires* in his long-stay wards, also produced the post-traumatic symptoms found among the predominantly male population of workplace and railway

---

15. Charcot, lecture XVIII, "Concerning Six Cases of Hysteria in the Male" in *Clinical Lectures on Diseases of the Nervous System*, vol. III : 230–32.

accident victims. "That a vigorous artisan, well-built, not enervated by high culture, the stoker of an engine for example, not previously emotional, . . . should after an accident to the train, by a collision or running off the rails, become hysterical for the same reason as a woman, is what surpasses our imagination" (Lecture XVIII, in Charcot 1889: 222). The analogy, between the operation of a suggestion under hypnosis and the operation of a psychical trauma involved in an accident, was made through the idea of an 'auto-suggestion,' which does not require the verbal statement from another person: "Your arm feels heavy, it is numb, you cannot move it, etc." A mere tap on the shoulder of a hypnotized subject, like the often minor impact of an accident, can operate as a suggestion in certain conditions:

> Upon the assumption of this hypothesis, the peculiar sensation felt . . . may be considered as having originated . . . the idea of motor paralysis of the member. But because of the annihilation of the *ego* produced by the hypnotism in the one case, and . . . by the nervous shock in the other, that idea once installed in the brain takes sole possession and acquires sufficient domination to realise itself objectively in the form of paralysis. The sensation, in question, therefore, in both cases plays the part of a veritable *suggestion*.[16]

Charcot's thesis of an *auto suggestion*, in which a subjective impression or idea, provoked by an impact in either a hypnotized state or one of shock or fright, acts as an objective force on the subject's functioning, takes him to the very border between neurology and psychology. The preliminary condition for the successful execution of any movement is, he argues, "the production of an image, or of a mental representation . . . of the movement to be executed." The formation of this executive image is inhibited by "the fixed idea of motor weakness" that is suggested by the numbness or local physical effects of the impact (ibid., 309–10). The hypnotized patient experiences in her shoulder the sensation of weight and feebleness, "as if *the member struck did not belong to her, that it had become strange to her*" (ibid., 304). However, for this fixed idea of motor weakness actually to have the power to inhibit movement and to produce paralysis, certain psychological conditions are necessary, namely, the loss of consciousness and what he

16. Lecture XXII, "On Two Cases of Hysterical Brachial Monoplegia in the Male (continued)," in Charcot 1889: 305.

calls "the annihilation of the ego." He restates this in more developed psychological terms when he argues that in these conditions "an idea or a group of associated ideas . . . freed from all control, all opposition, may become developed into an autonomous condition which acquires by that very fact an enormous force, and a power of realisation which is almost without limits."[17] Charcot is here positing a *condition seconde*, a set of ideas or a psychical group that exists and acts outside the awareness and control of the ego. This is the dawning recognition of the work of a properly psychical unconscious.

A closely parallel description can be found in Charcot's account of the operation of hypnotic suggestion in a state of catalepsy:

> Consequently the idea, or group of ideas suggested, are met with in a state of isolation, free from the control of that large collection of personal ideas long accumulated and organised, which constitute the conscience [*sic*] properly so-called, the *ego*. It is for this reason that the movements which exteriorly represent the acts of unconscious cerebration, are distinguished by their automatic and purely mechanical character. Then it is truly that we see before us the *human machine* in all its simplicity, dreamt of by De la Mettrie." (Charcot 1889: 290)

The English 'conscience' is a mistranslation of the French *conscience*, more properly translated by the English 'consciousness' in this context. Charcot makes the striking connection here between unconscious ideas "free from the control of . . . the ego" and the "human machine," in which we might recognize an anticipation of the motif of repetition that Freud is to reformulate as first 'the return of the repressed' and later the 'repetition-compulsion.'

To summarize: two key elements of Charcot's work on hysteria are taken over by Freud and reworked: the *attitudes passionelles* or scenes of passionate movement with their hallucinatory acting out of past but still active events and the conception of executive mental schemas necessary for bodily movement, which have become inhibited by unconscious ideas that have escaped the control of the ego and that determine the body's functions and processes.

---

17. Appendix I: "Two Additional Cases of Hystero-Traumatic Paralysis in Men," in Charcot 1889: 383.

*From Neurology to Psychology: Freud's Exit*

In what is often considered the urtext of psychoanalysis, Freud and Breuer's "On the Psychical Mechanism of Hysterical Phenomena: Preliminary Communication" (1893a), and, even more explicitly, in its twin text of the same month, a lecture with the same title delivered by Freud alone, the notion of trauma and the traumatic neurosis is both the starting point and central focus for an argument that exits from the terrain of neurology entirely in order to formulate precisely what Freud calls the *psychical* mechanism for the production of hysterical symptoms.[18] The second of these twin texts, Freud's solo lecture, begins with a celebration of Charcot's work as the source of "all the modern advances made in the understanding and knowledge of hysteria" (1893h, 27). In particular, it singles out Charcot's work on the post-traumatic hysterical paralyses for the highest commendation, declaring that "it is precisely this work of which ours appears as the continuation" (ibid., 27). In fact, rather than a continuation, what is taking place through a reconfiguration of key elements in Charcot's work is a radical break from that work, and from the neurological tradition Charcot represents, in order to construct a *psychology* of hysteria.

Charcot had integrated the range of ideogenic and mimetic symptoms into the field of hysteria and then, by establishing experimentally their identity with the post-traumatic neuroses, by artificially inducing the same symptoms under hypnosis and demonstrating their ideogenic nature, he had included also the post-traumatic conditions as precisely 'hystero-traumatic.' In the 1893 texts Breuer and Freud make what might seem at first glance a similar gesture, but in fact it is the reverse of Charcot's. Appealing to a range of clinical experiences, Freud argues for *"an analogy between the pathogenesis of common hysteria and that of traumatic neuroses"* but an analogy that in fact justifies *"an extension of the concept of traumatic hysteria"* (1893a, 5). Instead of trauma along with its mimetic and ideogenic symptoms being assimilated to the preexisting field of hysteria, the latter is now subordinated to the idea of trauma. Common or constitutional (that is,

18. Sigmund Freud, "On the Psychical Mechanism of Hysterical Phenomena: Preliminary Communication" (1893a), *SE* 2; "On the Psychical Mechanism of Hysterical Phenomena" (1893h), *SE* 3.

inherited) hysteria is now to be understood on the model of the traumatic. Both the spectacular convulsive forms of the *grande attaque* and the non-convulsive stigmata of anesthesias and hyperesthesias, the standard paralyses and contractures, all held together by their common ideogenic as well as their 'imitative' character, are to be understood as products of the same psychical and traumatic causality.

To understand the break from Charcot and neurology that has taken place in these two inaugural texts of 1893, a brief detour is illuminating through another text of 1893 that had been in suspended animation since the mid-1880s, "Some Points for a Comparative Study of Organic and Hysterical Motor Paralyses," together with a later text of 1896, "Heredity and the Aetiology of the Neuroses."[19] On Freud's departure from Paris in February 1886, he tells us in the first of these papers that he took with him a task entrusted to him by his teacher Charcot. That task, given in the title, of a comparative study of organic and hysterical paralyses, is an exemplary neurological project, continuing if not replicating the work of Charcot on the apparent similarities and more radical discontinuities of the two kinds of paralysis. As James Strachey, Freud's translator, points out in his editorial introduction to the paper in the *Standard Edition*, it consists of four parts of which the first three were finished by August 1888, after which a five-year silence ensued before the final fourth part was completed in 1893. The first three parts are a summa of all that the anatomo-clinical method can tell us of the anatomical and functional differences between the two kinds of paralysis, and they end with a consideration of the aporia of Charcot's neurology of hysteria: the postulation of a dynamic or functional lesion for which no appreciable tissue changes can be found postmortem. The delayed fourth part offers a solution to this aporia by transposing it onto the ground of a psychical trauma and its effects. Split three-quarters of the way through by its five-year suspension, this is preeminently a transitional text, a text of the break.

It was first published originally in French in Charcot's journal, *Archives de Neurologie*, and it appeared in July 1893, two weeks before his sudden

19. Sigmund Freud, "Some Points for a Comparative Study of Organic and Hysterical Motor Paralyses" (1893c), *SE* 1; "Heredity and the Aetiology of the Neuroses" (1896a), *SE* 3.

death.[20] It reads like a payment of old debts to his former teacher, a discharge of obligations and a settling of scores with his own formation as a neurologist. Freud is concerned, first, to demonstrate the precise determination of the two kinds of *organic* motor paralysis, the periphero-spinal and the cerebral, by the differences in the anatomical structure of the nervous system. The former, the *periphero-spinal*, is determined by the nature of the conductive fibers that run from the periphery (e.g., hands and feet) to the spinal cord, the latter, the *cerebral*, by those that run from the spinal cord to the cerebral cortex. The anatomical difference between these two sets of conductive fibers, and their positioning vis-à-vis each other, is expressed in the clinical difference between the periphero-spinal, which is "*a paralysis 'détaillée'*" and the cerebral, which is "*a paralysis 'en masse'*" (1893c, 160). In the former, each muscle can be paralyzed individually and in isolation, and it is the precise location and extent of the lesion that determines which peripheral element is affected. By contrast, cerebral paralysis affects a large section of the periphery, a whole limb or a complex motor apparatus, never an individual muscle. The only exception Freud points out are where "muscles . . . perform by themselves a function of which they are the sole instrument" (ibid., 161). In cerebral paralysis the distal segments are more adversely affected than the proximal, the hand more than the shoulder; "there is no such thing as an isolated cerebral paralysis of the shoulder with the hand retaining its motility," while the reverse case, in which the hand is paralyzed but not the shoulder, is often found.

In periphero-spinal paralysis each element of the periphery corresponds to an element in the spinal cord in which it terminates: "the periphery is, so to say, projected upon the grey matter of the cord, point by point and element by element," which leads Freud to label it "projection paralysis" (ibid., 161). By contrast, because of the reduced number of fibers in the second part of the nervous system running from the spinal cord to the cortex, there is not a second point-by-point projection of the periphery upon the cortex. "We must suppose that the fibres running from the cord to the cortex no longer each represent a single element of the periphery but rather a group of them, and even, on the other hand, that one element of

20. "Quelques Considérations pour une Étude Comparative des Paralysies Motrices Organiques et Hystériques," *Archives de Neurologie* 26 (July 1893): 29–43.

the periphery may correspond to several spino-cortical conductive fibres" (ibid., 161). Because of this anatomical change from one section of the conductive fibers to the next, the spino-cortical relations are not those of "faithful reproduction" or "true projection"; it is, instead, Freud argues, a relation by means of what he calls "representative fibres," hence he labels cerebral paralysis a "representation paralysis." While periphero-spinal paralysis when extensive or total may result in paralysis *en masse*, spino-cortical paralysis is *always* a representation paralysis *en masse*.

It is clear from this analysis that the possibility of a paralysis of isolated or individual elements follows from the nature of the first set of spino-peripheral fibers (one-to-one projection), whereas the 'representative' character of the second set of spino-cortical fibres determines the paralysis of larger functional complexes *en masse*. It is also very striking that the overlapping of the more numerous peripheral elements onto the fewer cortical fibers that 'represent' rather than simply reproduce them exactly prefigures the model of 'overdetermination' that Freud is later to develop in his analysis of dreams. Overdetermination specifies the relations between the separate multiple elements of the latent dream-thoughts and the much-reduced manifest elements of the dream scene. This reduced number of manifest dream elements 'represents' the dream-thoughts through the dream-work's processes of condensation and displacement rather than simply reproducing them point for point.

The significance of this strictly neurological analysis becomes apparent when Freud states that "hysteria never simulates periphero-spinal or projection paralyses; hysterical paralyses only share the characteristics of organic representation paralyses" (ibid., 162). That is, hysterical paralyses are always paralyses *en masse*. However, in their imitation of organic cerebral paralyses, they deviate significantly, for in hysteria the proximal parts, shoulder, hip, or thigh, may be found to be totally paralyzed, while the distal segments, fingers, hands, and feet, remain unaffected. This "contradiction to the rules of organic cerebral paralysis" leads Freud to conclude provisionally that while "hysterical paralysis is also a representation paralysis," it is "a special kind of representation whose characteristics remain to be discovered" (ibid., 163).

Freud also cites other features that indicate the functional rather than the anatomical basis of hysteria; absolute paralyses of the arm or leg appear in isolation from each other in hysteria, whereas they tend to be associated with the paralysis of larger sections on the same side of the body in organic paralyses (i.e., hemiplegias rather than isolated monoplegias). Significantly, hysterical aphasia (speech loss) can affect the use of a particular language while not affecting the reception and use of another (so Anna O. loses the use of her native German for certain periods and can speak only English or French). Similarly, hysteria can produce "the total abolition of a function (e.g., in abasia [loss of capacity to walk—JF] and astasia [loss of capacity to stand—JF]) while another function performed by the same organs remains intact" (ibid., 164). Hysteria has a capacity to dissociate one segment from another or one function from another (and Freud remarks in passing that in organic paralyses the loss of the more complex functions, the ones that have been acquired last, comes first, whereas the hysterical loss of function is *not* determined by the developmental sequence of acquisition). Moreover, what he calls "the hall-mark of the neurosis" is that it is "a disease of excessive manifestations," which "tends to produce its symptoms with the greatest possible intensity" (ibid., 164). Where hysteria produces profound anesthesia or absolute paralysis, by contrast, in organic paralysis, paresis (or partial paralysis) is more frequently found. Hysteria then combines both precise limitation with excessive intensity, while these two qualities are mutually exclusive in organic paralyses where isolated paralyses or monoplegias are only of moderate intensity; when they intensify toward absolute paralysis, they tend to spread to adjoining areas, a paralysis of the arm developing to include the leg or face on the same side of the body and to lose its delimitation.

Freud ends the third part of his essay with the conclusion that "since there can only be a single cerebral anatomy that is true, and since it finds expression in the clinical characteristics of the cerebral paralyses, it is clearly impossible for that anatomy to be the explanation of the distinctive features of hysterical paralyses" (ibid., 168). By contrast, in organic paralyses the anatomical structure of the nervous system, with its different relations of projection or representation between its two different sets of conductive fibers, is the primary determinant, while the localization and the extent of the lesion play a secondary part subject to the structural conditions set by the primary determinant. This has implications for Charcot's organizing thesis that poses the whole question of hysteria within the framework of neurology: the thesis of a dynamic or functional lesion that leaves no traces for postmortem analysis. Freud is explicitly critical of Charcot's attempt to localize the 'hysterical lesion' by analogy with the organic lesion, thus reading back from the imitated organic symptoms to their hysterical imitations, as we saw Charcot proposed to do in his 1881 inaugural lecture. So Freud concludes the neurological section of his argument by meticulously pushing the founding propositions and the analyses of Charcot's anatomico-clinical method into contradiction, exposing the aporia on which they are based:

> I, on the contrary, assert that the lesion in hysterical paralyses must be completely independent of the anatomy of the nervous system, since *in its paralyses and other manifestations hysteria behaves as though anatomy does not exist or as though it had no knowledge of it.* (Freud 1893c, 169)

If, in Freud's striking proposition, "hysteria is ignorant of the distribution of the nerves, and that is why it does not simulate periphero-spinal or projection paralyses," then localization of lesions within the structure of fibers, muscles, and nerves as revealed by anatomy becomes irrelevant. If "the leg is the leg as far up as its insertion into the hip, the arm is the upper limb as it is visible under the clothing," as Freud puts it, invoking what has been called the 'glove and stocking' pattern of hysterical paralyses, then it is to these conceptions of "the organs in the ordinary, popular sense of the names they bear" (ibid.) that we must turn when looking for the determination of hysterical symptoms. It is as if Freud is drawing out the implication of Charcot's recognition that the symptoms of traumatic hysteria are idea-based, the implication *contra Charcot* that in hysteria anatomical localization is therefore neither possible nor pertinent.

The fourth part of Freud's essay is explicit in its exit from neurology: "I only ask permission to move onto psychological ground" (ibid., 170). However this radical move is cast in hesitant and provisional terms—Freud "asks permission" and throughout he gives the impression of being implicitly in anxious dialogue with Charcot himself. Of Charcot's hypothetical "functional lesion," he writes, "I do not say that I will show what it *is* like; it is merely a question of indicating a line of thought that might lead to a conception which does not contradict the properties of hysterical paralysis" (ibid., 169). In fact, Freud continues to use Charcot's vocabulary while giving a quite different signification to it. Freud thus reformulates Charcot's hypothesis: "I shall take the phrase 'functional or dynamic lesion' in its proper sense of 'alteration in function or dynamics'—alteration of a functional property," giving as an example "a diminution of excitability" (ibid., 169). This lesion will be at the level of "the everyday, popular conception of the organs and the body," based on "our tactile and above all our visual perceptions." "The lesion in hysterical paralysis will therefore be an alteration of the *conception*, the *idea*, of the arm, for instance" (ibid., 170)—in other words, *not a lesion at all*.

> Considered psychologically, the paralysis of the arm consists in the fact that the conception of the arm cannot enter into association with the other ideas constituting the ego of which the subject's body forms an important part. The lesion would therefore be *the abolition of the associative accessibility of the arm*. The arm behaves as if it does not exist for the play of associations. (Freud 1893c , 170)

Taken thus far, Freud's formulations have a distinct resemblance to Charcot at his most 'psychological,' that is, in his account of hypnotic suggestion or traumatic autosuggestion as they operate in hysterical paralyses. These operate at the level of the executive mental representations or schemas necessary for any mobilization of the bodily organs, representations that have been inhibited by the implanted or self-suggested idea of motor weakness or incapacity. This inhibiting counter-representation has the power to paralyze, according to Charcot, because it is outside the control of the ego, originating in an unconscious hypnoid state. Freud also focuses on the withdrawal of the representation of the arm from "associative accessibility" to the ego. Here, with both Charcot and Freud, we have a 'representation paralysis' in a different sense from that of the organic cerebral paralyses Freud had in mind earlier, where the peripheral elements reproduced in the spinal cord are then 'represented' in the cerebral cortex; here it is a case of paralysis by means of *mental* representations and of their relation not to the cortex but to the ego, a psychological entity, not a neuro-anatomical one.[21]

---

21. We might see here the seed of Freud's later conception of the ego, especially his analogy of the primitive body-ego originating in "a mental projection of the surface of the body" with "the 'cortical homunculus' of the anatomists," and thereby distinguished from it. See *The Ego and the Id* (1923b), *SE* 19, 26.

Freud moves beyond Charcot by invoking the outline elements for a model of the ego and what he is soon to call 'the psychical apparatus.' This is the model of a closed homeostatic entity, the breach of whose boundaries from the outside will entail fluctuations in energy levels that need to be restored. This is the principle of constancy. In particular, any increase in excitations will need to be discharged or 'abreacted,' otherwise the accumulated, undischarged excitations will act as a psychical equivalent of a trauma. Freud is in fact giving the notion of trauma as a breach or breaking of boundaries a quantitative or economic dimension. We can then conclude that "the special kind of representation whose characteristics remain to be discovered," (ibid., 163) mentioned in part one of the essay, is now revealed as a *mental representation charged with affect.*

What distinguishes Freud's account of a *psychical* representation paralysis from Charcot's conception is his development of the role of affect and his conception of psychical trauma in terms of accumulated, undischarged affect. Affect for Charcot was the state of fright accompanying the physical trauma, which constituted a quasi-hypnotic precondition and medium in which paralyzing autosuggestions could arise. For Freud, affect is an active causal agent conceived as a "quota of affect" regulated by the principle of constancy.

> Every event, every psychical impression is provided with a certain quota of affect (*Affektbetrag*) of which the ego divests itself by means of a motor reaction or by associative psychical activity. If the subject is unable or unwilling to get rid of this surplus, the memory of the impression attains the importance of a trauma and becomes the cause of permanent hysterical symptoms. (Freud 1893c, 171–72)

The psychical trauma is constituted by the undischargeable surplus of affect, an excess that prevents the psychical system from returning to its optimum equilibrium or state of constancy prior to its disruption by the traumatic event. The traumatic affect becomes fixated by association to the mental conception of the arm or other bodily organ affected by the trauma, an organ that is "saturated in a subconscious association with the memory of the event, the trauma, which produced the paralysis" (ibid., 172). This entails the consequence, according to Freud, that the conception of the arm "is not accessible to conscious associations and impulses" (ibid., 170).

He illustrates this idea of a fixation that renders the fixated organ withdrawn from normal functioning with the comic anecdote of the loyal subject, who refused ever to wash his hand once the king had touched it. "The relation of his hand to the idea of the king seemed so important to the man's psychical life that he refused to let the hand enter into any other relation" (ibid., 170). Freud's argument is highly condensed and is elaborated more fully in the "Preliminary Communication" with Breuer, also published in 1893, which he references. The relations between fixated affect and traumatic memory are alluded to but not spelled out. What is important is that the idea of abreaction as a therapeutic outcome is entailed by the general psychological theory of the ego and of psychical functioning (the principle of constancy entailing some notion of discharge or abreaction), even though it is only gestured toward as a therapeutic practice: "the paralysed organ or the lost function . . . involved in a subconscious association . . . is liberated as soon as this quota of affect is wiped out" (ibid., 171).

Freud concludes by offering his psychological reformulation of Charcot's neurological thesis as shaped "under M. Charcot's instruction": "The lesion in hysterical paralyses consists in nothing other than the inaccessibility of the organ or function concerned to the associations of the ego," and this "functional alteration" is the result of the psychical operation of the memory and affect of a precipitating trauma (ibid., 172). The latter proposition raises the larger question of etiology, which Freud is only to address explicitly after Charcot's death in his 1896 paper on heredity.

*Heredity and Causality*

Many of the elements of Freud's psychological theory were present in Charcot's work: the ideogenic basis of hysterical symptoms, the dissociation of operative ideas from the ego and conscious functioning, and of course the presence of trauma. Indeed, Freud and Breuer explicitly affiliate their work to Charcot's theory of traumatic hysteria. What enables Freud to reorganize these elements into a radically different theory is the question of etiology, or the *causal* theory of hysteria, not just as a field of ideogenic and mimetic symptoms, however well delimited, but as an underlying generative condition. The latter for Charcot is a question of nervous heredity: "a special morbid predisposing condition inherent in the individual" (Charcot and Marie 1892, 628). All other causes are occasional, secondary, mere agents provocateurs, in a favorite metaphor of Charcot's, which simply activate what is inherited and latent in the individual's constitution. From the 1880s Charcot worked within the framework of the hereditarian and degeneration theory that was so dominant in nineteenth-century medicine. In this framework a particular diathesis or predisposition was transmitted from one generation to another. The La Salpêtrière school developed a special version of this with the doctrine of the *famille névropathique*, a particular 'family' or grouping of nervous diseases—epilepsy, locomotor ataxy, hysteria—that alternate through a transformational series from generation to generation. This was elaborated further with a psychopathic family of diseases and an arthritic family, both alternating in sequences with each other. In particular, Charcot and his colleagues were involved in an intellectual battle over the etiology of locomotor ataxy (or *tabes dorsalis*), a battle in which they opposed their hereditarian theory to the Erb-Fournier thesis that the condition was the result of syphilis as a primary cause and was not inherited. The Erb-Fournier thesis, definitively established through laboratory work, was vindicated soon after Charcot's death. What was at stake in that controversy was the eventual replacement of hereditarian and degeneration theory as a whole by the emergence of germ theory and the revolution brought about by the work of Louis Pasteur. It was the weakness of Charcot's work on hysteria with regard to the question of etiology—the problem of 'the missing lesion,' as it was called, his failure to identify and localize his hypothetical functional lesion, together with his reliance on the unverifiable and overgeneralized claims of heredity—that was responsible for the rapid dismemberment of Charcot's model of hysteria after his death, as Mark Micale has persuasively argued.[22]

Freud had initially accepted Charcot's insistence on the primacy of heredity, as his 1888 article on hysteria, where he is impeccably orthodox, makes clear. However, he increasingly came to argue for the importance of

22. "But it was precisely the etiological elusiveness of these concepts of hysteria, the lack of a strong causal theory to hold them together, that would allow for their swift symptomological dissolution in the future;" see Micale, "On the 'Disappearance' of Hysteria," 504.

*acquired* nervous illness, due to specific causes, without verifiable evidence of heredity. In his translation of Charcot's *Tuesday Lectures*, Freud had added notes that were critical of Charcot's hereditarian position, championing the Erb-Fournier thesis and rejecting the doctrine of the *famille névropathique*, and he received a letter of rebuke from Charcot over the matter (although a number of Charcot's students and colleagues had done the same).[23] It was, however, only in his 1896 paper that Freud addressed the question of heredity and etiology systematically. Here he outlines a model of causality in which he proposes different sets of causes. He distinguishes between "preconditions" which are indispensable but "of a general nature and are met equally with in the aetiology of many other disorders," "concurrent causes," also of a general nature but not indispensable for the particular disease and common to many others, and "specific causes," which are indispensable "but are of a limited nature and appear only in the aetiology of the disorder for which they are specific" (1896a, 147). Freud is happy to assign heredity to the category of preconditions that are necessary but cannot by themselves produce the particular disease: "The action of heredity is comparable to that of a multiplier in an electric circuit, which exaggerates the visible deviation of the needle, but which cannot determine its direction" (ibid., 147). Freud's example here, however, seems rather unsatisfactory, as a multiplier that merely exaggerates a given direction is purely quantitative and hardly an indispensable precondition. While the direct transmission of the same disease from one generation to another without other etiological factors in 'similar heredity' (Huntingdon's chorea, Thomsen's disease, etc.) is relatively unproblematic, Freud's critique bears on the claims of 'dissimilar heredity' made by the La Salpêtrière school in which different diseases, said to be of the same disease family, leapfrog each other down the generations. This doctrine was unable to establish a law determining the replacement of one disease by another, or

23. Sigmund Freud, "Preface and Footnotes to Charcot's *Tuesday Lectures* (1892–94), 139–40, 142–43; Toby Gelfand, "'Mon Cher Docteur Freud': Charcot's Unpublished Correspondence to Freud, 1888–1893," translation with annotation and commentary, *Bulletin of the History of Medicine* 62 (1988): 563–588; Toby Gelfand, "Charcot's Response to Freud's Rebellion," *Journal of the History of Ideas* 50, no. 1 (1989): 293–307; Goetz, Bonduelle, and Gelfand, "The Cause of Diseases," in *Charcot: Constructing Neurology*, 258–63.

why one member of a family falls ill while other members do not, or why they should choose one nervous illness rather than another (the 'choice of neurosis' was to become a key issue for Freud in his etiological and structural explanations of the neuroses). Perhaps the most damaging argument against the hereditarian paradigm was that once the possibility of acquired nervous illness without hereditary predisposition was allowed, no one earlier instance of illness in a previous ancestor could escape the suspicion of being acquired, and so could no longer count as incontrovertible evidence of a hereditary diathesis at work in the family line.

With this backgrounding (and virtual discrediting) of heredity, the specific causes that result only in the particular disease in question are foregrounded as of key etiological importance. In a nosographical field newly realigned and redescribed by Freud, each of the neuroses has as its immediate and specific cause "one particular disturbance of the economics of the nervous system," while their common source is the subject's sexual life (1896a, 147). Subdivided into the actual neuroses and the psychoneuroses of defense, the actual neuroses have as their specific cause supposedly dysfunctional sexual practices in contemporary adult life (one set of practices, masturbation, for neurasthenia and another, coitus interruptus, for anxiety neurosis), while the psychoneuroses are rooted in premature sexual experiences in childhood (hysteria in passive experiences of abuse and obsessional neurosis in actively pleasurable experiences). The nosographical categories and subdivisions are no longer defined in a purely descriptive way, simply as a complex of observable symptoms, as in Charcot's account of hysteria, but are differentiated through a structural correlation between a symptomatic complex and an etiology specific to that complex. For hysteria, a particular temporal structure of causation is described, with post-puberty sexual events being classified as concurrent causes, that is, as nonspecific agents provocateurs, and infantile sexual trauma being the determining, specific cause rather than an inherited hysterical constitution.

What is important for my argument here is not the introduction of sexuality (which we will consider later) but the displacement of the nonspecific general condition of an hereditary disposition as the prime determinant of hysteria by different categories of specific but contingent causes. In the case of the psychoneuroses, these specific causes are traumas whose specificity is now considered determinant for the particular form taken by neurosis (e.g., neurasthenia as against anxiety neurosis or hysteria as against obsessional neurosis), and which thereby become the object of clinical interrogation. As commentators have observed, in Charcot's clinic both the content of the hysteric's delirious discourse in the third stage of the hysterical attack, the *attitudes passionelles*, and the details of the physical accidents in traumatic hysteria were recorded, meticulously and at length. While the connection of the events spoken of to the symptoms examined was recognized, the events themselves were not assigned any causal or determining power in the production of the hysteria, being merely noted as occasions for the onset of the symptoms. De Marneffe notes of the figure of Augustine, one of the leading hysterical stars of the *Iconographie Photographique de la Salpêtrière*, that her traumatic history of sexual harassment, rape, and exploitation is recorded in detail, as were seven pages of her delirious discourse, referred to as *bavardage* or chatter. While these were filled with references to her traumatic experiences, they remained unanalyzed and uninterpreted (the reviewer in the *British Medical Journal* protested at the publication of such lubricious material!).[24] It is as if these deliria were the verbal equivalent of the bodily by-products that were so conscientiously collected, measured, and recorded by her medical observers, a kind of logorrhea or verbal flow. Charcot's hereditarian etiology, however, and his focus on the mapping of anatomical symptoms and physiological malfunctions had actually precluded the interrogation of this traumatic material for its causal and form-giving significance. It was Freud's rejection of the hereditarian doctrine that released the idea of trauma from its relegation to one among many agents provocateurs and enabled its generalization as the single specific causal psychical mechanism for all forms of hysteria (indeed, for a time, for all forms of psychoneurosis), and whose clinical interrogation was therefore to perform a central therapeutic function.

24. de Marneffe, "Looking and Listening," 87. She comments: "What amazes me about the *Iconographie* is the wealth of visual information it presents and the poverty of interpretation" (104).

# Freud's Hysteria: "Scenes of Passionate Movement"[1]

If we return now to the "Preliminary Communication" of 1893, which was first published separately and then reprinted as the opening chapter of Breuer and Freud's *Studies on Hysteria*,[2] we can see in the retrospective light of Freud's 1896 critique of heredity that Freud is already in 1893 shifting the whole causal paradigm inherited from Charcot. His movement of thought, as I have argued, is not, as Charcot did, to assimilate the preexisting field of traumatic neuroses to the ideogenesis previously identified in 'constitutional' or inherited hysteria but the reverse, that is, to subsume the whole symptomatic field of the hysterias under the reign of a generalized traumatic causality. Freud indicates explicitly that the "causal relation" with which he is concerned is not, as in Charcot, one in which "the trauma acts like an *agent provocateur* in releasing the symptom, which thereafter

---

1. Sigmund Freud, "Hysteria" (1888b), *SE* 1: 43.
2. Josef Breuer and Sigmund Freud, *Studies on Hysteria* (1895d), *SE* 2.

leads an independent existence"; rather, the psychical trauma or its memory "acts like a foreign body which long after its entry must continue to be regarded as an agent that is still at work" (Freud and Breuer1893a, 6). Against Charcot's favorite metaphor of the agent provocateur, Freud counterposes the idea of the foreign body, whose mode of presence and efficacy is altogether different. Rather than the aftereffects of the agent provocateur as a now-absent precipitating cause, there is "an agent that is still at work," and, for our purposes, this "agent still at work," the "foreign body," takes us back to the action of scenes in the present, of voices "as though . . . from a phonograph," with which this book began. For Freud, the question of causal agency and its distinctive mode of operation directly connects to the question of therapeutic treatment, and initially both are connected to the role of hypnotism.

For Charcot, who rehabilitated hypnotism as a medium of experimental inquiry, artificially producing hysterical symptoms and demonstrating their psychogenetic character and identity with traumatic symptoms, it had no implications for therapeutic treatment, and he increasingly warned against its misuse. He considered it an artificial form of hysteria and applicable only to hysterics (he formulated a model of the *grande hypnotisme* in three stages like the schema of the hysterical *grande attaque*). For his main opponents, the Nancy school of Bernheim and Liébault, hypnotic potentiality was universal and based on the power of suggestion. It was not specific to hysteria, they argued, and hypnotic countersuggestion by the physician could be used therapeutically to eliminate a range of psychological symptoms. However, they displayed no more interest than Charcot in the content of the patient's discourse under hypnosis, and no interest in its implications, either for the etiology of hysterical symptoms or for constructing a general psychology. It was Breuer's contribution in the first of the case studies on hysteria, the case of Anna O. (whom he had treated from 1880–82), to realize that under hypnosis the patient could recall the forgotten provoking causes of her or his state and that "the attempt at discovering the determining cause of the symptom was at the same time a therapeutic manoeuvre" (Freud 1893h, 35). Hypnosis for Breuer and Freud was thus a medium both for inquiry into the hysteria's specific causes and for therapeutic catharsis. The patient's discourse here becomes central, which it was not for Bernheim's practice of 'suggestion theory,' where it was the discourse of the all-powerful physician that was center stage, 'suggesting away' the patient's symptoms or even forbidding them.[3] For Breuer and Freud, by contrast, etiology and therapy were intimately connected because the latter became the test of the former: "The moment at which the physician finds out the occasion when the symptom first appeared and the reason for its appearance is also the moment at which the symptom vanishes" (ibid., 35).

However, the discovery of a cause is not a purely cognitive achievement. Freud warns, "Recollection without affect almost invariably produces no result" (1893a, 6). Psychical trauma is essentially a matter of affect, and this determines its peculiar mode of presence and its direct causal agency. For the unearthing of the traumatic cause to be therapeutic, its action in the therapy must be *of the same kind* as its action as a trauma. Freud's most striking statement of this occurs in the 1893 lecture:

> When, for instance, the symptom presented by the patient consists in pains, and when we enquire from him under hypnosis as to their origin, he will produce a series of memories in connection with them. If we can succeed in eliciting a really vivid memory in him, and if he sees things before him in all their original actuality, we shall observe that he is completely dominated by some affect. And if we compel him to put this affect into words, we shall find that, at the same time as he is producing this violent affect, the phenomenon of his pains emerges very markedly once again and that thenceforward the symptom, in its chronic character, disappears. . . . It could only be supposed, that the psychical trauma does in fact continue to operate in the subject and maintains the hysterical phenomenon, and that it comes to an end as soon as the patient has spoken about it. (Freud 1893h, 35)

The causal relation between the event being remembered and the symptom seems to be confirmed by the fact that the symptom in question, first, is intensified and, then, disappears after the event and its associated affect are

---

3. Suggestion as a technique of excising or banishing memories and the impulses that arise from them is in fact a use of hypnotism that is antithetical to the cathartic technique in which pathogenic memories and associations are worked through and integrated into the patient's preconscious memory system. Initially Freud seems to have attempted the former on some occasions, as in the case of Emmy von N., but abandoned it for the latter. See the discussion of the elimination as against the integration of memories in Ruth Leys, *Trauma: A Genealogy* (Chicago: University of Chicago Press, 2000), esp. chap. 3.

"put into words." The words, however, do not perform just a purely refer-
ential function, reporting on a past event; rather, they in some sense reproduce the lived experience of that event. As Breuer and Freud describe the
process, in the equivalent passage of the "Preliminary Communication":
"The psychical process which originally took place must be repeated as
vividly as possible: it must be brought back to its *status nascendi* and then
given verbal utterance" (1893a, 6). The patient's speech comes not from the
present moment but from the traumatic experience in its condition or state
of emergence, its moment of origin. The domination by affect entails the
quasi-hallucinatory acting out of the scene of the symptom's emergence;
but this must be put into words, the event and its emotional logic verbalized, with the result that, as Freud is later to say in the *Studies on Hysteria*,
"the symptom joins in the conversation" (1895d, 296), intensifying only to
disappear. The enactment of affect in the present, in these 'scenes of passionate movement,' characterizes both the afterlife of the trauma (either
directly in the *attitudes passionnelles* of the hysterical attack or by conversion
in the chronic bodily symptoms or stigmata) and the scene of therapy.
"Where what we are dealing with are phenomena involving stimuli (spasms,
neuralgias and hallucinations) these re-appear once again with the fullest
intensity and then vanish forever. Failures of function, such as paralyses
and anaesthesias, vanish in the same way" (ibid., 6–7). What distinguishes
the 'blind' acting out of the hysterical attack or the chronic symptom from
the reproductions of therapy is explained by Freud in terms of his theory of
abreaction. Therapeutic reproduction "brings to an end the operative force
of the idea," the idea behind the symptom, derived from the traumatic
event and acting outside the ego's consciousness or control. It does so "by
allowing its strangulated affect to find a way out through speech; and it
subjects it to associative correction by introducing it into normal consciousness" (ibid., 17). The 1893 lecture explicates this by adding that the
release of "strangulated affect," whose undischarged presence constituted
the psychical trauma, is based on "one of the dearest of human wishes—the
wish to be able to do something over again." Freud states, "We get him to
experience [the psychical trauma] a second time . . . and we now compel
him to complete his reaction to it" (1893h, 39). With the delayed discharge
of the affect, the operative power of the idea, its capacity to generate symptoms, disappears.

*Causes and Effects*

In the "Preliminary Communication" and its twin lecture Freud tends to assume a relatively straightforward relation between cause and symptom, which might seem plausible enough in the case of the traumatic hysterias consequent upon a physical trauma such as an accident. By contrast, in common, apparently 'nontraumatic' hysteria, what is at stake is "not a *single* major event . . . but rather a *series* of affective impressions—a whole story of suffering" (ibid., 31), which attains the status of a trauma through summation. Even though the latter might be accessible only under hypnosis, it acts "not *indirectly*, through a chain of intermediate links, but as a *directly* releasing cause." This leads to the famous proposition that "*hysterics suffer mainly from reminiscences*" (1893a, 7). Freud's tacit argument here is with Charcot's hereditarian model, which reduced the trauma to being simply an occasion, a precipitating cause or vanishing agent provocateur, that merely releases or activates the pregiven, hereditary condition (Charcot uses the—to us, ludicrous—example of a blow on the knee that produces a tubercular inflammation in someone with a disposition to tuberculosis). Against this conception Freud invokes what he calls "another kind of causation— namely, *direct causation*." He pictures this as "a foreign body, which continues to operate unceasingly as a stimulating cause of illness, until it is got rid of" (1893h, 35), a metaphor that has resonances with the new germ theory that was to displace the dominance of hereditarian explanations.[4] This attribution of full causal dignity to the trauma reproduced and acted out under hypnosis, however, tends to collapse the very distinction between the precipitating cause in the moment of the symptom's first emergence and the determining cause (a pregiven complex which for Charcot was heredity and for Freud remained to be elaborated). The specificity of the symptom is determined by the specificity of the traumatic moment of its emergence, for example, a man watching his brother having his hip joint extended under an anesthetic hears the crack as the joint gives way and instantly feels a pain in his own hip that lasts for a year. Even where the determining rela-

---

4. For a discussion of the new germ theory in relation to the development of Freud's etiological theories, see K. Codell Carter, "Germ Theory, Hysteria, and Freud's Early Work in Psychopathology," *Medical History* 24 (1980): 259–74.

tion is metaphorical or symbolic—vomiting produced by moral disgust, a headache by a piercing stare—the symptom finds its cause in a single originary moment. This may be complicated by the phenomenon of delay, the belated appearance in traumatic hysteria of paralysis after an incubation period, but this is usually referred back by the patient to the previous accident; so despite the delay, Freud considers the causal connection direct.

These two texts of 1893, in both their examples and their general statements, offer the model of a direct cause-and-effect relation between a symptom and a traumatic event or an emotional sequence. They do this by raising the trauma from its status as merely a releasing cause or an agent provocateur to that of a direct cause or still active foreign body. They thereby evict a general nonspecific heredity from its place in Charcot's schema as a prime determinant. Causal agency is concentrated in a single event or closely connected sequence—"a single story of suffering" (1893a, 6). This seems to be confirmed by the patient's affective acting out in the present, in the *attitudes passionnelle*s or 'scenes of passionate movement' we considered in the previous chapter, which when verbalized appear to liquidate the symptom. The sensory and emotional intensity of the event in the present and its therapeutic liquidation of the symptom are taken by Freud as the guarantor of its historical identity with the originary trauma in the past. The historical accuracy of the patient's memories is assumed to be authenticated by therapeutic success, and both are correlated with the immediacy of the reproduced scene, dominated by a set of emotions that are alive and active in the present just as they were in the past. Breuer's account of Anna O. and Freud's account of Emmy von N. seem to exemplify just this direct causal relation. Anna O. reproduced on a daily basis over a six-month period the traumatic experiences undergone on the exact same day of the previous year (a correlation confirmed by the entries in her mother's diary), while Emmy von N. relived the long-forgotten events of ten years previously. Even events of fifteen to twenty-five years previously, Freud assures us, "were found to be astonishingly intact and to possess remarkable sensory force" and to return "with all the affective strength of new experiences" (ibid., 10).

By the time of the publication of the whole *Studies on Hysteria* in 1895, however, the simple reference back to a unitary origin found in the formulations and examples of the "Preliminary Communication" has been complicated. In the case studies of Anna O., Elizabeth von R., and Emmy von N., the patient presents such a multiplicity of symptoms that the treatment requires a consequent complexity of references back to originating scenes and cumulative sequences of scenes, a whole memorial system of references, linked associatively to particular symptoms via what Freud calls "files of memories." In Breuer's case of Anna O., for example, the "theme of becoming deaf, of not hearing" was organized into "seven sets of determinants, and under each of these seven headings ten to over a hundred individual memories were connected in chronological series" (1895d, 288). Even in the two short cases of Lucy R. and Katharina, where the patient presents at any one time a single leading symptom, the simple model of a single unitary origin is complicated by the tendency of the analysis to uncover a sequence of scenes that cooperate to produce the symptom rather than a single moment.

### The Multiplication of Scenes: The Case of Miss Lucy R.

In the case of Lucy R., her suffering from a persistent condition of suppurative rhinitis privileged the sense of smell as the sensory medium for the presenting symptom, which was the persistent hallucinatory smell of burned pudding that was then replaced by the smell of cigar smoke. These were accompanied by a state of persistent depression and fatigue, loss of appetite and efficiency. Each of these olfactory hallucinations was the fixation of one sensory element of a painful scene that bore on her relations with the man who had employed her as the governess of his children. The treatment worked backward in time, dealing first with the presenting symptom of the persistent smell of burned pudding, a smell that intensified when she became emotionally agitated. Consideration of the smell led to the most recent scene in which the children, to whom she was strongly attached, hide a letter to her from her mother in order to be able to give it to her as their present for her birthday. While they are doing this, a pudding they were cooking is burned. Freud interprets this as the scene of a conflict of affects between her affection for the children and her determination to leave her situation and to return to live with her mother, due to slights she had received from the other domestic employees who had complained about her to her employer, and who she felt had not given her sufficient support. When asked if there was a particular reason for her affection for the children, she replied, "Yes. Their mother was a distant relation of my mother's, and I promised her on her deathbed that I would devote myself with all my power to the children, that I would not leave them and that I would take their mother's place with them. In giving notice I have broken this promise" (ibid., 115). The mother's letter does not just remind her of her decision to leave, but it connects to an earlier scene and to another mother, a deathbed scene in which the governess inherits the children and the place of the mother.

If the smell becomes the symbol of the scene with the children and its associated conflicts, the question for Freud remains why this should have led to hysteria and not "remained on the level of normal psychical life . . . why did she not always call to mind the scene itself, instead of the associated sensation?" (ibid., 116). The conversion of the emotional distress into a somatic symptom, the persistent smell, leads Freud to infer that "an idea must be *intentionally repressed from consciousness* and excluded from associative modification" (ibid.), and that this repression is the basis of the somatic conversion of excitation into the symptom. The repressed idea is an element of the trauma that she has sought to forget and to put out of her mind. Freud puts his interpretation to her quite bluntly: "I cannot think that these are all the reasons for your feelings about the children. I believe that really you are in love with your employer, the Director . . . and that you have a secret hope of taking their mother's place in actual fact" (ibid., 117). She acknowledges the truth of Freud's inference immediately, and in explanation of her silence on the matter, she responds: "I didn't know—or rather I didn't want to know. I wanted to drive it out of my head and not think of it again; and I believe latterly I have succeeded" (ibid.). Her acknowledgment leads to her recollection of another scene, a moment of rare intimacy with her employer in which the usually reserved man "unbent more and was more cordial than was usual and told her how much he depended on her for looking after his orphaned children; and as he said this he looked at her meaningly. . . ." (ibid., 118). Her love for him and hopes for the future, we are told, began at that moment, but the lack of any further scene of intimacy with him led to her decision to banish her feelings from her mind. She is persuaded by Freud, in retrospect, that "the look she had caught during their conversation had probably sprung from his thoughts about his wife" (ibid.). As they work through a range of associated memories and feelings, the persistent smell begins gradually to diminish.

On her return after the Christmas break, however, the smell of burned pudding had been replaced by another persistent smell, that of cigar smoke. Here a scene is gradually visualized in which her employer shouts angrily at an old accountant, a visiting family friend, when he tries to kiss the children good-bye. The governess comments: "I feel a stab at my heart; and as the gentlemen are already smoking, the cigar-smoke sticks in my memory" (ibid., 120). This response to a violence not directed at her is puzzling, until further exploration reveals yet another scene that Freud calls "the really operative trauma and which had given the scene with the chief accountant its traumatic effectiveness" (ibid.). Some months earlier a visiting lady had kissed the children on the mouth and the father had said nothing to her but on her departure had directed his anger at the governess. The father's response as recorded by Freud is itself symptomatically disproportionate, although Freud does not at any point explore or seek to interpret the father's highly charged contributions to the situation. "He said he held her responsible if anyone kissed the children on the mouth, that it was her duty not to permit it and that she was guilty of a dereliction of duty if she allowed it; if it ever happened again he would entrust his children's upbringing to other hands" (ibid.). The timing of the scene is significant, as it comes soon after the scene of intimacy with its meaningful look, when she was hoping for another such scene and a further development of their relations. Freud paraphrases the governess's response: "I must have made a mistake. He can never have had any warm feelings for me" (ibid.). He only comments that "it was obviously the recollection of this distressing scene which had come to her when the chief accountant had tried to kiss the children and had been reprimanded by their father" (ibid., 121).

Freud offers this short case of a "slight and mild hysteria" as a "model instance" of an *acquired* hysteria without any evidence of hereditary taint (ibid., 121, 122). He presents it as a temporal structure, in which a sequence of scenes, one behind another, operates in a relay to generate the two sensory symptoms, the later one masking the earlier. He makes a distinction between the traumatic scene and later auxiliary scenes in terms of his newly formulated theory of defense. Initially, this stood in uneasy alliance with

Breuer's postulation of spontaneously generated hypnoid states in which ideas are split off from normal consciousness and become traumatic, regardless of their content, due to the special properties of these states of consciousness (Breuer's position is very close to Charcot's account of hypnotic 'auto suggestion' in the wake of physical traumas, as discussed in the previous chapter). In the "Preliminary Communication" Breuer and Freud had argued that "the basis and *sine qua non* of hysteria is the existence of hypnoid states" (1893a, 12). In the first paper on "The Neuro-Psychoses of Defence" of 1894, 'defence hysteria' is one of three kinds of hysteria, alongside 'hypnoid hysteria' and 'retention hysteria.' By the time *Studies on Hysteria* appears, defense has become primary and is even, according to Freud (though not to Breuer), at the root of the appearance of hypnoid states. In this case study he characterizes the traumatic moment in terms of the emergence of an incompatibility between an intense idea and the ego. The differentiation between the different neuroses, Freud argues, rests on "the different methods adopted by the ego to escape this incompatibility" (1895d, 122). The hysterical method of defense "lies in the conversion of the excitation into a somatic innervation" (ibid.).[5] The incompatible idea is repressed from consciousness, which, however, from now on suffers from a 'physical reminiscence,' the result of conversion (the governess's persistent olfactory hallucinations), and from the affect that is lodged in those bodily parts and sensations and is bound to them.

The traumatic moment is the scene in which "the incompatibility forces itself on the ego and at which the latter decides on the repudiation of the incompatible idea" (ibid., 123). This results in a splitting of consciousness and the formation of "a nucleus and centre of crystallisation for the formation of a psychical group divorced from the ego" (ibid.). Freud identifies the traumatic moment in the case study as the moment of the employer's attack on the governess, after the children had been kissed by the lady visitor. This is the moment when she repudiates her feelings for him by denying

---

5. Laplanche and Pontalis usefully point out that the term *innervation* usually has an anatomical reference: "the route of a nerve on its way to a given organ. For Freud, however, innervation was a physiological process: the transmission, generally in an efferent direction, of energy along a nerve-pathway." Jean Laplanche and J-B. Pontalis, *The Language of Psycho-Analysis*, trans. Donald Nicholson-Smith (London: The Hogarth Press, 1973), 213.

that anything had happened between them: "I had made a mistake." However, the hysterical symptoms do not start here but in two later moments that Freud designates "auxiliary." What characterizes the auxiliary moment is that "the two divided psychical groups temporarily converge in it" (ibid.), as they do in the recovery of traumatic memories under hypnosis. This nonhypnotic convergence, however, is not elaborated by Freud and would seem to be less a moment of transparency in which what had been repressed is now momentarily accessible than an example of what Freud is later to call 'the return of the repressed.' This happens in *displaced* form as the repressed complex establishes links with certain features of the current situation and discharges its affect by proxy through that connection. The auxiliary scenes here are the two scenes of hysterical conversion from which the hallucinatory smells arise as the symptom that maintains the repression of the disturbing affect (desire for the father, pain at his repudiation) and its representations. There is the scene with the chief accountant in which her employer's violence against the visitor recalls his earlier violence *against her* in the traumatic scene. It is the traumatic scene that resonates within the details of the auxiliary scene: the memory of the father's earlier anger at her about the lady visitor's kissing of the children and his threat of dismissal is reactivated in his anger against the accountant's kissing the children, producing the "stab at my heart" and, according to Freud, the fixated smell of cigar smoke. Freud also applies his definition of an auxiliary scene to the scene with the children and the mother's letter that leads to the final form of the symptom, the smell of burned pudding, but without demonstrating how the logic of this most recent scene displays the convergence he posits. So Freud's etiological formula of traumatic scene plus auxiliary scenes (1 + 2) analyzes the hysteria into the original traumatic scene of the lady visitor kissing the children and the father's anger unfairly holding the governess responsible, followed by two later auxiliary scenes, first with the father's anger against the chief accountant that precipitates the smell of the cigar smoke and the stab at her heart and then the children's game with the mother's letter and the smell of the burned pudding.

This formal etiological analysis, however, leaves unspecified two further accompanying scenes, which I will call "originary" scenes, beyond the three designated as "traumatic" or "auxiliary," which nevertheless are essential preconditions for the development of the governess's hysteria. These are the *paternal scene* of the meaningful look between the governess and the children's father in which we are told her love for him begins and the earliest scene of all, which is produced in relation to the most recent scene of her mother's letter and the burned pudding, that is, the *maternal scene*, the deathbed scene of the children's mother and the governess's promise to "take their mother's place with them" (ibid., 115).

Consideration of the first of these supplementary scenes foregrounds the role of the father-employer in the whole story, a role that Freud's analysis tends to minimize. Surprisingly, he makes no comment on the disproportionate intensity of the father's phobia about the children being kissed, and its associated anger at the governess (she has not kissed the children, the visiting lady has) and his threat to dismiss her. Freud also assumes that the governess misreads the meaning of the look her employer gives her, as he tells her "how much he depended on her for looking after his orphaned children" (ibid., 118). The disproportionate intensity of the father's later reactions suggests that to kiss the children *on the mouth* is to take the place of their mother, and it looks very much like an energy of repudiation that arises in relation to the lady visitor but is displaced onto the governess (who has done nothing to deserve it, but who is held responsible for the lady's actions). If the governess has not kissed the children, she has, however, been the recipient both of the father's look and confession of dependency as well as of the dying mother's request. While looks can be ambiguous and easily misread, it is difficult not to feel that the father is repudiating the meaning of his own look with its implicit, if not unconscious, invitation to the governess to take the mother's place, not just with the children but also with him. Freud of course seizes on this phrase as a clue to the governess's as yet unadmitted desire—to take the mother's place with the father—and she readily admits her love for him, in response to Freud's rather precipitate guess. Clearly the role of the father has been crucial in the genesis of the governess's hysteria, both in his initiative toward her and in his repudiation of it (no one is to take the mother's place and kiss the children, but the governess is guilty if someone does—not the father). Freud does not consider whether the father might not still be in a state of mourning for his dead wife and so feeling guilty about his attraction to any other woman (the lady visitor, the governess) who might take her place by kissing the children.

The other *maternal* deathbed scene has even more originary force than the one with the father. Surprisingly, Freud makes very little of either the governess's promise or the connection between the dying mother and the governess's own mother (one, we are told, is a distant relation of the other). He does pick up, however, on the phrasing of the governess's promise to 'take the mother's place with them' and shrewdly but narrowly reads it as a clue to her feelings for the father, and to her wish to take up a particular place in the familial and marital scene. The relation back to the dead mother to whom the promise was made, and to her own still-living mother, remains uninterrogated by Freud; consequently, the complexities and nuances of her feelings for either maternal figure can only be guessed at. Regret, guilt, or some such strong emotion is clearly an important part of the conflict of affects in the scene of the mother's letter. Reading backward in light of later Freudian positions, a strong female oedipal situation seems to assert itself. The dying mother as a relation or representative of the living mother licenses an infantile oedipal wish to take her place, to occupy that place and with her blessing. One might, indeed, wonder whether the deathbed discourse of the mother had not framed the whole case history—and not least the figure of the father-husband—constituting him as the paternal object of the governess's specifically *oedipal* desire. Thus the paternal scene of the meaningful look and the speech about his dependency are overdetermined by that earlier maternal scene, where for a moment the wishes of all three seem to converge in the governess's accession to the coveted place that gives her both the older man and his children. Freud persuades his patient that "the look she had caught in their conversation had probably sprung from thoughts about his wife" (ibid., 118), but, given that earlier deathbed scene, thoughts about his wife could hardly exclude the governess, who is his dying wife's delegate and heir apparent.

Freud notes that, because the treatment deals with the scenes in the reverse order of their occurrence, the later symptom of the burned pudding smell masks the earlier smell of the cigar smoke. However, though the cigar smell references the earlier scene, it does not seem to have been experienced by the governess directly from its occurrence in that scene or in the interval between the two auxiliary scenes; it only appears clearly for the first time in the course of the analysis itself, after the dissolution of the later symptomatic smell of the burned pudding. Although Freud states that the conversion of affect into smell takes place during the scene it references (ibid., 124), in fact it only makes a *belated* appearance as if it were an artifact of the treatment. The governess says of the smell of cigar smoke: "It had been there earlier as well, she thought, but had, as it were, been covered by the smell of the pudding. Now it had emerged by itself" (ibid., 119). This implies that it had not been present as a separate symptom prior to the most recent scene of the letter and the burned pudding. The question is then posed of the relation between the two forms of the symptom, between the smell of the cigar smoke and that of the burned pudding. While the burned pudding references the recent scene of the letter from the governess's mother, its repressed signification, requiring the conversion of disturbing affect into hallucinatory smell, is suggested by the children's taking over the letter and re-presenting it as *their* present to the governess. In this context the living mother's letter ("Leave your post, come home") comes also to signify the children's dying mother and her message or request "to take their mother's place with them." Furthermore, as the children give it to her as their present, it might also be taken as signifying for the governess that this is their wish/message as well ("We love you, Miss Lucy. Please stay!").

Such a letter-wish, however, necessarily invokes but is contradicted by the father's intensely ambivalent inputs into the situation. These are signified by the cigar smoke with its sequence of scenes of paternal anger, and possibly behind them the father's implicit but repudiated invitation, which this smell both sums up and substitutes for. At the level of the sensory-perceptual signifier, the connection is made in both cases by the smell of something burning. The contradictory significations of the first hidden and then re-presented letter include the mother's invitation to the governess to return home because the father-employer has repudiated her, and also the governess's continuing desire to fulfil the dying mother's request to stay with the children. The cigar smoke as signifier only appears belatedly in the treatment after the partial clarification of the burned pudding smell, as I have argued above, and *not*, as Freud suggests, at the moment of the scene it references. The governess suggests that it had been present earlier along with but covered over by the later smell, but *not*, as Freud proposes, formed as a symptom from the time of that scene. This is important because the confusion and affinity of the two smells suggest that the cigar smell had also implicitly played a role in the conflicts of the later, second auxiliary scene, before being precipitated out in its own right as a separate symptom.

This conflict might be described as a conflict between two sequences or scenographies: that bearing on the mother and that bearing on the father. The re-presented letter signifies the two mothers, and the cigar smoke signifies the father. The smell of burned pudding seems like a bridge or compromise between the mother's explicit plea and the father's repudiated invitation. The letter's very doubleness as a message from the two mothers signifies both the mother's request and the governess's promise, on the one hand, and the giving of notice with its *broken* promise and the indifferent or hostile employer-father, on the other. It might be read as the governess's compromised attempt to subsume the burned smell of the father's violent repudiation (if anyone kisses the children on the mouth, the governess will be fired) into the scene of the letter where the mother's invitation still stands. However, it is the prior existence of the cigar smoke/"stab at my heart" linkage that determines the selection of the burned pudding smell as the overdetermined sensory element that will represent the painful conflicts of the later scene in the register of smell. While the first phase of the analysis partially uncovers some of these, it does not lift the governess's depression, and the burned-pudding-mother's-letter-deathbed maternal sequence makes way for the cigar smoke, now raised retrospectively from its position as latent signifier in the maternal sequence to a fully fledged separate symptom of the as yet unaddressed paternal sequence of scenes that are both signified and substituted for by its acrid persistence. This relay between earlier and later scenes calls for further clarification in terms of the later concepts of afterwardsness/deferred action (*Nachträglichkeit*) and of screen memories, which I will discuss in the next two chapters.

These absent dimensions in Freud's analysis consist of two key elements: the role of the other and the other's unconscious wishes and repudiations and, as well, the possibility that behind the sequence of contemporary adult scenes, each with varying traumatic force and part of a complex system of mutual references, there lies an originary childhood scene or oedipal configuration of wishes and identifications. This acts as a subjective template through which the later scenes of adult life are experienced and which they in turn translate and rework.

*From Symptom to Subjectivity*

Freud himself was aware of the therapeutic limitations of the cathartic method of abreaction that Breuer and he had pioneered. In the "Preliminary Communication" of 1893, he acknowledged that "we do not cure hysteria in so far as it is a matter of disposition" (1893a, 17). The cathartic method cannot prevent the emergence of hypnoid states or the replacement of hysterical symptoms that have been removed by fresh ones, especially in states of acute hysteria. They have been able, following Charcot, to uncover the *psychical mechanism* of hysterical symptoms but not "the internal causes of hysteria." "We have done no more than touch upon the aetiology of hysteria" (ibid., 17). However, by the end of the last chapter of *Studies on Hysteria*, Freud had moved from a narrowly symptom-focussed perspective to a mental cartography of the 'memory-files' associated with the symptoms being treated, and of the ways in which they are layered and organized into something like a psychical system. He states explicitly that a hysteria with one main presenting symptom, such as the cases of Miss Lucy R. and Katharina, is "an elementary organism, a unicellular creature" (1895d, 288), and even these do not refer back to just "a *single* traumatic memory or pathogenic idea as its nucleus," which we might be led to expect from the examples in the "Preliminary Communication." As we have seen in the previous discussion, behind the hallucinatory sensations of smell Freud describes a relay of traumatic and auxiliary scenes, and I have argued that at least two other originary scenes—the mother's deathbed appeal and the father's meaningful look—are contributory preconditions for the operation of the sequence Freud describes, each organizing what one might call a maternal and a paternal sequence or scenography.

What we discover are "*successions* of *partial* traumas and *concatenations* of pathogenic trains of thought" (ibid., 288), and these "successions" and "concatenations" form a terrain that is organized in peculiar ways. Freud addresses this peculiar organization of what he calls "the pathogenic material" under three different headings that specify different kinds of arrangements of the material and that map out a series of lines of force and interconnection, as well as a therapeutic pathway that traverses them. This psychical system organizes a large amount of material around "a nucleus consisting in memories of events or trains of thought in which the traumatic factor has culminated or the pathogenic idea had found its purest manifestation" (ibid.). The first heading refers to the different "files of memories" grouped under certain leading themes, as in the example taken from the case of Anna O., where the theme of "becoming deaf, not hearing" was divided into seven subheadings, each of which could contain anything up to one hundred or more memories. Each of these groupings is filed chronologically like "a dossier that had been kept in good order" (ibid.), and Freud claims that the memories are always reproduced in reverse order to the one in which they occurred, from the most recent to the earliest and most obscure.

These linear sequences that embody key themes are also organized in a second way—"stratified concentrically around the pathogenic nucleus" (ibid., 289). Each stratum is characterized by an equal degree of resistance that varies as a function of its distance from the pathogenic nucleus, the resistance increasing with the strata nearer the nucleus and lessening with those at the periphery. The 'resistance co-efficient,' as it were, of each stratum creates a zone in which there is "an equal degree of modification of consciousness" (ibid.). So the memory files at the periphery are easily remembered and have always been available to consciousness. By contrast, at the nucleus, where the resistance is greatest, Freud writes, "We come across memories which the patient disavows even in reproducing them" (ibid.). This paradox raises questions about what counts as a memory and what the nature of that reproduction is. If memory references a past moment, it is also the possession of a subject in the present—"my memory of . . ." What Freud seems to be alluding to here are emotive, affect-laden scenes that are reproduced "as though . . . from a phonograph"[6] but that are never acknowledged by the subject as *his* memory. The paradoxical emotional force of these scenes in the present is active unconsciously in the hysterical attack, or active through conversion in the hysterical symptom, and, even more puzzlingly, active in the reproduction in consciousness of a scene that is, nevertheless, disavowed as memory. This dismantles the commonsense problematic of remembrance. Instead of a subject-centered process, "I re-

6. Jeffrey Moussaiff Masson, trans. and ed., *The Complete Letters of Sigmund Freud to Wilhelm Fliess 1887–1904* (Cambridge, Mass.: Harvard University Press, 1985), 226.

member that event," we need a formulation more like, "This scene is remembered or remembers itself in me," or even, "This scene remembers me." This paradox is to haunt Freud throughout his clinical and theoretical development, from the seduction theory through the theory of transference and acting out to the late paper on "Constructions in Analysis" (1937d).

The third kind of arrangement of the pathogenic material that Freud describes is more elusive. It is an arrangement by thought-content, "the linkage made by a logical thread which reaches as far as the nucleus and tends to take an irregular and twisting path, different in every case" (1895d, 289). While the first two arrangements, Freud says, could be represented spatially by continuous lines, curved or straight, tracing the radial, thematic connections of the chronological memory files or the lateral connections of the different zones of resistance, here the twisting and roundabout path of Freud's logical thread or chain, moving from surface to depth and back, is compared strikingly by him to "the zig-zag line in the solution of a Knight's Move problem, which cuts across the squares in the diagram of the chess-board" (ibid., 289). This seems less like a pregiven arrangement of the material than a particular pathway through it taken by the analysis, determined by the rhythm and pattern of the patient's free associations. This is borne out by his statement that it has "a dynamic character, in contrast to the morphological one of the two stratifications mentioned previously," and that it advances "from the periphery to the central nucleus, touching at every intermediate halting-place" (ibid.).

Confusingly, Freud then shifts his metaphor from the zigzag line of the Knight's Move that seems to indicate a dynamic movement through a stratified field of force to yet another mode of arrangement of the material being traversed. This centers on an idea crucial to Freud's mapping of the associational field of dreams, that of the nodal point "at which two or more threads meet and thereafter proceed as one." This corresponds to "a ramifying system of lines and more particularly to a converging one" (ibid., 290), which leads Freud to make what is to become his standard point about all formations of the unconscious—symptoms, dreams, parapraxes—that the symptom is 'overdetermined,' that is, the symptom is the convergence point of a number of different threads of association and a number of different lines of force produce it, like a resultant force in physics. If traced back, these separate lines of connection "debouch into the nucleus" (ibid., 290), which seems also to be a convergence point.

Perhaps Freud's most significant move is to interrogate his preferred metaphor of the foreign body previously counterposed to Charcot's agent provocateur. Hitherto he had posited that the pathogenic material acts like a foreign body, and so the treatment would operate like "the removal of a foreign body from the living tissue" (ibid.). Where, medically, the foreign body remains separable from the living tissue, Freud now argues:

> Our pathogenic psychical group . . . does not admit of being cleanly extirpated from the ego. Its external strata pass over in every direction into the ego; and, indeed, they belong to the latter just as much as to the pathogenic organisation. (Freud 1895d, 290)

Here the whole problematic of the unconscious as a pathological formation produced by the trauma, and so in principle reducible and open to thera-peutic dissolution, is by implication being put into question. As Freud de-scribes the complex organization of memory files, of zones and degrees of resistance, of nucleus and periphery, of nodal points and points of conver-gence, it begins increasingly to look like a whole cartography of the subject, of the mental and affective organization of *subjectivity as such*, conscious, preconscious, and unconscious, is being laid out. Where the "external strata" of the pathogenic material belong as much to the ego as to the for-eign body, then we have a situation where the unconscious is permanent and structural, not temporary and removable. However, Freud still retains the element of 'foreignness,' insisting that "the interior layers of the patho-genic organisation are increasingly alien to the ego," even though no clear boundary where one takes over from the other can be demarcated. This prompts a radical shift of metaphor:

> In fact the pathogenic organisation does not behave like a foreign body, but far more like an infiltrate. In this simile the resistance must be regarded as what is infiltrating. (Freud 1895d, 290)

With this new metaphor of the resistance as "infiltrate," we can begin to see the oscillation between two different perspectives on "resistance" in Freud's thought, as described by Laplanche and Pontalis. The previous mapping of "zones of resistance" seemed to locate "the ultimate source of resistance in a repelling force derived from the repressed itself"[7] and which increased with the approach to the pathogenic nucleus.

Resistance as 'infiltrate,' however, is cognate with Freud's theory of pathological defense and its increasing centrality to the whole theory of the psychoneuroses. His letters to Fliess and his later papers oscillate over whether the form and specificity of the neuroses arise from the content of the original trauma or from the mode of defense that the ego brings to bear on it. The latter position tends gradually to predominate, but not exclusively, as a late work such as *Inhibitions, Symptoms and Anxiety* (1926d) re-affirms the resistance of the unconscious due to "the attraction exerted by the unconscious prototypes upon the repressed instinctual process."[8] Here, however, what gives the material the distinct pathogenic form of a symptom is precisely the infiltrating resistance brought to bear against it—by the ego. The therapeutic consequence immediately follows, that the treatment does not "consist in extirpating something" but "in causing the resistance to melt and in thus enabling the circulation to make its way into a region that has hitherto been cut off" (1895d, 291). The notion of an "infiltrating resistance" locates resistance as an ego defense and differentiates it from the second mode of organization of the pathogenic material, that is, the concentric zones of resistance with their increasing coefficient of resistance from the periphery to the nucleus. This anticipates later psychoanalytic debates about the place of the analysis of the ego and its resistances in the treatment as against the analysis of unconscious wishes and their associated fantasies.

Freud steps back from his choice of similes, noting their limitations and mutual incompatibility. However, the shift from foreign body to infiltrating resistance foregrounds the centrality of the ego's defense in the production of hysteria and the permanent inextricability of the ego from the material it represses. What is at stake is no longer a temporary pathological episode but the permanent modes of organization of both the ego and the unconscious material it excludes. Although not in the form of Charcot's hereditary '*tare nerveuse*', the question of a 'constitution' (this time psychical) is back on the agenda. As the psychoanalytic treatment increasingly

7. Laplanche and Pontalis, *The Language of Psycho-Analysis*, 395.
8. Sigmund Freud, *Inhibitions, Symptoms and Anxiety* (1926d), *SE* 20, 158–60.

addresses itself to the ramifying memorial system deposited by what at times looks like a virtual life history, as the relay of scenes and moments, of preconditions and auxiliaries, reaches further and further back toward the subject's childhood, then the object of psychoanalytic theory begins to shift from specific delimited pathologies to the constitution of subjectivity itself. Before this emergent development becomes fully fledged, however, Freud pushes his 'special case' theory of trauma to its limit in the theory of infantile seduction. Here the elaboration of a traumatic scenography, including scenes of memory and scenes of fantasy, plays a central role. This will be the starting point for the following chapter.

# Part II  Memorial Fantasies, Fantasmatic Memories

## THREE

# The Afterwardsness of Trauma and the Theory of Seduction

"The aim seems to be to arrive [back] at the primal scenes."[1]

As the previous chapter sought to show, in the period 1889–95 Freud's model of trauma inherited from Charcot was transformed from a neurological account with important psychological components into one that was fully psychological. At the same time its object was extended from hysteria to psychopathology in general, or what Freud in the years 1894–96 called 'the neuro-psychoses of defence.' What enabled this diagnostic ambitiousness was a double movement of unification and elaboration, which is evident as one reads through *Studies on Hysteria* (1895d) and the papers contempo-

---

1. Sigmund Freud, "Draft L," Letter to Fliess, May 2, 1897, *SE* 1, 248. Masson unfortunately translates Freud's key term *Urszenen* (originary or primal scenes) as "earliest [sexual] scenes," which loses Freud's conceptual and terminological consistency (*The Complete Letters of Sigmund Freud to Wilhelm Fliess 1887–1904*, trans. and ed. Jeffrey Moussaiff Masson, Cambridge, Mass.: Harvard University Press, 1985: 240, henceforth, Masson 1985a). This is the first appearance of the 'primal scenes' formulation in Freud's writing.

rary with its writing. The repositioning of various diagnostic categories in a newly unified field results from Freud's increasing insistence on the location of the originating trauma in certain sexual experiences, along with the centrality of the conflict between the ego's defenses and the incompatible sexual ideas and affects resulting from the trauma. Significantly, however, neither sexual experience nor the defensive conflict was a feature of either the ur-case of psychoanalysis, that of Anna O., whose treatment Breuer had begun fifteen years prior to the *Studies*, or the general model of trauma, advanced in the "Preliminary Communication" (1893a) and reprinted as its introduction. The same is true of the movement of conceptual elaboration by which the relatively simple cause-and-effect model, evident in the "Preliminary Communication" and, for all its proliferation of symptoms, in the Anna O. case as well, gradually evolves into a more complex time structure in which the initial traumatic scene is supplemented by a series of auxiliary scenes that orchestrate the production of symptoms. Freud's formulation of the seduction theory in the years immediately following the *Studies* combines two potentially contradictory tendencies. These are an increasingly exact specification of the sexual trauma involved (in the final unpublished version in the letters to Wilhelm Fliess, it will narrow down to the figure of the perverse and abusive father), combined with an elaboration of its temporal effectivity or mode of traumatic agency. As the multiplication of scenes, and the resulting complex memorial system that Freud maps out in the final chapter of the *Studies*, are driven back further and further into the individual subject's personal prehistory by the impasses and difficulties of his clinical practice, then a system of 'scenes,' a psychical scenography, is elaborated that is governed by a distinctive temporal logic. Freud's name for this is *Nachträglichkeit*. This has been translated in the *Standard Edition*, with a considerable narrowing of meaning as 'deferred action,' and more recently as 'afterwardsness,' an alternative translation suggested by Jean Laplanche (the French translation is *après coup*).[2] It is both central to Freud's seduction theory and, I will argue, also put at risk by it.

2. Jean Laplanche, "Notes on Afterwardsness," in *Essays on Otherness*, ed. John Fletcher (London: Routledge, 1999); *Problématiques VI: L'Après-coup* (Paris: Presses Universitaires de France, 2006). Freud turns an ordinary German word *nachträglich* (later, afterwards, subsequently, etc.) into an abstract noun *Nachträglichkeit*, which from its verbal

## Trauma and Its Auxiliaries

The schematic representation of an acquired hysteria in the *Studies*, as we saw in the previous chapter, consisted of an initial traumatic moment, one in which an excessively intense and incompatible idea confronts and threatens to overwhelm the ego, leading to its exclusion or repression from consciousness as a separate psychical group. This is followed by an auxiliary moment or moments where the split-off group of representations temporarily returns to or converges with consciousness. This paired set of terms, 'traumatic' and 'auxiliary,' and the distinction between them appear first and briefly in "The Neuro-Psychoses of Defence" (1894a) and then again in the two cases in the *Studies*, of Miss Lucy R. discussed in the last chapter and of Katharina. They are the beginnings of Freud's development of a temporal schema, but he gives their separate moments a different value in each instance. In the 1894 paper he locates the moment of defense and repudiation of the incompatible idea, along with the formation of the neurotic symptom, whether hysterical or obsessional, all in the initial traumatic moment itself. Freud describes a weakening of the powerful idea by the splitting off of its load of affect or excitation and the redeployment of this excitation, either by its conversion into a bodily symptom in hysteria or, alternatively, in obsessional neurosis, by its investment in an alternative set of obsessional ideas, associated by 'false connections' with the incompatible idea. "By this means the ego succeeds in freeing itself from the contradiction [with which it is confronted]; but instead, it has burdened itself with a mnemic symbol which finds a lodgement in consciousness, like a sort of parasite."[3] Both the moment of repression and the moment of symptom formation occur together in what Freud calls the traumatic moment. The later auxiliary moments are here conceived as repressions similar to the traumatic moment, which augment the separate psychical group already split off; this happens "whenever the arrival of a fresh impression of the same sort succeeds in breaking through . . . in furnishing the weakened idea with fresh affect and re-establishing for a time the associative link between

---

components—*nach*/after, *tragen*/*to bear or carry*, as in to bear a grudge—might be literally translated as 'carrying-after-ness.'

3. Sigmund Freud, "The Neuro-Psychoses of Defence" (1894a), *SE* 3, 52, 49.

the two psychical groups, until a further conversion sets up a defence" (1894a, 50).

In the two cases in the *Studies*, however, the distinction between traumatic and auxiliary moments is somewhat differently conceived. In the simplest of them, that of Katharina, the early confused experiences of sexual advances from her father,[4] which are rejected by her without a clear understanding of their significance, do not immediately result in a hysterical symptom, although Freud postulates that "an element of consciousness was created which was excluded from the thought-activity of the ego and remained, as it were, in storage."[5] This splitting off, however, does not amount to a full instance of repression with its accompanying symptom formation, for Freud characterizes this period between the traumatic and auxiliary scenes thus: "At that time she had carried about with her two sets of experiences which she remembered but did not understand, and from which she drew no inferences" (ibid., 131). The hysteria is only precipitated by the so-called auxiliary scene, where she witnesses her father lying on top of her cousin and reacts with the classic symptoms of the hysterical aura—breathlessness, a sensation of blankness, pressure on the eyes and chest, and a hammering and buzzing in the head. There follows what Freud calls "a short period of working-out, of 'incubation', after which the symptoms of conversion set in, the vomiting as a substitute for moral disgust" (ibid.). As she saw nothing clearly in the precipitating auxiliary scene, she could not tell Freud exactly what it was that she was so disgusted by, and which had produced such an intense reaction in her. Freud infers that it was not the obscure sight itself that provoked her disgust but a memory of one of the early advances from her father that it awoke, in particular, an occasion on which she "woke up suddenly 'feeling his body' in the bed" (ibid., 130). Freud's leading question—"What part of his body was it that you felt that night?"—gets no answer but an embarrassed smile, which leads him to infer "what tactile sensation it was she had learnt later to interpret" (ibid., 132).

Unlike the 1894 text, where the auxiliary moments seem merely to repeat and augment the effects of repression and symptom formation in the previous

---

4. He is described as the girl's uncle in the main body of the text, but Freud adds in a self-critical note in 1924 that he was in fact her father.

5. Joseph Breuer and Sigmund Freud, *Studies on Hysteria* (1895d), *SE* 2, 133.

traumatic moment, here the effects of the traumatic moment include a repudiation of the father's advances whose full consequences remain latent *until* the auxiliary moment. It is this later moment that is the moment of repression and symptom formation, of hysterical anxiety attacks and an inability to know what is causing them. In other words, *before* the process of repression and its consequent symptom formation can occur, an even earlier and more obscure inscription must have taken place, which is only later reactivated and plays its part in the deferred production of the hysterical symptom. It is this earlier moment that Freud now calls the traumatic moment. The auxiliary moment has its effect only after an interval during which it acts back on the first moment interpreting its significance in a new context. Freud compares this interval to Charcot's account of "the 'period of psychical working-out' [*élaboration*]" (ibid., 134) between the traumatic event and the deferred appearance of symptoms in his accident cases (although this is something of a false analogy, as Freud is concerned with the interplay of two events, whereas Charcot describes the postponed aftereffects of a single event).

In considering the status of this traumatic precondition, Freud notes that it is characterized by virginal ignorance rather than by repression, as in the case of Lucy R. and her repudiated feelings for her employer. He goes on to assert, however, that "the case of Katharina is typical," as in all cases of hysteria, analysis finds that "impressions from the pre-sexual period which produced no effect on the child attain traumatic power at a later date as memories" (ibid., 133). We have here the germ of the concept of *Nachträglichkeit*, as Strachey's editorial footnote registers. What is striking is that Freud goes on to wonder whether the splitting of consciousness caused by ignorance—the exclusion of something that "remained, as it were, in storage"—is not all that different from that due to repression, and "whether even adolescents do not possess sexual knowledge far oftener than is supposed or than they themselves believe." The implication here is that what we take to be ignorance in adolescents is in fact the work of repression, one that is not a pathological exception but "a normal process of adolescent development" (ibid., 134). So Katharina's deferred traumatic reaction is typical not just of the processes of hysteria but of normal development itself. Freud's formulations are ambiguous, combining the commonsense background assumptions of an infantile 'pre-sexual period' with the contrary suggestion of a pre-adolescent sexual knowledge, with its aftereffects of psychical disturbances in normal development, therefore, a sort of 'normal disturbance.' Well before Freud's recognition and theorization of infantile sexual drives, normal development is here implicated in both an unspecified precocious sexual knowledge and in the temporality peculiar to the action of a trauma. A similar generalization takes place in the case of Emma in "Project for a Scientific Psychology" (1895), as we shall see.

Freud notes, however, that the scene where Katharina sees her father and her cousin lying together is also a traumatic moment in its own right and "on account of its own content and not merely as something that revived traumatic experiences" (1895d, 134). The auxiliary scene here is not just an occasion for the emergence of an already formed entity, as with Charcot's analogy of the agent provocateur that Freud had repudiated in order to give a properly causal force to the scene of the symptom's formation over the predestined power of heredity. Freud insists on both Katharina's retrospective interpretation of the "tactile sensation" of her father's body, deferred from the earlier scene, and on the disturbing content of the scene itself as a fully sexual scene. Causal power or effectivity is attributed to each scene in the relay of scenes, although the traumatic force of the auxiliary second scene in its own right is not explored in any detail due to its obscurity. The latter scene's *doubling* as both auxiliary to the first scene and yet traumatic in its own right does not for Freud call into question his conceptual distinction between these terms, or his postulation of a first scene whose full implication and force is only precipitated in a later scene, although the processes by which this happens remain to be specified.

## Miss Lucy R Revisited

The case of Miss Lucy R. has been discussed at length in the previous chapter, mainly with respect to the two supplementary parental scenes described by the analysand, which lie *outside* the etiological formula of a traumatic scene plus two auxiliary scenes that Freud proposes. I do not wish to repeat the arguments made previously about the complexities of this only apparently simple case. I will comment solely on Freud's etiological formula itself. Freud states the main distinction as one between a traumatic scene, in which a splitting of consciousness takes place in response to a distressing incompatibility, and a further auxiliary scene, in which the split-off psychical group is reconnected with the conscious mainstream of the ego. Unlike the case of Katharina, the distressing idea in the traumatic scene is described as "repressed into the unconscious" (1895d, 123). However, the relay between these scenes displays a similar structure of deferral, as in the Katharina case, with the scene designated traumatic having its hysterical aftereffects only in the later scenes. Although Freud does not explicitly designate the later auxiliary scenes as also traumatic in their own right, as in the Katharina case, it follows from my previous analysis of the case that, in fact, this is so.

The designated traumatic first scene is the moment when the children's father attacks their governess because the lady visitor has kissed them on the mouth, and where he threatens to dismiss her if it happens again. This provokes her repudiation and repression of her romantic feelings for him evoked in their earlier scene of intimacy. *However, the two later auxiliary scenes also have each their own traumatic force and effects.* The first auxiliary scene, where the father attacks the accountant and family friend for the same reason (kissing the children on the mouth), produces, the governess tells Freud, "a stab at my heart" (ibid., 120), a violence she experiences as directed at her and her feelings, "at my heart." Clearly this first auxiliary scene of paternal aggression both reactivates the previous traumatic scene and, as has already been argued at length in the last chapter, also produces its own deferred symptom, but only in the later second auxiliary scene of the mother's letter. The governess's presenting symptom of the smell of burned pudding dates from and references this second auxiliary scene of the letter and its emotional conflicts, which themselves date back to the memory of the children's mother and the governess's promise at her deathbed. After its dissolution in the analysis, the burned-pudding smell is replaced by the second smell of the cigar smoke that references the first auxiliary scene with the accountant and the "stab at my heart." This scene did not release its symptom straightaway, as Freud seems to assume. The cigar smell was first present mixed in with the smell of the burned pudding, according to the governess, but not perceived as such in the later scene of the letter. It is only in the course of the analysis that it appears in its own right. This first auxiliary scene with the accountant would also give good grounds for being judged to be *both* a moment of deferred reactivation of the traumatic scene with the lady visitor and, given the father's emotional violence and the governess's distressed response, a traumatic scene in its own right with its own process of deferred symptom formation in the second auxiliary scene of the letter.

The third and latest scene of the letter might appear to be relatively innocent and lacking in the emotional violence of the earlier scenes, but it is more than a mere occasion or agent provocateur for the release of preexisting material. It has its own effectivity, both in the action of the governess's mother in writing to her and agreeing to her leaving her post and coming home, and in the action of the children in appropriating the letter, thus making it *their* present to the governess and so the bearer of their affection for her. The letter is thus arguably overdetermined by the memory that the governess instantly produces of their mother's deathbed request that she stay to "take their mother's place with them" (ibid., 115). In other words, the letter functions as a letter from *both* mothers: from the governess's living mother allowing her to leave her post, and from the dead mother *via her children*, reminding the governess of her promise to stay. Consequently, in both cases where this etiological formula is deployed by Freud, all the scenes have a variable traumatic force and initiate a process of symptom formation that is at once deferred and retrospective.

*The Pathology of Defense*

While the terminological distinction between 'traumatic' and 'auxiliary' scenes disappears after *Studies on Hysteria*, the conceptual distinction is taken up in the development of the concept of *Nachträglichkeit*. This is laid out with schematic clarity in Part II of the unfinished and only posthumously published "Project for a Scientific Psychology" (1950a [1895]), which was begun in the months after the publication of the *Studies* and shown only to Wilhelm Fliess as part of Freud's long correspondence with him. Part I is an attempt to formulate a *general* psychology of mind that is, nevertheless, neurologically based on the postulation of three different kinds of neurones, the fundamental units of the nervous system (what Freud called in a letter to Fliess his 'Psychology for Neurologists'[6]). His

6. Freud, April 27, 1895, Masson 1985a: 127.

concern in Part II (entitled "Psychopathology of Hysteria") is with the pathological nature of defense in hysteria as contrasted with the mind's normal defensive strategies when faced with distressing or unpleasant phenomena. His argument about hysterical defense implicitly engages with the issues raised by the distinction between traumatic and auxiliary moments in the earlier texts: the relay and interplay between scenes or moments, the nature and place of defense or repression, and the nature and status of the originary traumatic moment. The distance traveled from the "Preliminary Communication," where the hysterical symptom could be readily traced back under hypnosis to its moment of first emergence (thought thus to be the causal moment) and so resolved, is striking. By contrast, Part II of the "Project" begins with precisely the *inexplicability* of the hysterical symptom as an "excessively intense idea" that resists resolution by reference to its apparent object or occasion.[7] Freud proposes that the "*hysterical compulsion is* (1) *unintelligible*, (2) *incapable of being resolved by the activity of thought*, (3) *incongruous* in its structure" (ibid., 348). He contrasts this hysterical compulsion with what he calls "a simple neurotic compulsion." His example of the latter displays the same direct causality he had described in the early trauma model of the "Preliminary Communication": "For instance, a man may have run into danger by falling out of a carriage, and driving in a carriage may after that be impossible for him" (ibid.). We are back in the world of travel and railway traumas and Charcot's traumatic hysteria. Freud comments that the compulsion is intelligible because we know its origin, and that it is congruous with its cause because the accident justifies the connection between fear and driving in carriages. What it has in common with hysterical compulsion is that it is not able to be resolved by thought, that is, the rational calculation of the likelihood of further accidents. It persists regardless of such calculation. Normally such compulsions gradually lessen and eventually disappear. Its persistence points to its being what Freud calls a simple neurosis. By contrast, the hysterical compulsion is incongruous— its object and occasion do not justify the subject's intense reactions, which seem absurd. These reactions do not point to an obvious cause or origin.

Freud expresses this in a schematic example. *A* is an intense idea. The subject weeps at *A* but cannot explain why nor prevent it. Analysis reveals

---

7. Sigmund Freud, "Project for a Scientific Psychology" (1950a [1895]), *SE* 1, 348.

the existence of another idea, $B$, which justifiably leads to weeping. Freud then postulates an event in which $B+A$ occurred together. $B$ was the appropriate cause of the emotional effect, but in memory "it is as though $A$ had stepped into $B$'s place. $A$ has become a substitute, a *symbol* for $B$. Hence the incongruity: $A$ is accompanied by consequences which it does not seem worthy of, which do not fit in with it" (ibid., 349). Again, Freud contrasts this hysterical symbol formation with normal symbolism in which a soldier risks his life for a piece of colored cloth on a pole or a knight fights for his lady's glove. Both the soldier and the knight know the significance of the flag or glove as symbol—they are not prevented from thinking of what they symbolize or acting on it in other respects. By contrast with them, "the *hysteric*, who weeps at $A$, is quite unaware that he is doing so because of the association $A-B$, and $B$ itself plays no part at all in his psychical life. The symbol has in this case taken the place of the *thing* itself" (ibid.). Freud's conclusion is that $A$ is compulsive, $B$ is repressed; for every compulsion there is a corresponding repression. The economic dimension of this hysterical or amnesiac symbolism entails that "something has been added to $A$ which has been subtracted from $B$. The pathological process is one of *displacement*, such as we have come to know it in dreams—a primary process therefore" (ibid., 350).

The amnesiac nature of this displacement, the fact that it transfers all its quantity of affect or excitation from $B$ to $A$, leading to the eclipse of $B$ from consciousness, qualifies it as a primary process. This would lead us to assume that it is a process characteristic of the unconscious—to use later terminology, an id-process. However, it is both a pathological displacement but also "an ego-process" (ibid., 353), that is, a form of defense by the ego. It produces a hysterical symptom in the form of a compulsion to weep in response to the innocuous idea $A$, while it involves a repression of the actually distressing idea $B$. Repression is brought to bear against the release of distressing affect but succeeds only in banishing the distressing idea and transferring the affect to an innocuous idea. What differentiates it from an ordinary unconscious process is that it is "a defensive process emanating from the *cathected ego*" but one that results in hysterical repression and a corresponding compulsion (ibid., 351). We have the paradox of an ego-process that acts blindly like an unconscious primary process, as well as a repression that targets ideas that are both distressing and arise from sexual life. The latter specification cannot just be because sexual ideas are more distressing than other ideas. Freud cites the example of remorse over bad actions that cannot be repressed and replaced by symbols (he had yet to develop a theory of guilt and the superego). Freud's claim, that clinical observation indicates that only ideas connected to sexual life are subject to repression, points to a further precondition for pathological defense, a "special psychical constellation in the sexual sphere" (ibid., 353). It is in this context of the enigma, as Freud calls it, of pathological defense, that this "special psychical constellation" of afterwardsness (*Nachträglichkeit*) is presented through the case of Emma.

### Afterwardsness: The Time of the Trauma

The case of Emma exemplifies the scenic structure we have been encountering in previous cases, in this instance a sequence of two scenes with a certain interplay between them. The traumatic consequences of the first scene are only released in the form of a hysterical symptom as a result of the retrospective action of the second scene that reactivated memory traces of the first. Emma's presenting symptom is a phobia, a compulsive inability to go into shops *alone*. She traces this to a scene when she was twelve years old where she went into a shop and saw two shop assistants laughing together, and then ran away in a state of fright. About this scene she reports that she thought that the shop assistants were laughing at her clothes and that one of them had pleased her sexually. None of the components of the scene as remembered make much sense put together. That the twelve-year-old's clothes were laughed at then, should not later on have deterred the young adult from going into shops, nor would the presence of a companion make any difference to the risibility or otherwise of her dress. Nor, as Freud remarks, does she seem in need of protection, for, as in agoraphobia, the presence even of a small child was enough to make her feel safe. Furthermore, none of these elements seem to have any connection with the fact that one of the assistants pleased her. By contrast with the simple model of trauma in the "Preliminary Communication," here neither the phobic compulsion nor the form taken by the symptom seems to be explained by the scene in which it first appears and to which it is an inexplicably disproportionate response. However, analysis revealed an earlier scene, where at the age of eight she had gone to a shop to buy sweets and the shop-keeper had grabbed at her genitals through her clothes. She had gone back a second time "as though she had wanted in that way to provoke the assault." Freud comments that "a state of 'oppressive bad conscience' is to be traced back to this experience" (ibid., 354), and the single quotation marks around the phrase indicate the patient's own description of her mental state. This suggests that the inference as to her motive is her own. Emma herself seems to have inferred that her guilty feelings resulted from her return to the scene. The anomalies and disconnections between the elements of the later 'innocent' scene, its puzzling traumatic force and resultant phobia, can only be understood by interpolating the elements of the earlier scene, which runs parallel to them. Freud does this in a rather confusing diagram for which I will substitute an alternative presentation of the components of the two scenes. Although Emma denied having the earlier scene in mind during the later one, nevertheless, it is the associative links between the two scenes that explain the puzzling traumatic effectivity of the later one. The links consist in the elements of laughter (the assistants' laughter recalled for her the grin with which the shopkeeper carried out his assault) and the similarity of her situation—she is again by herself in a shop with the man behind the counter. The key difference between the two scenes for Freud is that by the later one she had reached puberty and hence he draws the conclusion that "the memory aroused what it certainly was not able to at the time, a *sexual release*, which was transformed into anxiety. With this anxiety, she was afraid that the shop-assistants might repeat the assault, and she ran away" (ibid., 354 ).

Of the traumatic process that produces the hysterical symptom, Freud comments that the memory of the first scene was in a quite different state from that of the second scene. The relation between the two scenes is mapped out along the lines of his schematic representation of hysterical repression and compulsion in the previous sections of the "Project," discussed earlier. The puzzling sequence of the later scene, Idea *A*:

shop assistants—laughing—clothes—sexual release—fright—phobia

remains in consciousness, but it is unintelligible and incongruous. The scene of the symptom's emergence does not explain the symptom. The

outcome of flight from the danger of assault and the subsequent fear of being in a shop alone, Freud comments, are rationally constructed, except
that the only element from the earlier scene that entered consciousness was
the clothes. Consequently, Emma constructed a series of false connections
between the puzzling elements of the later scene: the assistants were laughing *at her clothes* and it was *one of them* who had aroused an excitation. The
sequence that makes up the earlier scene, Idea *B*:

shopkeeper—grinning—assault—clothes

is, through a process of displacement, substituted for by the apparently innocuous but overdetermined element of the clothes. The clothes act as a
bridge between the two parallel situations of being in a shop alone with the
grinning shopkeeper and being in a store with the laughing shop assistants,
transferring the significance of the first situation, whose memory is only
*now* repressed, to the second.

Freud argues that the process of repression, accompanied by pathological symbol formation (the clothes as the condensed symbol of the now repressed early scene), is provoked by the deferred sexual release made possible
by the advent of puberty. He asserts that the sexual release was not part of
the child's experience of the original assault. Hence we have the paradox
of "a memory arousing an affect which it did not arouse as an experience,
because . . . puberty had made possible a *different understanding* of what was
remembered" (ibid., 356). This is the psychical constellation peculiar to
sexual life that determines the nature of hysterical repression: "a memory is
repressed which has become a trauma by *deferred action*" (ibid.). "Deferred
action" is Strachey's translation as a noun in the *Standard Edition* of the
adjective-adverb *nachträglich*. Its inadequacy is clear from its suggestion of a
merely forward linear progression and postponement, as in the old idea of
abreaction, whereas the logic of Freud's argument entails a belated precipitation of the sexual affect and meaning of a primary scene by the retrospective interpretation and *"different understanding* of what was remembered"
(ibid. emphasis added). While Freud claims that, as with the case of Katharina, this is typical of repression in hysteria, he also generalizes this logic of
deferral and retrospection by claiming that "every adolescent individual has
memory-traces which can only be understood with the emergence of sexual
feelings of his own," hence everyone carries "the germ of hysteria" (ibid.).

What distinguishes the small number of actual hysterics from the majority of people is that "they have become *prematurely* sexually excitable owing to mechanical and emotional stimulation (masturbation)"—presumably by others—or due to "innate disposition" (ibid., 357). Here Freud tells us that the weight must fall on the *prematureness* of the sexual release as the factor that provokes the hysterical repression. Freud's reasoning here is significant: "It cannot be maintained that sexual release in general is an occasion for repression; this would once again make repression into a process of normal frequency" (ibid., 357). It is clear that at this point Freud is still working with the notion of repression, and so by implication of the repressed unconscious, as a pathological phenomenon that is not "normal," and that what provokes this temporary pathological mechanism that creates the hysterical symptom is what he calls a "premature sexual release" specific to hysterics. However, this constitutes a puzzling aporia in Freud's argument. He postulates both a deferred sexual release (from scene 1 with the grinning shopkeeper to scene 2 with the laughing assistants) and a premature sexual release (which can only mean in scene 1, prepuberty) as the determinants of hysterical repression. These contradictory statements are repeated cheek by jowl at the beginning of section 6 as if they were consistent with each other: "(1) that the sexual release was attached to a memory instead of to an experience, (2) that the sexual release took place *prematurely*" (ibid., 357). The first statement claims that the sexual release occurred after puberty, while the second statement claims that it occurred before puberty.

However, it is the first statement of *deferred* release, rather than the thesis of prematureness, that is central to Freud's attempt to explain how repression—the "disturbance of thought by affect" (ibid.,)—works. In the final section of Part II Freud returns to his larger argument about defense that enables an understanding of how the isolated memory of the first scene of assault overcomes the ego's defenses. In the wake of a painful or distressing experience, he says, "It is the ego's business not to permit any release of affect, because this at the same time permits a primary process" (ibid., 358). The ego's usual strategy for avoiding this is the mechanism of attention, which inhibits the influx of fresh perceptions that might awaken the distressing memory traces. In the case of Emma, clearly a defensive isolation of the first scene had already taken place. However, the rhyme between the two scenes, together with the various associative connections between them, had enabled this defensive isolation of the first scene to be breached. Freud describes the result:

> Attention is [normally] adjusted towards perceptions, which are what ordinarily give occasion for a release of unpleasure. Here, [however, what has appeared] is no perception but a memory, which unexpectedly releases unpleasure, and the ego only discovers this too late. It has permitted a primary process because it did not expect one. (Freud 1950a, 358)

The reactivation of the memory traces of the first scene allows a sexual release in the new context of puberty, with its new physiological powers and understandings. However, like the Fall of Singapore, where defenses that were trained on an enemy approaching from the sea were overtaken by an approach overland from behind, here the exciting and distressing representation occurs in the form of a memory and so from within. Like Singapore, the ego is taken by surprise and from behind. Its defensive reaction against this unexpected traitor within the gates is to strike out the offending memory from consciousness, while partly transferring the sexual release, now intensified in the new context of puberty and its developments, onto the homologous but 'innocent' later scene (from the grinning shopkeeper to the pleasing assistant), and partly transforming it into anxiety and the apparently unmotivated fear of going into shops alone. As Freud points out: "A repression accompanied by symbol-formation has taken place," together with the hysterical symptom of the phobia (in which, puzzlingly, the symbol of the clothes plays no part, that is, the phobia does not attach itself to the clothes, although they remain an occasion for anxiety as the object of the laughing/grinning male gaze), hence the paradox of a secondary ego-process of defense that behaves in the blind, amnesiac manner of a primary id-process.

This argument about the operation of hysterical repression is premised on the deferred release of sexual feeling produced by the reactivation of an unconscious memory, and the contrary emphasis on the *premature* sexual release seems to play no part in it. We are still left, however, with this striking but unremarked contradiction in Freud's argument between the deferred and the premature. This is all the more puzzling because Freud insists in the case of Emma on the absence of any sexual release in the earliest remembered scene. Now there would seem to be an empirical question as to whether the case materials support such a claim. Freud's own report of Emma's two visits to the molesting shopkeeper, her quoted words about "a state of 'oppressive bad conscience'" (ibid., 354), and her self-reproaches over her second visit "as though she had wanted in that way to provoke the assault," all suggest that she had in fact experienced a sexual excitation of some kind in the first scene (not necessarily pleasurable), had sought to repeat it, and had then developed guilty feelings about this, well before the later moment of the hysterical symptom. This would, of course, be in keeping with the later psychoanalytic account of infantile sexuality that would indicate that a child of eight would have passed through a variety of phases of infantile sexual development.

Freud's theoretical insistence on the necessary *prematureness* of sexual release as a precondition for hysterical repression (otherwise repression would be normalized as a response to sexual feeling in general), while denying it in the case of Emma, is puzzling. This can be partly explained due to the fact that his formulation of afterwardsness is, at this point in the development of his thought, tied up with a special emphasis on puberty as a crucial threshold before which the sexual preconditions for neurosis must be laid down. This goes with the assumption that prepuberty is a presexual period, an assumption that will be overturned by the postulation of a distinctively infantile sexuality in the *Three Essays in the Theory of Sexuality* (1905d). It is on these grounds that Strachey, in a contradictory editorial note to this section of the "Project," dismisses Freud's "special psychical constellation" as obsolete: "The whole idea had the ground cut from under it by the discovery a year or two later of infantile sexuality and the recognition of the persistence of unconscious instinctual impulses" (ibid., 356, n. 1). Nevertheless, however important Freud's emphasis on puberty as a threshold was, the temporal structure of afterwardsness is not tied *intrinsically* to a conception of the infantile as asexual. Rather, it is a preliminary description of a temporal dialectic of deferral and retroaction, which can operate between different developmental periods and resulting strata of the mind quite *other* than puberty. Consequently, it has a pertinence in other contexts, as Strachey in effect admits by noting the reappearance some twenty years later of the motif of afterwardsness in the case of the Wolf Man (1918b [1914]), where Freud locates it without any relation to puberty, as operating between the ages of one and a half and four years. This reappearance of the term and concept will be discussed extensively in Chapters 9 and 10.

So also the recognition of a premature sexual release or affect in Emma's response in the first scene need not detract from Freud's formulation of the logic of afterwardsness in play between the two scenes. Indeed, the possibility of its sexual valency postpuberty, it might be argued contra Freud, depends precisely on its having had a sexual impact in the moment of its occurrence, albeit of a kind and intensity appropriate to the child's then premature state of development. Freud's contradictory insistence on the absence of sexual excitation or affect in the first scene of the Emma case is perhaps due to his concern with the complexity of the activity in the second, 'innocent' scene, and to a desire to affirm its determining power, in order for it to be more than merely an agent provocateur, merely activating an already existing complex or inherited predisposition as with Charcot.

However, it remains possible to maintain Freud's formulation that the first scene had an effect as memory, acting unconsciously from scene 2 onward, which it did not have as an experience, *without* it entailing the assumption of childhood asexuality. The structure of deferral bears not on the absolute absence or presence of a sexual release as such in scene 1 but on the belated production of the traumatic drama and its hysterical outcome in scene 2. As we have seen with the 'auxiliary' scenes of the *Studies*, it is only in this second moment that, simultaneously, repression sets in and the phobic symptom appears from then on, as a defensive transformation of a postpuberty sexual release connected to the revived memory traces of the first event. The significance of Freud's emphasis on puberty is not just the assumption that puberty initiates the biological advent of sexuality in a previously nonsexual being. This was already being challenged by his awareness of the 'germs of hysteria' in the prepuberty child. More important is that *new understandings and ideas* come into play at puberty that retrospectively transform and reinterpret the memories of the first event. Along with the process of deferral goes the process of retrospection and translation, such that *both* scenes are given a determining power in the production of the traumatic outcome, even with such an apparently 'innocent' scene as that of the laughing shop assistants.[8]

---

8. One may wonder just how nonsexual the later scene actually was, as the young Emma might well have been reacting not just to a parallelism of situations but to the

The status of the first scene in the interval between the two scenes remains unexplored in Freud's account. Jean Laplanche, who was the first psychoanalytic writer to recognize the seminal nature of the Emma case and the larger argument about defense of which it is part, comments:

> "We may legitimately ask what the psychical status of the first scene is . . . it would seem that for Freud it persists neither in a conscious state, nor, properly speaking, in a repressed state; it remains there, waiting in a kind of limbo, in a corner of the "preconscious"; the crucial point is that it is not linked to the rest of psychical life."[9]

Although the experience gave rise to "a state of 'oppressive bad conscience'" (Freud 1950a [1895], 354), in Emma's own words, it has not been repressed and so does not return in symptomatic form. The memory of this first scene persists, in a defensively isolated state—"in a kind of limbo," or "in storage," as Freud says of Katharina—as an untranslatable, unassimilated foreign body. It is then reactivated by the second scene with its connections and homologies, which translates it into a new postpuberty context, where it becomes actively present and thus provokes its repression by the ego.

### The Impasse of the Seduction Theory (1896–97)

I have interpreted the contradiction between the 'deferred' and the 'premature' in the Emma case as resulting from the different gravitational pulls exerted by the different scenes and moments within the temporal schema of afterwardsness. Beginning with a simple model of trauma that privileged the moment of the symptom's emergence as the *determining* moment, Freud encounters a multiplication of scenes that complicates the question of etiology in unexpected ways. However, he addresses these issues in the framework of an etiological model that he inherits from Charcot and from his quarrel with Charcot's hereditarian theory, and this etiological framework

---

sexually appraising or provocative gaze of the laughing young men—a common enough situation.

9. Jean Laplanche, *Life and Death in Psychoanalysis*, trans. Jeffrey Mehlman (Baltimore and London: The Johns Hopkins University Press, 1976), 41.

acts as a constraint on his own discovery and exploration of afterwardsness, and on the temporality of trauma entailed by that very multiplication of scenes.

As we saw in the previous chapter, Charcot posited an unlocatable functional lesion, the result of a physical trauma with its psychological effects of fright and dissociation, in his account of the formation of hysterical symptoms. He then downgraded the causal status of the trauma to that of a mere agent provocateur in relation to hysteria understood as an inherited, constitutional predisposition. There is a tension, if not an outright contradiction, here between Charcot's account of symptom formation through suggestion or autosuggestion in a fright-induced hypnoid state and the primacy he gave to heredity. The trauma is reduced to being a mere precipitating occasion that activates a preexisting constitutional hysteria. By contrast, in the first of his three published 1896 papers on the so-called 'seduction theory,' Freud demotes heredity to being a mere precondition. This is sometimes said to be necessary but nonspecific, being common to a number of disorders, and sometimes heredity is held to be superseded altogether by the postulation of an entirely *acquired* hysteria due to a category of specific contingent causes of a traumatic kind. Even where hereditary predisposition is still said to be a factor, without the operation of these specific causes it can produce nothing. In dethroning heredity from its central causal role and relegating it to being a nonspecific factor $x$, Freud promotes the traumatic genealogy of symptoms to the role of an indispensable *specific* cause that is found in no other pathological condition and can be absent in no instances of the condition. He also postulates a category of *concurrent or auxiliary* causes, which are the stock agents met with in many conditions— "emotional disturbance, physical exhaustion, acute illnesses, intoxications, traumatic incidents, intellectual overwork."[10] These act as intensifiers of the specific causes and where the latter are quantitatively weak may hence act as *precipitating* causes. It is clear that in this etiological framework the search for a specific cause, one that is uniform with respect to all instances of the pathological condition in question, has the effect of relegating all other categories of cause—the concurrent/auxiliary causes and the precipitating causes—to a merely accessory quantitative role, lacking any specific

10. Sigmund Freud, "Heredity and the Aetiology of the Neuroses" (1896a), *SE* 3, 148.

or form-giving capacities. This search for a specific etiology is presented in all three of the 1896 papers that put forward the hypothesis of infantile seduction and it results in a constant move backward in time to the earliest years. The uniform specific cause is declared to be *"a precocious experience of sexual relations with actual excitement of the genitals, resulting from sexual abuse committed by another person"* and occurring before the cutoff point of eight to ten years. *"A passive sexual experience before puberty*: this, then, is the specific aetiology of hysteria" (ibid., 152). The tendency in all three seduction theory papers is to attribute overwhelming determining power to this first causal scene and so to drain it from the other scenes that orchestrate its effects.

The tension here results from a particular etiological model, derived from Aristotle,[11] which assigns a hierarchy of determining causes in which the specific cause takes primacy over preconditions, as well as over both auxiliary and precipitating causes. Consequently, it interferes with the temporal schema of afterwardsness that Freud developed in *Studies on Hysteria* and the Emma case, with their multiplication of scenes and consequent overdetermination. The more Freud's theory is based on the primacy of the single specific cause, the more the complexity and richness of the model of afterwardsness is put at risk, even though it is also, paradoxically, affirmed in all three papers.

This fault line in Freud's thinking of afterwardsness is produced by the tension between two conceptual models that we have detected at work in the previous texts discussed. There is, first, the model of the foreign body that is explicitly counterposed by Freud to Charcot's metaphor of the agent provocateur. It is the expression of Freud's clinical experience of the reproduction by his analysands of a traumatic scene "as though it came from a phonograph" (Masson 1985a, 226), acting directly in the present like a current event; and there is, second, the model of defense and, in particular, that of repression, expressed in the shift of metaphor from the foreign body to the infiltrate, in which "the resistance must be regarded as what is infiltrating" (1895d, 290), which we noted in the last chapter. This fault line can also be seen at work in the presentation of the Emma case with its two

---

11. See Sulloway's brief discussion and sourcing of Freud's etiological equation in *Freud: Biologist of the Mind* (Cambridge, Mass: Harvard University Press, 1992), 92.

contradictory emphases, on the *premature* release of sexual affect, privileging the first moment of implantation of the foreign body, as against the *deferred* sexual release, privileging the later moment of defense and repression, where the claims of the two moments in the schema of afterwardsness to exercise determining power seem to be in competition with each other. However, the Emma case belongs to the larger Part II of the unpublished "Project for a Scientific Psychology" of 1895, which centers on the problematic of defense and, in particular, repression, conceived as a pathological form of defense in hysteria. As a result, Freud focuses at length on the complexity of the activity that takes place in the second moment, as we have seen, which involves both the factor of puberty and the ego's defensive operations. The scene of the two laughing shop assistants both reactivates the earlier scene of molestation and represses it, producing Emma's anxiety phobia as a new symptom that from now on persists. Although in Freud's account it was deemed to be nonsexual in itself, the second moment is, nonetheless, the scene of the release of the sexual affect generated by the reactivated memory traces of the first scene with the shopkeeper. The release of sexual feeling is one of the effects of puberty, which Freud tells us "had made possible a new understanding of what was remembered" (1950a, 56). Much then happens in the busy second moment of Freud's temporal dialectic as elaborated in the Emma case.

With the three 1896 papers that formulate the seduction theory, the focus of attention shifts overwhelmingly to the first scene, and to its determining power as a specific cause within the framework of the etiological theory.[12] Working through them, one can see Freud mapping this etiological model onto the temporal schema of afterwardsness. In the first of these papers, "Heredity and the Aetiology of the Neuroses" (1896a), which begins with an explicit critique of Charcot's hereditary etiology, the etiological model is dominant, and the formulation of afterwardsness is translated into its terms. Nevertheless, Freud reaffirms the central proposition that "due to puberty, the memory will display a power which was completely lacking from the event itself. *The memory will operate as though it were a contemporary event.* What happens is, as it were, a *posthumous action by a sexual trauma*" (1896a,

---

12. "Heredity and the Aetiology of the Neuroses" (1896a), *SE* 3; "Further Remarks on the Neuro-Psychoses of Defence" (1896b), *SE* 3; "The Aetiology of Hysteria" (1896c), *SE* 3.

154). Accompanying this reaffirmation of afterwardsness, however, there is once again the same implausible assertion of infantile sexual indifference or apathy faced with the first scene of abuse. Furthermore, the role of puberty is now reduced to being a purely *physiological* one, the developed "reactions of the sexual organs," whereas in the Emma case the emphasis was on "a different understanding of what was remembered" (1950a, 356), which is a process of translation of a memory into new circumstances and a new language. The core remains, however: the strange nature of that repetition in which a memory is lived out "as though it were a contemporary event." The result is a 'posthumous' trauma in a second moment where, Freud claims, there had been no such trauma in the first moment.

Rather than exploring the complexities of the interaction between the two scenes as he had done previously, Freud's conviction that he had made "the discovery of a *caput Nili* in neuropathology,"[13] the source of the Nile as regards the psychoneuroses, leads him to privilege a single scene of infantile sexual abuse as the *sole* specific cause of psychopathology.

> All the events subsequent to puberty to which an influence must be attributed upon the development of the hysterical neurosis and upon the formation of its symptoms are in fact only concurrent causes, *agents provocateurs*, as Charcot used to say, though for him nervous heredity occupied the place which I claim for precocious sexual experience. (Freud, 1896a, 155)

We can see here that, despite the eviction of Charcot's heredity by a specific infantile trauma, Freud retains Charcot's etiological model of a single privileged cause reducing all other factors to being mere catalysts or "agent provocateurs." He enforces this with the statement that the later postpuberty events, mere "accessory agents," only enjoy "a pathogenic influence" due to their awakening "the unconscious psychical trace of the childhood event" (ibid.). The *auxiliary* scene with its power to codetermine the *form* of the symptom—as in the case of Miss Lucy R. —is through a slide on the word 'auxiliary' conflated with the very different category of 'concurrent or *auxiliary* causes,' mere quantitative intensifiers of the primary specific cause; but an 'auxiliary scene' is not the same thing as an 'auxiliary cause.' This diminution of the determining power of the later scenes, their reduction to being

---

13. Freud, "The Aetiology of Hysteria" (1896c), *SE* 3, 203.

mere precipitating occasions or intensifying factors, under the influence of the etiological model, characterizes all three published papers that put forward the so-called seduction theory. This is in effect a regression to the single-scene model of the "Preliminary Communication."

In the third and longest of the three papers, "The Aetiology of Hysteria" (1896c), however, it is striking that in the opening section Freud begins by explicitly dramatizing the inadequacy of the expectations based on his earlier single-scene model of trauma. The readily remembered scene either lacks appropriateness of form and theme—Why should a railway accident give rise specifically to *vomiting* as a hysterical symptom rather than to any other expression of affect?—or, it lacks traumatic force—Why should merely eating a rotten fruit lead to *hysterical* vomiting? A chain of memories leads to a succession of scenes, having either force without appropriateness of form, or vice versa, or lacking either. Freud maps out again the territory of the 'memory files' that he had described previously in the *Studies*. In his backward movement into the increasingly remoter past, he once again describes a memorial system of scenes that he begins by describing in terms of inoperative linking scenes and determining operative scenes, but which proliferate in ways that cannot be contained by this simple opposition. Indeed, he admits that some of these intermediate scenes have both traumatic force and appropriateness, recall of which leads to the dissolution of the symptom in question. However, it is clear that it is the memorial system itself that must be traversed in all its 'by-paths and indirect crooked ways,' missing out no significant link or interconnection, in order to gain access to the earliest traumatically operative infantile scenes. There can be no shortcuts. Freud represents the memorial system in terms of the ramifying interconnections of "the genealogical tree of a family whose members have intermarried" (ibid., 198), for from a single scene two or more memories are reached, and these in turn produce side chains whose links connect back to the main chain; or a single scene may be called up a number of times in the same chain exhibiting both direct and indirect relations to a scene that is arrived at later on. Freud also specifies again what he calls 'nodal points,' where the genealogical tree of one symptom intertwines with that of another in a scene shared by both, or scenes where two different genealogical trees converge in different details of a single scene in the field of sexuality, first of all in experiences at puberty and then in earliest childhood.

There are moments in the essay where the memory of the model of defense and repression appears briefly under the rubric of an "auxiliary aetiology" (ibid., 210), only to be subordinated to the primacy of the single specific cause. In a moment of rhetorical self-criticism, Freud announces: "I am afraid that I may have misled you into over-estimating their power [that of 'infantile sexual scenes'] to form symptoms" and goes on to assert that "every case of hysteria exhibits symptoms which are determined, not by infantile but by later, often recent, experiences" (ibid., 214). However, instead of following through this line of thought, he is immediately diverted into further descriptions of the all-pervasive drama of the single specific scene of infantile seduction.

Within the dominant perspective of this third fullest statement of the seduction theory (originally given as a lecture before the Vienna Society for Psychiatry and Neurology with Krafft-Ebing in the chair), which privileges the determining power of the first infantile scenes, there are nevertheless shifts in emphasis provoked by the anomalous form of repetition Freud is struggling to conceptualize. He asserts: "None of the later scenes, in which the symptoms arise, are the effective ones; and the experiences which *are* effective have at first no result" (ibid., 213). Reversing the emergent model of trauma in the case studies of 1895, Freud seems determined here to strip the later scenes of the symptom's emergence of any determining power, and at the same time to reduce the collaborative power of the whole memorial system and its companion thesis of overdetermination; and yet the anomaly persists: the trauma and the hysterical symptom do not appear as such until these later scenes.

Freud appeals to his previous distinction between "the *mechanism* of the formation of symptoms" and "the causation of those symptoms," the first of which he assigns to the later scene in which it appears and the latter to the infantile scene (ibid., 214). This distinction was first made in the *Studies* where he considered Breuer's cathartic method as a symptomatic but not a causal method, one effective against hysterical *symptoms* but not against "the underlying causes of hysteria: thus it cannot prevent fresh symptoms from taking the place of ones that have been got rid of" (1895d, 261–62). By 1896, Freud was now able to address the underlying *causes* of hysteria as a condition (as distinct from its "psychical mechanism"), and these he now identified with the earliest scenes of infantile sexual abuse, which lay behind the later scenes of the symptom's first appearance. However, it was the mode of their operation that posed such an enigma: "We are not accustomed to the notion of powers emanating from a mnemic image which were absent from the real impression" (1896c, 213). The paradox of afterwardsness was that it was neither the immediate action of either infantile or later scenes that explained the symptoms but "the powers emanating from a mnemic image," an image that belonged exclusively to neither scene but derived from both. The effect of afterwardsness depended on the articulation of both scenes (or whole sequences of them) and included the crucial role of defense and repression. Freud acknowledges this in passing but then sets it aside (ibid., 213, 216). As a result, the necessary *overdetermination* of the symptom, "called up by a combination of several factors and . . . aroused from various directions simultaneously" (216), is marginalized by the drive to identify the earliest infantile scene as the sole specific cause responsible for the hysterical *disposition* as such.

Despite the various calls to order and momentary reminders of the complexity and overdetermined nature of the process of afterwardsness, Freud's conviction of his momentous discovery of the 'source of the Nile' tends to produce, in his descriptions of the infantile scenes that he is prioritizing, a regression to the earlier notion of a *single*-scene trauma whose effects are merely delayed, as in the model of abreaction in the "Preliminary Communication." In particular, the twin thesis of infantile indifference or mere fright in response to the first scene of seduction, and of the scene's traumatic effectivity being tied to its repressed, unconscious status—consciously remembered scenes could not be responsible for later hysteria, Freud insists—runs up against the actual descriptions he gives of those scenes. This lack of fit between the infantile scenes of sexual trauma and the requirements of the theory has been remarked on by other commentators.[14] Freud gives very little in the way of illustration of the clinical materials obtained from his analyses. Mostly he provides summary standard situations and anecdotes. The most extended is the case of paranoia, discussed in the second of the

14. Jean G. Schimek, "Fact and Fantasy in the Seduction Theory: A Historical Review,, *Journal of the American Psychoanalytic Association* 35 (1987): 937–65; Kurt Eissler, *Freud and the Seduction Theory: A Brief Love Affair* (New York: International Universities Press, 2001), esp. Chap. 5: "Inconsistencies and Incongruities in Freud's 1896 Papers on the Seduction Theory."

three essays.[15] He summarizes the severest of his thirteen analyzed cases as involving "grave sexual injuries" and a bewilderingly large cast of abusers (strangers, nursemaids, governesses, domestic servants, teachers, and elder brothers, but no fathers) for his small number of cases (1896b, 164). In the third paper he devotes an eloquent, page-long paragraph to both the perverse sexual practices involved—the adult's sexual abuse of the child's mouth and anus—and, more significantly, the psychological dynamics of the power relations in play between "the ill-matched pair":

> On the one hand the adult, who cannot escape his share in the mutual dependence necessarily entailed by a sexual relationship, and who is yet armed with complete authority and the right to punish, and can exchange the one role for the other to the uninhibited satisfaction of his moods, and on the other hand the child, who in his helplessness is at the mercy of this arbitrary will, who is prematurely aroused to every kind of sensibility and exposed to every disappointment, and whose performance of the sexual activities assigned to him is often interrupted by his imperfect control of his natural needs—all these grotesque and yet tragic incongruities reveal themselves as stamped upon the later development of the individual and his neurosis, in countless permanent effects which deserve to be traced in the greatest detail. (1896c, 215)

In this poignant account, Freud's emphasis falls on the "incongruities" of "the ill-matched pair"—disparities of authority and power and their arbitrary if not sadistic exercise, as well as incongruities between the child's bodily functioning and the sexual demands of the adult, incongruities that "will reveal themselves as stamped upon the later development of the individual . . . in countless permanent effects." While Freud's account is a summary of general characteristics and not a particular case study, it is clear that the child of this description is *not* indifferent or subject merely to fright but "prematurely aroused to every kind of sensibility," a subject of sexual feeling, however premature or incongruous, and not at all asexual. The "grave sexual injuries" that result from the abuse of the child's body and "sensibility" are described as "permanent effects" of a virtually developmental or constitutional kind. It is hard to see these as being subject to the logic of deferred action or retrospection, any more than the memories

---

15. "Further Remarks on the Neuro-Psychoses of Defence" (1896b), *SE* 3.

of such injuries might be subject to wholesale repression. In his impassioned empathy for the child's sufferings, Freud seems to have forgotten the key requirements for his model of hysteria.

This is the case with many of the summary examples he gives elsewhere in the three essays, most notably the seven out of his thirteen cases which involved child—usually brother–sister—couples: "These relations sometimes continued for years, until the little guilty parties reached puberty" (ibid., 152). This is the case as well with his account of adult–child relations in which the adult caregiver "has initiated the child into sexual intercourse and has maintained a regular love relationship with it—a love relationship, moreover, with its mental side developed—which has often lasted for years" (1896c, 208). It is clear that such relations flagrantly contradict the description only a few pages later of "sexual experiences which show no immediate effect" (ibid., 212). If the thesis of the child's sexual indifference is obviously unsustainable, the question of *repressed* scenes is also problematized when what is in question is a love relation of many years "with its mental side developed." However, one should note that the one case Freud presents in the three essays, that of the paranoid woman, does show a loving brother–sister relation euphemistically remembered with its earliest sexual scenes plausibly subject to censorship and repression, although these are scarcely explored or presented in much detail. The explanation offered in the Emma case of a scene defensively isolated in the preconscious and only subject to repression at a later date might have a certain explanatory purchase here.

These kinds of childhood experiences—years-long relationships with adults or siblings—would seem to have both an immediate as well as a long-lasting effect, and to give rise to—no doubt isolated—memories, but ones available to conscious, if reluctant and extremely distressing, recall. While they testified to the presence of premature sexual experience in the childhood of his patients, they cannot be the 'specific cause' required by his theory. In his critique of the seduction theory, Jean Schimek argues that Freud's descriptions cannot refer to the "uniform early trauma . . . that was never remembered by the patient but had to be reconstructed from partial, indirect 'reproductions' and whose existence was demanded by the 'logical necessity' of the structure of the present neurosis" (Schimek 1987, 947). Schimek is here referring to the various 'proofs' Freud had adduced in defense of the authenticity of the early scenes he had uncovered. The latter were like missing pieces in a child's picture puzzle, in Freud's analogy, "indispensable supplements to the associative and logical framework of the neurosis, whose insertion makes its course of development for the first time evident" (1896c, 205). Of these missing supplementary scenes, Schimek comments, "It seems likely that Freud, in reconstructing the original scenes, made use of the patient's direct reports (dealing mostly with later years of childhood) and the contents of enacted 'reproductions' in the treatment situation" (Schimek 1987, 947).

These "original scenes" did not arrive, then, through a process of ordinary recall. They had to be reconstructed. The material from which they were reconstructed is precisely the paradoxical form of repetition with which this book began, a scene that is acted out with all the force of a present event, even in the form of some kind of attack—"epileptiform convulsions" or hallucinatory reenactments, as described in the letters to Fliess commented on in the Prologue. These "reproductions" (Freud's preferred term) carry with them the apparent signs of their authenticity—"they [the patients] suffer under the most violent sensations, of which they are ashamed and which they try to conceal" (1896c, 204), from which one infers that these "violent sensations" include sexual sensations and their physiological expression. The clinical paradox is that, nevertheless, "even after they have gone through them once more in such a convincing manner, they still attempt to withhold belief from them, by emphasizing the fact that, unlike what happens in the case of other forgotten material, they have no feeling of remembering the scenes" (ibid.). As we have seen, Freud had confronted this paradox in *Studies on Hysteria* when describing the intensification of resistance as the analysis approached the pathogenic nucleus of the memorial system: "We come across memories that the patient disavows even in reproducing them" (1895d, 289).

For Freud this constituted a further sign of authenticity, "conclusive proof" that the patients had not fabricated such scenes, for he asks, "Why should patients assure me so emphatically of their unbelief, if what they want to discredit is something which . . . they themselves have invented?" (1896c, 204). The same appeal to the emotional, even the hallucinatory, enactment of scenes as a criterion of their authenticity as memories is made by Freud to counter the objection that such scenes are produced by the patient at the suggestion of the analyst: "I have never yet succeeded in forcing on a patient a scene I was expecting to find, in such a way that *he seemed to be living through it with all the appropriate feelings*" (ibid., 205, emphasis added).

In fact, apart from brief comments in the case of female paranoia in the second 1896 paper, Freud offers no reconstruction of a specific infantile scene in the three published seduction theory papers. It is to the case of Emma, already discussed, and to the unpublished letters to Fliess, that we must turn for glimpses of such reconstructions and the materials they are based on. It is also in the Fliess correspondence that we will find Freud further complicating his theory in such a way as to introduce a key term—fantasy—that helps explain the refusal of recognition, by Freud's patients, of the reconstructed scenes as memories. The introduction of the role of fantasy offers an approach to these paradoxical scenes that undo the commonsense model of memory as my possession—"my memory now of that scene then . . ."—and that, as I suggested in the previous chapter, seem to require a description more like "a scene is being remembered in me" or even "this scene remembers me."

## FOUR

## Memory and the Key of Fantasy

"Fantasy as the key holds fast."[1]

These two terms, memory (or the real event of which it is the subjective record) and fantasy, have unfortunately been polarized as mutually exclusive
alternatives in most of the retrospective commentary on Freud's seduction
theory, including Freud's own. In the letter of the so-called turning point
(September 21, 1897), Freud gives Fliess as one of his four reasons for questioning his theory: "There are no indications of reality in the unconscious,
so that one cannot distinguish between truth and fiction that has been cathected with affect. (Accordingly, there would remain the solution that the
sexual fantasy invariably seizes on the theme of the parents)" (Masson 1985a,
264–65). However, in the period between the last of the seduction theory
papers of 1896 and Freud's private rejection of his theory to Fliess in Sep-

1. Freud to Fliess, January 30, 1899, in Jeffrey Moussaiff Masson, trans. and ed., *The
Complete Letters of Sigmund Freud to Wilhelm Fliess 1887–1904* (Cambridge, Mass.: Harvard University Press, 1985), 342. Hereafter Masson 1985a.

tember 1897, Freud elaborated an account of the role of fantasy as *part* of his theory of traumatic seduction rather than as an alternative to it.

### The Letters to Fliess: The Discovery of Fantasy

In one of the earliest indications of the emerging significance of fantasy in the letters to Fliess (April 6, 1897), Freud significantly couples fantasy with the deferred logic of afterwardsness:

> The point that escaped me in the solution of hysteria lies in the discovery of a different source, from which a new element of the product of the unconscious arises. What I have in mind are hysterical fantasies which regularly, as I see it, go back to things that children overhear at an early age and understand only subsequently [*nachträglich* JF]. The age at which they take in information of this kind is, strangely enough, from six to seven months on! (Masson 1985a, 234)

The articulation of the two terms, fantasy and afterwardsness (*Nachträglich-keit*), is as yet unclear, except that auditory elements ("information") are acquired in a first moment and are understood in a later one, while hysterical fantasies result somehow from this process. Barely a month later, Freud is attempting to clarify these interrelations in Drafts L, M, and N and their accompanying letters. Throughout May 1897 Freud returns again and again in his letters to Fliess to the role of fantasy, which assumes increasing importance in relation to what he calls "my protohysteria scenes" (May 2, 1897, ibid., 239).

> Everything goes back to the reproduction of scenes. Some can be obtained directly, others always by way of fantasies set up in front of them. The fantasies stem from the things that have been *heard* but understood *subsequently* [*nachträglich*, JF] and all their material is of course genuine. They are protective structures, sublimations of the facts, embellishments of them, and at the same time serve for self-relief. Their accidental origin is perhaps from masturbation fantasies. (Masson 1985a, 239)

In this passage and the accompanying Draft L, there is the same imperative, characteristic of the 1896 seduction theory papers, "to reach the earliest [sexual] scenes" (Draft L, ibid., 240). Freud's term in both the letter and the draft is *Urszenen*, translated in the *Standard Edition* as 'primal scenes' and used here for the first time in Freud's work. Unlike its current psychoanalytic usage to refer to a particular *content*, the scene of parental intercourse either directly witnessed, overheard, or imagined by the child, here *Urszenen* signifies the first originary sexual scenes, regardless of specific actors or actions. While in a few cases the scenes can be accessed directly, access to them seems mainly to require "a detour via fantasies. For the fantasies are psychic facades produced to bar access to these memories" (ibid.). They are both "protective structures" with the function of defense *against* the memories and also a site of sexual excitation and discharge. Freud stresses again their deferred relation to things heard as well as their hybrid nature, combining "things experienced and heard, past events (from the history of parents and ancestors), and things that are seen by oneself" (ibid.). Both Draft M (May 25) and Draft N (May 31) also stress the role of fantasy as the mediating facade of memories. The Draft L letter (May 2) had proposed that the building blocks or fundamental elements of all three neuroses—hysteria, obsessional neurosis, and paranoia (as it was then categorized by Freud)— were "memory fragments, *impulses* (derived from memories) and *protective fictions*" (ibid., 239). It had sought to differentiate the neuroses by deriving them structurally from whichever of these three elements is the site of the return of the repressed and the formation of symptoms (like a classic structuralist combinatory of elementary terms). In Draft N, however, under the heading of "Relation between Impulses and Fantasies," Freud raises by contrast the possibility of assigning an originary power to fantasy itself:

> Memories appear to bifurcate: one part of them is put aside and replaced by fantasies; another accessible part seems to lead directly to impulses. Is it possible that later on impulses can also derive from fantasies? (Masson 1985a, 250)

Where the Draft L letter had proposed "impulses that derive from primal scenes" (ibid., 239), here Draft N postulates impulses that derive from fantasies. It is Jean Laplanche who has recognized the potential significance of this sequence and its implied conceptual model, "sketched out but left in his bottom drawer by Freud himself."[2] It implies an alternative causal sequence to both a realist conception of traumatic memory:

$$\text{event } 1 + \text{event n} \ldots > \text{memory} > \text{repression} > \text{symptom}$$

2. Jean Laplanche, "The Drive and Its Source-Object" (1992a), in *Essays on Otherness*, ed. John Fletcher (London: Routledge, 1999), 125.

and the later biological determinism:

$$\text{somatic source (biological need + instinctual reflex)} \\ > \text{instinct/drive} > \text{fantasy}$$

where fantasy is the expression or efflorescence of the drives, arising from their somatic sources. Instead we have here the sequence:

$$\text{event} > \text{memory} > \text{fantasy} > \text{impulses} > \text{repression} > \text{symptoms}$$

In a period prior to the elaboration of a theory of the drive (*Trieb*) in the *Three Essays* of 1905, Freud's term '*Impulse*' (translated into French as *pulsion* or drive) marks the site of a proto-drive, a wishful impulse whose source would be neither a traumatic memory as such nor a biological need but a fantasy whose action it would be.[3]

Freud also stresses the fantasy as a hybrid formation, analogous to the overdetermined nature of the dream that he is systematically formulating in the same years: "It is possible to follow the path, the time, and the material of the formation of fantasies, which then closely resembles the formation of dreams" (Draft L, ibid., 242). However, the materials of the fantasy are memory elements and fragments, and the fantasy is conceived in intimate relation to the memories it both reworks and stands in for. In "Draft M" (May 25, 1897), Freud writes:

> Fantasies arise from an unconscious combination of things experienced and heard, according to certain tendencies. These tendencies are toward making inaccessible the memory from which symptoms have emerged or might emerge. Fantasies are formed by amalgamation and distortion analogous to the decomposition of a chemical body which is compounded with another one. For the first sort of distortion consists in a falsification of memory by fragmentation in which it is precisely the chronological relations that are neglected. . . . A fragment of the visual scene then combines with a fragment of the auditory one into the fantasy, while the fragment set free links up with something else. Thereby an original has become untraceable. As a result of the formation of fantasies like

3. "To state things in a lapidary formula, one could say that from a certain point in Freud's thought the unconscious will arise from the drive, then the drive from the somatic, but that before 1897 it is the drive which arises from the unconscious." See Jean Laplanche, "The Unfinished Copernican Revolution" (1992b), in *Essays on Otherness*, 63, esp. n. 24.

this . . . the mnemic symptoms cease. Instead, unconscious fictions are present
which have not been subjected to defence. (Masson 1895a , 247)

Here fantasy emerges from an unconscious process of decomposition and
recombination of the materials of memory in which the original chronological relations are lost. The tendency governing this process is defensive,
and Freud's account reads like a development of his previous description of
defensive pathological displacement in "Project for a Scientific Psychology" (1950a), discussed in the previous chapter. The fantasies or "unconscious fictions" take the place of what Freud calls "mnemic symptoms," and
this cryptic phrase perhaps refers to traumatic memories and their repetition, which are substituted for by the production of fantasies that have not
themselves been repressed.

What is striking, by contrast with both Freud's account of dreams and
his later account of fantasy, is the absence at this early point of any emphasis on the function of fantasy as direct wish-fulfillment. While Freud connects the production of symptoms to the repression of fantasies that had
become too intense—"a symptom is generated through a [process of] pushing the fantasy back to its constituent memories" (Masson, 247)—fantasies
are conceived at this point *mainly in terms of the management of memories.*
Freud has hopes of elaborating a typology of fantasies as he had with dreams
and memory scenes.

> There is the soundest hope that it will be possible to determine the number
> and kind of fantasies just as it is possible with scenes. A romance of alienation
> (cf. paranoia) is found regularly and serves as a means of illegitimizing the
> relatives in question. Agoraphobia seems to depend on a romance of prostitu-
> tion, which itself goes back once more to this family romance. Thus a woman
> who will not go out by herself asserts her mother's unfaithfulness. (Draft M,
> Masson 1985a, 248)

Reading backward through a process of interpreting typical symptoms:

symptom     =     phobia of public spaces
                  ↑
fantasy      =     scene of prostitution, of being a 'public woman'
                  ↑
memory      =     mother's unfaithfulness.

Rather than fantasy being an *alternative* to memory, it is understood as being an ultimate defensive *outcome* of memory, from which the latter might be inferred and reconstructed. We have the germ of the notion of the *screen memory* that Freud was to elaborate systematically within the next few years. Although the fantasy of prostitution implies the dramatization of a sexual wish, Freud interprets it as an assertion, through an implied process of identification, about the fantasist's mother and her sexuality. Behind the fantasy is a memory fragment involving the figure of the mother and the mother's desire. The relation to the other is still in play.

## The Sins of the Fathers

Paradoxically, during the same period in which Freud is elaborating a theory of the fantasy–memory relation, his account of the originary infantile sexual scene is, in an apparently separate development, becoming more and more tightly specified. In the great letter to Fliess of December 6, 1896, full of burgeoning insights and incipient hypotheses about the stratification of the psyche and the translation processes between its various strata, Freud writes:

> It seems to me more and more that the essential point of hysteria is that it results from *perversion* on the part of the seducer, and *more and more* that heredity is seduction by the father. Thus an alternation emerges between generations:
> 1st generation—perversion
> 2nd generation—hysteria. . . .
> Accordingly, hysteria is not repudiated sexuality but rather *repudiated perversion*. (Masson 1895a, 212)

In successive letters over the next six months or so, the figure of the perverse father proliferates in one lurid clinical vignette after another, as Freud maps the transmission and reproduction of perverse symptoms, referencing oral and anal sex acts, from one generation to another, explaining the appearance of heredity by a perverse paternal legacy and its poisonous aftereffects (in the letter of January 11, 1897, he maps out a pattern of

transmitted perversions across two generations). His summary slogan contra
Charcot is "heredity is seduction by the father" (212). On January 3, he ex-
claims ironically over one family symptomology, *"Habemus Papam!,"*[4] while
on January 24, he writes, "In hysteria I recognize the *pater* in the high demands made in love, in the humility in relation to the lover, or in the inability to marry because of high ideals. The reason for this is, of course, the
height from which the father lowers himself to the child" (220, 228). On
February 8, he ruefully remarks: "Unfortunately, my own father was one of
these perverts and is responsible for the hysteria of my brother . . . and
those of several younger sisters. The frequency of this circumstance often
makes me wonder" (ibid., 230–31). However, the unease on Freud's part to
which this highly specific, perverse paternal scenario gave rise also grows
and increasingly accompanies his references to it. April 28 finds Freud simultaneously confessing, "I am still in doubt about matters concerning
fathers," while going on to welcome "a lucky chance this morning" that
"brought a fresh confirmation of paternal etiology" (237). On May 31, he
even confesses an incestuous dream about his eldest daughter, Mathilde,
which he interprets as "the fulfilment of my wish to catch a *Pater* as the
originator of neurosis and thus [the dream] puts an end to my ever-
recurring doubts" (249). By August 18, he is "tormented by grave doubts
about my theory of the neuroses" (261). After a vacation in northern Italy,
he writes a month later on his return home his famous letter of repudiation on September 21, 1897, a repudiation "that had been slowly dawning
on me in the last few months": "I no longer believe in my *neurotica* [theory
of the neuroses]" (264).

This double development in the first nine months of 1897, the narrowing down of the originating sexual trauma to the figure of the perverse father, together with a theory of fantasy in intimate connection to traumatic
memory as one of its *sequellae*, might seem initially very puzzling. Jean
Schimek comments that the hypothesis of a *necessary* paternal seduction
"became less and less plausible if it had to rest on actual events, external
accidents of individual history. The universal role of the father could only
be maintained by switching from accidental real events to inner deter-

4. The official Latin proclamation from St. Peter's in Rome on the election of a Pope:
"We have a Pope (Father)." Masson (1985a), 220.

mined fantasies."[5] However, at this point, Freud is not postulating a "universal" paternal seduction but simply its necessity in the earliest years for all cases of psychopathology. Furthermore, this opposition of inner fantasy and real event, which Freud himself adopts in his letter of repudiation, ignores the specific role of fantasy that Freud had been elaborating, as precisely a defense, a protective fiction *against* traumatic memory and, crucially, one that is formed out of a rearrangement of the materials of that very memory. It also leaves unexplained the question as to why if the *event* of paternal seduction is not guaranteed the *fantasy* of it should be, especially if there is no paternal provocation to arouse it.

However, in these two opposed developments taking place in these months, we can see another version of the tension that has inhabited Freud's model of afterwardsness from the beginning and threatened its complexity. Freud refers to this in the letter of January 24, 1897, where he raises again the question as to which moment determines the choice of neurosis (between hysteria, obsessional neurosis or paranoia). Here he confesses that "the decision keeps on oscillating between the period in which it originated and the period in which repression occurs (which is what I presently prefer)" (ibid., 228). The period immediately leading up to the letter of repudiation of the seduction theory in September 1897 is dominated by this tension between an increasingly strict specification of a necessary first moment, in which the actions of a perverse father are the sole specific cause, and a later moment of defensive fantasy, which forms the symptomology of a specific neurosis, through analysis of which access to the prior moment is possible. It is clear that Freud's favoring once again the later defensive moment (involving repression and substitutive fantasy) will gradually challenge the privileging of the first moment as a single specific cause or *caput Nili*.

*Seduction and Its Vicissitudes*

When it comes, Freud's repudiation of his seduction theory is based on both clinical considerations and what one might call the epidemiology of

5. Jean Schimek, "Fact and Fantasy in the Seduction Theory: A Historical Review," *Journal of the American Psychoanalytic Association* 35 (1987): 953.

abuse, as well as the internal developments of his metapsychology. He gives four headings under which he groups his objections. The first is that of *clinical failure*—the complaint repeated to Fliess throughout the previous months of being unable to bring a single treatment to a successful conclusion. Given the nature of Freud's therapy, the regressive backward movement from scene to scene, further and further into the patient's past, where scenes are reached that appear temporarily to clear up particular symptoms only to have them replaced by others, or where little or no improvement follows the appearance of a memory, it is not surprising that his clinical reports alternate between premature claims to success (as in the 1896 papers) followed by despair over the persistence of the patient's condition. Freud cites treatments abandoned by patients "who for a period of time had been most gripped" and, rather more cryptically, "partial successes" that could be explained "in the usual fashion" (ibid., 264).

The second heading addresses the role of the father and the *epidemiological implications* of infantile abuse. Freud expresses "surprise that in all cases, the *father*, not excluding my own, had to be accused of being perverse." The already surprising frequency of hysteria would then imply an even greater and improbable degree of "perversions against children" (ibid.), for the population of hysterics would require an even larger population of those who had been sexually abused, because hysteria as a condition requires an accumulation of such events and their subsequent repression; abusive events that had not been repressed were not hysterogenic (though it needs to be stressed were still profoundly damaging as Freud recognized).[6]

The third heading brings up the question of *fantasy*, but as I have had occasion to note, it does so as an *alternative* to the idea of truthful representation and as a skeptical response to the "decomposition" of memory and its recomposition into fantasy (as elaborated previously in Draft M): "There are no indications of reality in the unconscious, so that one cannot distinguish between truth and fiction that has been cathected with affect" (ibid., 264–65). Freud had concluded in Draft M that "an original has become untraceable," but this reworking of memory into fantasy had not, at that point, undermined Freud's clinical confidence in being able to reconstruct

---

6. See Freud's description of their effects in "The Aetiology of Hysteria" (1896c), *SE* 3, discussed in Chapter 3.

the rearranged materials of memory. Now the untraceable original leads Freud to a despairing skepticism about the possibility of distinguishing fiction charged with affect from truth-telling memory. His earlier appeal, in the long paper on the etiology of hysteria (1896c) to the emotional living out of scenes as a criterion of their authenticity, seems now to fail him in the face of the evolving function of fantasy: protective fictions as well as truth can be "cathected with affect." To Freud's question posed in the 1896 papers—"Why should patients assure me so emphatically of their unbelief, if what they want to discredit is something which . . . they themselves have invented?" (1896c, 204)—an answer now presents itself: "Accordingly there would remain the solution that the sexual fantasy invariably seizes upon the theme of the parents" (ibid., 264–65).

The fourth heading confirms the *skeptical conclusion* of the third. Not only is the clinician not able to tell the difference between fiction and truth, but from the patient's point of view the moment of recognition and cathartic recall never seems finally to come: "In the most deep-reaching psychosis the unconscious memory does not break through, so that the secret of childhood experiences is not disclosed even in the most confused delirium" (265). This reformulates Freud's epistemological skepticism about the indistinguishability of truth (memory) and fiction (fantasy), since both are charged with affect, such that affect, emotional acting out, can no longer function as an indicator of reality. The epistemological skepticism, however, does not become an ontological skepticism. Behind the unreliability of phenomenal forms there is a *noumenon*—"the unconscious memory . . . the secret of childhood experiences," an *x*, the *Ding an sich* of traumatic reality—that does not manifest itself as such. If "the unconscious never overcomes the resistance of the conscious," if after the return of the repressed there is always still an unconscious remainder, then Freud's disappointed clinical hopes, that the opposite would happen "to the point where the unconscious is completely tamed by the conscious," make clear, as Jean Laplanche has pointed out, the assumptions about the nature and status of the unconscious with which Freud was working. The unconscious based on traumatic memories was conceived by Freud as pathological, temporary, and reducible; memory could be restored and the unconscious tamed or liquidated. Consequently, Freud's clinical and metapsychological aspirations here founder on an unconscious that is irreducible, permanent, but encountered only through its epistemologically unreliable derivatives.

At this point Freud does not have an alternative account of either fantasy or the unconscious. Bereft of "the complete resolution of a neurosis and the certain knowledge of its etiology in childhood," Freud comments, "Now I have no idea of where I stand because I have not succeeded in gaining a theoretical understanding of repression and its interplay of forces" (ibid.). I take this to be an allusion to the temporal complex of afterwardsness with its overdetermining moments, one of which is repression. With this apparently in ruins the only alternative conceptual scheme is the one Freud had rejected and had been thinking *against*:

> It seems once again arguable that only later experiences give the impetus to fantasies, which [then] hark back to childhood, and with this the factor of an hereditary disposition regains a sphere of influence from which I had made it my task to dislodge it—in the interest of illuminating neurosis. (Masson 1895a, 265)

The ghost of Charcot beckons in the wings, for with the collapse of any certainty about the earliest infantile scenes, two things happen: the fantasies can only be grounded in later experiences that are more readily available to memory (and to cross-checking with relatives) and that borrow the childhood scene for their own purposes; Charcot's hereditary disposition now returns to fill the space that had been occupied by these earliest infantile scenes that Freud had reconstructed from his patients' hallucinatory or transferential 'reproductions.' His now doubtful reconstructions had been conceived by Freud as the replacement for Charcot's heredity. They would constitute the long-term etiology of hysteria as a condition (as distinct from the localized 'psychical mechanism' for particular symptoms).

Within a matter of weeks Freud writes to Fliess on October 15 with an outline of what is later to be called the Oedipus complex, complete with references to Sophocles's *Oedipus* and Shakespeare's *Hamlet*: "A single idea of general value dawned on me. I have found, in my own case too, [the phenomenon of] being in love with my mother and jealous of my father, and I now consider it a universal event in early childhood" (ibid., 272). With this "universal" childhood event, Freud has found a potential alternative ground for his memorial fantasies and fantasmic memories, and hence an—as yet undeveloped—explanatory hypothesis to replace his paternal etiology.

However, along with a changed explanation is a change in the *object* of explanation, for "a universal event in early childhood" implies a general model of infantile psychic development rather than a narrowly conceived traumatic model of hysteria or even neurosis in general. This move from the pathological and particular to a developmental theory of "universal events" had already been latent within some of his earlier suggestions. In the letter of December 6, 1896, the concern with perversion pointed to the figure of the orally and anally abusive father, but it also pointed in a very different direction: "Furthermore, behind this lies the idea of abandoned *erotogenic zones*. That is to say, during childhood sexual release would be attainable from a great many parts of the body. . . . In this differentiation and limitation [would thus lie] progress in culture, and moral and individual development" (ibid., 212). This idea of abandoned erotogenic zones, which Freud would develop later into an account of infantile polymorphous perversity, decisively undermines the thesis of infantile sexual indifference or apathy. The germ of the later theory of infantile *pregenital* sexuality and its sublimation is here, which together with the "universal event" of the Oedipus drama will constitute the two major axes of the classical Freudian theory of sexuality.

## Freud's Self-Analysis

The aftermath of this moment of crisis, however, is not at all what one might have expected. There is not just a smooth transition from an abandoned hypothesis of infantile sexual abuse to a new one of infantile sexuality. The power of scenes and the temporal logic of afterwardsness survive the eclipse of the perverse father, and even he is not entirely banished. This is clear in the letter of October 3, less than two weeks later, where Freud has turned to his self-analysis, "which I consider indispensable for the clarification of the whole problem" (ibid., 268). Here he retracts his earlier attribution of sexual abuse to his father, indicating that "the old man plays no active part in my case," but adds that "in my case the 'prime originator' was an ugly, elderly but clever woman, who told me a great deal about God Almighty and hell and who instilled in me a high opinion of my own capacities" ( ibid.). He concludes:

I have not yet grasped anything at all of the *scenes* themselves which lie at the
bottom of the story. If they come [to light] and I succeed in resolving my
hysteria, then I shall be grateful to the memory of the old woman who
provided me at such an early age with the means for living and going on living.
(Masson 1895a, 269, emphasis added)

While the recent narrow paternal etiology is dismissed, there is still the
figure of the somewhat mysterious "prime originator," his nurse, and the
conviction that the coming to light of "the scenes themselves" is what will
determine the resolution of "my own hysteria." The welling up of feeling
for this shadowy woman moves Freud to comment to Fliess: "As you see,
the old liking is breaking through again today." As if to confirm the connection between this enigmatic figure and Freud's fundamental self-confidence
in his intellectual capacities, he immediately adds: "I cannot convey to you
any idea of the intellectual beauty of this work." His old feeling for "the
prime originator" and his new enthusiasm for the "intellectual beauty" of
what he is doing now are intimately connected. This seems less a break from
than a further complication of the problematic of seduction and its accompanying scenography.

The long postscript to the letter (October 4) with its analysis of the following night's dream would seem to confirm this. Freud's analysis is selective, but the role of the "prime originator" is further developed with the
cryptic addition that from "the strangest disguises" in the dream he could
infer that "she was my teacher in sexual matters and complained because I
was clumsy and unable to do anything" (ibid.). The startling juxtaposition
in this sentence might make one wonder exactly what the clumsiness in
question was, and what he was being required to do that he could not. Is
Freud implying that he had been sexually seduced or abused by his nurse?
His phrasing seems to echo the formulation from the impassioned passage
in the 1896 essay about the child "whose performance of the sexual activities assigned to him is often interrupted by his imperfect control of his natural needs" (Freud 1896c, 215). Did Freud's moving sympathy for the exploited
child arise from more than the analyst's attention to his abused patients?
However, Freud is more concerned to link the theme of clumsiness and incapacity to his later feelings of "neurotic impotence" with its "sexual substratum," whether of the fearful child at school or "my present impotence as a

therapist" (ibid., 269). His gratitude to his nurse in the previous day's letter, for "his high opinion of my own capacities" that enables him to go on living, would appear to be contradicted or reversed here in the following night's dream (which may be an indication of her contradictory legacy to him). As if in response to the previous day's letter to Fliess, Freud's dream produces one of "the scenes themselves." However, he does not give us a detailed account of the manifest content of the dream. He writes of "the paper ten-florin notes that I saw in the dream as Martha's weekly house-keeping money" (ibid.) and this, as Didier Anzieu argues,[7] must be connected to the dream fragment commented on in *The Interpretation of Dreams*:

> I took out a subscription in S and R's bookshop for a periodical costing TWENTY FLORINS *a year.* Source: My wife had reminded me the day before that I still owed her *twenty florins* for the weekly household expenses.[8]

In a further fragment, "the dream picture was a memory of my taking money from the *mother* of a doctor—that is, wrongfully" (ibid., 271, emphasis added), which appears to allude to a patient of Freud's sent to him by Fliess: "Mrs. Q., whose remark you reported to me: that I should not take anything from her, as she was the wife of a colleague (he of course made it a condition that I should)" (ibid., 270). The manifest dream, then, seems to have at least two moments or scenes, one involving Freud in a bookshop spending twenty florins of his wife's housekeeping money, and the second a scene of him taking money "wrongfully" from a doctor's mother, each scene alluding separately to his wife and his colleague's wife. Setting aside Freud's slippage from wife to mother (no doubt with its own significance), his interpretation of these fragments points to their common connection in the taking of money wrongfully from a wife/mother and the theme of "bad treatment," which "makes the most mortifying allusions to my present impotence as a therapist," taking money from patients whose hysteria he cannot cure. Behind this composite dream narrative with its contemporary allusions, Freud locates the archaic figure of the nurse about whom he makes two apparently factual claims: that "she washed me in reddish water

7. Didier Anzieu, *Freud's Self-analysis*, trans. Peter Graham (London: The Hogarth Press, 1986), 237.
8. Sigmund Freud, *The Interpretation of Dreams* (1900a), *SE* 4, 166.

in which she had herself washed," and that "she made me steal zehners (ten kreuzer coins) to give them to her" (ibid., 269).

Freud tells us that there is "a long chain" of associations that goes from the "paper ten-florin notes" that he sees in the dream, rightly belonging to his wife, Martha, for the household expenses (instead of being spent on his own interests and pursuits) to the zehners that his nurse made him steal from his mother to give to her. In the following letter of October 15, we learn that Freud turned to his mother for information about the nurse and had the broad outlines of his interpretation confirmed: except that his old nurse had stolen the coins herself rather than having made little Sigmund steal them. Freud's corrected interpretation goes: "I = she, and the mother of the doctor equals my mother. So far was I from knowing she was a thief that I made a wrong interpretation" (ibid., 271). This would seem to imply that Freud's first account of the stealing of the money was a retrospective inference or reconstruction from the manifest dream scene, rather than a visualized scene of theft in its own right offering itself as a memory.

None of this relates to or explains, however, the disturbing scene of the little boy being washed in the nurse's reddish bath water. There is no chain of associations provided by Freud for this element, which does seem to present itself as a visualized scene. However, the status of this grotesque scene is not clear. Is it part of the manifest dream scene, or is it a scene that emerges from the free associations released in the analysis of the manifest scene? The latter is probably more likely, for it seems to be the case that the dream makes use of more recent events or 'day's residues' from Freud's adult life to form the dream scene. Freud comments: "The interpretation is not difficult: I find nothing like this in the chain of my memories; so I regard it as a genuine ancient discovery" (ibid., 269). Two points can be considered here: that the scene itself does not belong to his store of conscious childhood memories, and that its meaning is only understood subsequently (*nachträglich*) by the adult Freud and not by the child in the scene itself. Freud never states his interpretation of the scene, but his later question— "Where do all patients get the horrible perverse details which often are remote from their experience as from their knowledge?" (ibid., 270)—appears to confirm the authenticity of the scene as a (newly emergent) memory by appealing to the naïve and unknowing reproduction of details whose "horrible, perverse" significance the infantile subjects are ignorant of. The belated interpretation of the scene, "not difficult" for the adult Freud, is presumably that the nurse had washed the child in water colored by menstrual blood from her own washing. If this is perverse, then it is obscurely perverse: What impulse could she have been acting on in doing that? It is clear that for Freud its perverseness points to the active role of the "prime originator," to the innocence of her object, the young Sigmund, and to the authenticity of the scene as memory, as "a genuine ancient discovery."

Freud's conviction that he has recovered a genuine memory fragment hitherto unknown to him is restated at the end of the letter where he invokes it to settle the intellectual impasse of the September 'repudiation' letter: "A harsh critic might say of all this that it was retrogressively fantasied instead of progressively determined. The *experimenta crucis* must decide against him. The reddish water indeed seems to be of that kind" (ibid., 270). But is it? The "harsh critic" is, of course, Freud himself of just over a month ago: "It seems once again arguable that only later experiences give the impetus to fantasies, which [then] hark back to childhood" (265). The harsh critic is momentarily confounded by Freud's "genuine ancient discovery" and its testimony to the reality of "the prime originator." However, the conceptual opposition Freud invokes here of regressive fantasy versus a progressively determining real event already forgets both the deferred and retrospective double logic of afterwardsness, part of which is the role of fantasy in mediating and binding belatedly traumatic memories. Indeed, the very enigmatic nature of the scene in all its perverseness might suggest its overdetermined and composite nature.

What Freud leaves unspecified is the relation between this scene and his inference from the dream's "strangest disguises" that "she was my teacher in sexual matters" (269) and hence, presumably, "the prime originator" of his hysteria, if not a lot more. If this was so, then the remoteness of the "horrible perverse details" from either the experience or the knowledge of little Sigmund might not have been as great as the adult Freud assumes. With such a partial reporting of both the dream's manifest content and the network of associations that lead to its latent dream thoughts, any commentary can be only speculative. That said, it is striking that there are two female figures in the letter that appear to have no connection with each other—at least none that Freud cares to make—the mother the sight of whose nakedness, Freud infers, aroused his libido toward her and the nurse, dubbed "prime originator" and "my teacher in sexual matters." Even as Freud alludes to his mother's nakedness, he manages to veil it loyally, like the good Jewish son he is, in the decent obscurity of italicized Latin: "*matrem . . . nudam.*" At the same time he exposes from "under the strangest disguises" the thieving pervert, ugly, clever, and old, who was his nurse. It is also striking that, in his attempts to interpret his sequence of dreams (and the one in question is part of a series), Freud turns to whom else but his mother for the truth about his nurse. If truth of the nurse lies with the mother, then the desexualized, Latinized "*matrem . . . nudam,*" the object of the little Sigmund's newly aroused libido, is once again being decently veiled behind the figure of the nurse. One can only wonder whether this doubly veiled figure is not a more likely candidate for the role of "prime originator" and "teacher in sexual matters" than the abjected figure of the nurse with her reddish water.

Freud's turn from the one to the other, their substitution, would also suggest that the appeal to the testimony of relatives in the attempt to settle the fantasmatic/memorial status of scenes might not necessarily provide the exit from fantasy and access to objectivity that Freud had hoped for. Also his mother's narrative of the nurse as reported by Freud is not entirely plausible: "It was discovered she was a thief, and that all the shiny new kreuzers and zehners and that all the toys that had been given to you were found in her possession. Your brother Philipp himself fetched the policeman; she then was given ten months in prison" (ibid., 271). The editor of the letters informs us that a zehner was "a coin of little value" (270, n. 2), however shiny, and Freud himself notes that one was worth ten kreuzers. So a nurse was found in possession of the virtually worthless small change that a young child might accumulate, together with her young charge's toys: How incriminating was that? Would it warrant the immediate calling of a policeman, let alone a ten-month prison sentence? The disproportion between crime and punishment, if it can even be seen as a crime, and the consequent implausible nature of the whole 'explanation' is confirmed by Didier Anzieu's information that the nurse was one Monica Zajic, the forty-year-old daughter of the Zajic family "who owned, and shared, the Freuds' house in Freiburg" (Anzieu 1986, 238). It seems even more unlikely that, for the sake of some valueless coins and children's toys, the Freud family would have called in the police to arrest the adult daughter of the

family from whom they rented their shared house, one they were on sufficiently good terms with to have employed as a nurse. Something else is not
being said in this narrative that sounds like a collective family fable;
whether that something was connected to Freud's conviction that she was
his sexual initiator (which might have justified the policeman and the ten-
month sentence) it is, of course, impossible to establish on the basis of his
letters alone.

There are grounds, then, for thinking that neither element in Freud's
dream—the scene of taking money wrongfully and the scene of bathing in
reddish water, connected by the theme of "bad treatment"—can be taken
simply as either a newly aroused memory scene or even a purely defensive
transformation of one. It is striking, however, that in the letters immediately following the September repudiation of his paternal etiology, including that of October 15, where he first proposes the idea of a universal
oedipal event in early childhood, Freud remains committed to both the
primacy of "the scenes themselves that lie at the bottom of the story," that
is, to a continuing scenography of trauma, and to the seductive role of a
"prime originator." The problematic of seduction is still in place.


## The Persistence of Scenes

The letters to Fliess are marked by repeated resurgences of confidence in
both the determining power of scenes in general and even the narrower
paternal etiology. On December 12, 1897, Freud writes: "My confidence in
paternal aetiology has risen greatly. Eckstein . . . obtained from her [pa-
tient], among other things, the identical scenes with the father." The significance of this finding lies in the fact that Emma Eckstein, Freud's former
patient, now practicing as an analyst, had not "given the slightest hint of
what would emerge from the unconscious" (ibid., 286), unlike Freud's habit
of giving advanced warnings or indications of what he expected. On December 22, three months after the September repudiation, Freud writes out
the long clinical anecdote with which this book began about the hallucinat-
ing woman and her small daughter, with its repetitive traumatic aftereffects of a violent and sexually abusive husband and father. It is the most
complex and elaborately scripted scenography of trauma in the entire

Fliess correspondence, with its description of a repetitive process that involves transmission to another person. It is clear in this case that Freud's retrospective analysis of the shadowy primal scene of marital rape, a scene that is repeated in the mother's hallucinatory attack and relayed in the daughter's unknowing account (as discussed in the Prologue), is *a different kind* of intellectual operation from the gathering of biographical data about the patient's childhood, and the corroborative evidence of the father's sexual abuse of both mother and child that accompanies the clinical anecdote. Freud's analysis is an interpretation of the *scene* of sexual violence that is being reenacted in the present moment of the mother's hysterical attack, albeit unrecognized as such in her daughter's narration of it.[9]

The predominance of the father figure and the question of the narrow *paternal* etiology in all these instances is, however, misleading, as it displaces attention from the larger questions of the memorial/fantasmic nature of the reproduced scenes and the temporal complex of afterwardsness with its primal and subsequent scenes. The figure of the father drops away over the next two years in the letters to Fliess of 1898–99, but these other two questions persist with as much urgency as before.

The letter of January 16, 1898, shows Freud remodeling hysteria more closely on the dream—"dream and hysteria fit together ever more neatly"—which leads to his definition of happiness: "Happiness is the belated [*nachträglich*] fulfilment of a prehistoric wish" (ibid., 294). He develops this primacy of "the prehistoric" on March 10.

> Biologically, dream-life seems to me to derive entirely from the residues of the prehistoric period of life (between the ages of one and three)—the same period which is the source of the unconscious and alone contains the etiology of all the psychoneuroses. . . . This formula suggests itself to me: What is *seen* in the prehistoric period produces dreams; what is *heard* in it produces fantasies; what

---

9. The biographical data bearing on the daughter's memory is itself, however, also organized as a sequence of scenes, beginning in earliest childhood:

> When the girl was six to seven months (!!!) old, her mother was lying in bed, bleeding nearly to death from an injury inflicted by the father. At the age of sixteen years she again saw her mother bleeding from the uterus (carcinoma), which brought on the beginning of her neurosis. The latter breaks out a year later when she hears about a haemorrhoid operation. Can one doubt that the father forces the mother to submit to anal intercourse?"(Masson 1985a, 289)

is *experienced sexually* in it produces the psychoneuroses. The repetition of what was experienced in that period is in itself the fulfilment of a wish; a recent wish only leads to a dream if it can put itself in connection with material from this period, if the recent wish is a derivative of the prehistoric one or can get itself adopted by one. (ibid., 302)

We can see here the influence of the model of the dream where the latent dream-thoughts take primacy over the manifest dream scene that draws its material mainly from the residues of the day before or from derivatives of more contemporary material. The latent thoughts organize the later material according to the templates of 'prehistoric' experience, infantile wishes encoded in the form of scenes with a strongly visual component. Later wishes and their imagined fulfillment acquire their ability to produce dreams (or, more generally, "happiness") because they stand in for and represent a prehistoric wish and its fulfillment by proxy. This primacy of the prehistoric is closely connected to the problematic of seduction as the role of the "unforgettable, prehistoric other person who is never equalled by anyone later" (December 6, 1896), the adult "prime originator" (October 3, 1897), gives ontological weight and objectivity to the psychic representations in which it is encoded. However, this invocation of the prehistoric other does not solve the problem of the *composite* status of the scenes in which that other is registered and of the other's fantasmic as well as memorial double nature.

Freud's oscillation continues throughout 1898. Of a male patient Freud comments on September 27: "Now, a child who regularly wets his bed until his seventh year . . . must have experienced sexual excitation in his earlier childhood. Spontaneous or by seduction? There it is" (ibid., 329). On July 7, Freud repeats this model of the alignment and substitution of earlier and later scenarios but this time giving the initiative and weight to the later scenes. A propos of C. F. Meyer's novel *The Monk's Wedding*, Freud describes the process of fantasy formation in that work: "A new experience is in fantasy projected back into the past so that the new persons become aligned with the old ones, who become their prototypes. The mirror image of the present is seen in a fantasied past, which then prophetically becomes the present" (ibid., 320). Here the past is the fantasmatic delegate of the present and its reality. This neatly *reverses* the dream model, where the recent representations are subordinated to and organized by the power of the repeated wishes and scenes from the past.

The power of fantasy and retrospect is recurrently reasserted throughout 1898 and early 1899 with various affirmations of "the key of fantasy" (ibid., 340, 342). On January 3, 1899, he writes to Fliess:

> In the first place, a small bit of my self-analysis has forced its way through and confirmed that fantasies are the products of later periods and are projected back from what was then the present into earliest childhood. The manner in which this occurs also emerged—once again by a verbal link.
>
> To the question "What happened in earliest childhood?" the answer is "Nothing, but the germ of a sexual impulse existed." (Mason 1895a, 338)

This seems not only to privilege the later moments over the earlier but to abandon yet again the whole problematic of seduction in favor of retrospective back projection and the childhood germs of sexuality that he had first postulated in *Studies on Hysteria* in 1895.

Nevertheless, the power of scenes, and their memorial value, continues to structure Freud's clinical practice right up to the publication of *The Interpretation of Dreams* in 1900 and beyond. At the very end of 1899, in the letter of December 21, Freud announces triumphantly of patient E ("You can well imagine how important this one persistent patient has become to me"):

> Buried deep beneath all his fantasies, we found a scene from his primal period (before twenty-two months) which meets all the requirements and in which all the remaining puzzles converge. It is everything at the same time—sexual, innocent, natural, and the rest. I scarcely dare believe it yet. It is as if Schliemann had once more excavated Troy, which had hitherto been deemed a fable. At the same time the fellow is doing outrageously well. (Masson 1895a, 391–92)

The archaeological metaphor refers to Schliemann, the great excavator of Troy and the vindicator of the truth of what "had hitherto been deemed a fable"; it suggests that for Freud some version of his abandoned theory seemed now vindicated. Even at this late stage, we have the primacy of remembered scenes, although remembered scenes in conjunction with defensive–protective fictions, "buried deep beneath all his fantasies." It is not clear what the content of this scene is, whether it is a scene of sexual abuse or seduction in the old sense or not, although Freud's description— "sexual, innocent, natural and the rest"—might suggest that it was nontraumatic. However, it is a sexual scene involving others and part of a relay of such scenes, as the letter of a few weeks later (January 8, 1900) indicates: "In E's case, the second scene is coming up after years of preparation; and it is one that may *perhaps* be confirmed objectively by asking his elder sister. Behind it a third, long-suspected scene approaches" (ibid., 395). Although the paternal etiology is now abandoned, and the sexual scene being "innocent, natural and the rest" implies that it involves the expression of infantile sexuality and its "germ of a sexual impulse," nevertheless, it is, once again, the power of memorial scenes, as distinguishable from the fantasies that disguise them, that is being reaffirmed.

Despite the gradual settling of certain secondary issues such as the gradually disappearing role of the perverse father, this oscillation continues in Freud's thought. Sometimes this is presented in terms of a mutually exclusive polarization between fantasy and memory, or fantasy and the real event, as in the September repudiation letter of 1897, and unfortunately this simplification of Freud's thought has set the terms in which most later commentary operates, even such a thoughtful return to sources as Rand and Torok's essay that traces precisely this oscillation in Freud's thinking.[10] However, the question of memory and fantasy persists (and it is definitely a matter of 'and' with all its complex interrelations, rather than 'or,'). Under the force of his development of a theory of fantasy, Freud's understanding of memory changes and this can be seen in his formulation of the concept of screen memories, which was a by-product of his continual wrestling with these issues.

## Screen Memories and the Critique of Memory

In May 1899 Freud sent off for periodical publication his paper on "Screen Memories" in which the concept is first formulated. It emerges directly out of his struggle with the fantasy–memory relation and is an attempt to articulate these terms in a way that refuses their simple opposition. He begins with a reaffirmation of the power of the 'pre-historic,' "that the

---

10. Nicholas Rand and Maria Torok, "The Concept of Psychical Reality and Its Traps," in *Questions for Freud*, (Cambridge, Mass.: Harvard University Press, 1997), pp. 24–44.

experiences of the earliest years of our childhood leave ineradicable traces in the depths of our minds."[11] However, these experiences are not represented *as such* in the archives of preconscious memory. The outcome of a direct interrogation of our memories is, disappointingly, "either nothing at all or a relatively small number of isolated recollections which are often of dubious or enigmatic importance" (ibid., 303). Continuous memory of a connected chain of events begins only with the sixth or seventh and often only the tenth year, leaving what only a year before he had called in a letter to Fliess the crucial "pre-historic period of life . . . which is the source of the unconscious and alone contains the etiology of the psychoneuroses" (January 16, 1898; Masson 1985a, 302), lost in the obscurity of a general infantile amnesia. It would appear at first that the general rule for adult memory, that emotionally significant experiences are retained and able to be recollected, does not obtain for the earliest years. Consequently, Freud addresses the enigmatic phenomenon of

> people whose earliest recollections of childhood are concerned with everyday and indifferent events which could not produce any emotional effect even in children, but which are recollected (*too* clearly, one is inclined to say) in every detail, while approximately contemporary events, even if, on the evidence of their parents, they moved them intensely at the time, have not been retained in their memory. (1899a, 305–6)

Focusing on this common subspecies of memory, the vividly recalled childhood scene that appears to lack emotional significance or any reason for its retention, let alone its clarity or sensory intensity, Freud elaborates an account that ends up calling into question the veridical transparency of all childhood memories. Drawing on research done in 1895 by V. and C. Henri based on responses by 123 subjects to a questionnaire about their earliest memories, Freud cites, as an exemplary instance of these enigmatic early scenes, that of a professor of philology whose earliest memory, from his fourth year, was of a table set for a meal with a basin of ice. This coincides with the death of a much-loved grandmother, which distressed him greatly but of which he had no recollection at all. Another man reports his earliest memory as a scene in which he breaks off a branch from a tree in

11. Sigmund Freud, "Screen Memories" (1899a), *SE* 3, 303.

the presence of other people, one of whom helped him. "He thinks he can still identify the spot where this happened" (ibid., 306).

If the enigmatic childhood scene is a torso, as Freud puts it, then its restoration will show that it does obey the rule of adult memories that the most important experiences are retained. As we have seen in the letters to Fliess on the memory–fantasy relation, the model Freud increasingly deployed to understand these mysterious and only apparently arbitrary fragments of memory is the one he had recently developed to analyze dreams and symptoms. He summarizes this as "conflict, repression, substitution involving a compromise" (308). It is a model that goes back to his earliest account of pathological defense in hysteria in "Project for a Scientific Psychology," which we considered in Chapter 3. There, schematically, an experience composed of two elements, A+B, is fragmented such that the innocuous element A takes the place of the emotionally charged element B: "The hysteric, who weeps at A, is quite unaware that he is doing so because of the association A–B, and B itself plays no part at all in his psychic life" (1950a [1895], 348). The last phrase needs amending as the repressed, substituted-for B does play a crucial role in the hysteric's *psychic* life, although not in his conscious life, as is clear from the role Freud accords such amnesiac defense in the second moment of his schema of afterwardsness in the case of Emma. The enigmatic childhood memory is shown to exemplify the same psychical mechanism as the "excessively intense idea" (ibid.) over which the hysteric unaccountably weeps, as do the symptoms of obsessional neurosis and paranoia, as well as the nonpathological phenomenon of the dream. However, the model of a simple substitution of A for B has been complicated by the notion of a compromise formation that results from a conflict of mental forces in which neither cancels out the other: "Instead, a compromise is brought about, somewhat on the analogy of the resultant in a parallelogram of forces" (1899a, 307). In the conflict between the force that seeks "to fix important impressions by establishing reproducible mnemic images" (ibid., 307) and the resistance to that force, what results is not a direct reproduction of the experience but an image to some degree associatively displaced from it. It will lack the emotionally significant but disturbing elements that provoked the resistance and hence will appear trivial or insignificant, but with its sensory elements fantasmatically enhanced and intensified. Its retention is due not to its own content but to its relation with the disturbing elements that have been excluded. Freud cites the old saying about counterfeit coins, that "they are not made of gold themselves but have lain beside something that *is* made of gold" (ibid., 307).

As Freud himself remarks, this schematic representation of the screen memory turns on a metonymical relation of displacement by contiguity, making use of two elements from a simultaneous ensemble, as in the A + B schema in the "Project." However, this forecloses the temporal dimension so crucial to the process of afterwardsness, but which nevertheless returns with all its problems in the extended example that he goes on to present. As is obvious from a knowledge of Freud's biography, and especially from his dream material in *The Interpretation of Dreams*, as well as the Fliess letters, the clinical example of a screen memory analyzed at length here in the form of a Socratic dialogue with a fictionalized patient is based on Freud's own memories. The dialogue is between Freud-the-analyst and the undisclosed 'Freud'-the-analysand ("who is not at all or only very slightly neurotic" [ibid., 309]). It enables him to dramatize something of the oscillations that have characterized his theoretical struggles over the previous years as we have followed them in this chapter. As Rand and Torok propose: "The essay is a dramatization of an internal debate; as in a play two interlocutors represent opposite points of view" (Rand and Torok 1997, 33). What is implicitly at stake here in the clinical dialogue is the temporal structure of the memory–fantasy relation, and, although it is not acknowledged as such, the logic of afterwardsness.

What had plagued Freud in the seduction theory was both the status to be given to certain focal scenes (memory or fantasy) and the relation between early and later moments of the dialectic of afterwardsness. Despite a tendency to polarize the priority of the early scene, as the site of memory and the progressive determination of later moments by earlier ones (the much vaunted 'source of the Nile'), over against the priority of the later scene, as the moment of back projection and retrospective fantasy, we have traced a fugitive if richer and more complex understanding of their asymmetrical interdependence. For the logic of afterwardsness entailed the inscription of an excess that resisted integration and binding into the ego and its archives but that was reactivated and reworked in a later moment. Its paradox was "the notion of powers emanating from a mnemic image which were absent from the real impression."[12] The hysterical symptom was not the immediate result of either the earlier infantile or later adult scenes, but, as we saw in Chapter 3, it was a composite image—memorial fantasy, fantasmic memory—that derived from both. Freud approaches this again in the form of the screen memory, which he explicitly compares with the production of the hysterical symptom. Unfortunately, it turns out to be something of a missed encounter.

Briefly, the enigmatic memory that 'Freud'-the-analysand presents stages a lush meadow full of yellow dandelions where three children, the young 'Freud' and two cousins, a boy and a girl, are playing and gathering flowers. The little girl has the best bunch, so the two boys "fall on her and snatch away her flowers." She runs in tears up the meadow to a cottage where a peasant woman gives her a big slice of black bread and butter. The two boys throw away their flowers and run up demanding to be given some bread too: "The peasant-woman cuts the loaf with a long knife. In my memory the bread tastes quite delicious." 'Freud' comments that there is "something not quite right about the scene" that he recalls, as the intensity of the yellow of the flowers and the taste of the bread "seem to me exaggerated in an almost hallucinatory fashion" (1899a, 311–12).

One of the functions of the dialogue between Freud-the-analyst and 'Freud'-the-analysand is to accommodate an emphasis on both early and later moments. The analysis begins by establishing that the memory (as distinct from the scene remembered) does not itself date back to early childhood but was first awoken at the age of seventeen when 'Freud' was visiting the rural scenes that feature in it and experiencing his first love. This gave rise to a set of fantasies that "were not concerned with the future but sought to improve the past" (ibid., 313), centering on the fifteen-year-old daughter of the old family friends with whom he was staying. Marriage to her represented an alternative and happier life history than the one that had followed his family's departure for the city, due to the collapse of his father's business. He comments, "I can remember quite well for what a long time afterwards I was affected by the yellow colour of the dress she was wearing when we first met, wherever I saw the same colour elsewhere" (ibid.). This clearly signals retrospective fantasy as the driving force in the

12. Sigmund Freud, "The Aetiology of Hysteria" (1896c), *SE* 3, 213.

production of the memory. Three years later, at the age of twenty, 'Freud' revisits the now grown-up cousins who figure as the other children in the fantasy. Here he does not fall in love with his female cousin from the childhood scene, but his uncle and father plan a possible marriage between them that would involve 'Freud' giving up his studies and joining his uncle's successful business. The fantasy shared by both the fathers, as well as the son's earlier one, aimed "to make good the loss in which the original catastrophe had involved my whole existence" (ibid., 314).

Freud-the-analyst pinpoints the amalgamation of these two later fantasies—marrying the girl in the yellow dress (associated with the chain—dark yellow Alpine flowers/light yellow lowland flowers/yellow dandelions of the memory scene) and marrying his cousin and joining the family business (exchanging the flowers of his academic interests for a prosperous 'bread-and-butter' occupation): "You projected the two fantasies onto one another and made a childhood memory of them." The screen memory thus constructed represents the fantasies of a later date through symbolic and associative (metaphoric and metonymic) connections. His alter ego replies: "But if that is so, there was *no* childhood memory, but only a phantasy put back into childhood. A feeling tells me, though, that the scene is genuine" (315). Two issues are at stake here: the familiar one of the authenticity of memory as against its retrospective construction and the question of motive: Why was it necessary to represent adult or adolescent fantasies (especially fantasies that had the stamp of paternal approval) by childhood scenes?

The reply to the latter involves the explication of a sexual dimension to the 'innocent' early scene. The taking of flowers from the girl – "the two boys fall on her and snatch away her flowers" – makes use of the traditional symbolism of 'deflowering' to represent a sexual wish. This sexual fantasy is the prolongation of the conscious one of marrying into an improved past and prosperous present, but one that has to remain unconscious because

> the dominating mood of diffidence and of respect towards the girl keeps it suppressed. So it remains unconscious . . . and slips away into a childhood memory. . . . It is the coarsely sensual element in the phantasy which explains why it does not develop into a *conscious* phantasy but must be content to find its way allusively and under a flowery disguise into a childhood scene. (Freud 1899a, 316–17)

Freud-the-analyst also formulates this as a general principle: "The slipping away of repressed thoughts and wishes into childhood memories" happens invariably with hysterical patients. He adds that there is always "some pleasurable motive" for the recall of the remote past (317)—a potential theory of remembrance as wish fulfillment parallel to the theory of dreams.

At this point the essay appears to be firmly aligned with the 'retrospective fantasy' position that derives from the September 1897 letter of repudiation and the much more recent January 1899 letter of a few months previously, quoted earlier (the latter a product of his self-analysis, as is the screen memory analyzed here). As a result, 'Freud' the alter ego responds:

> I cannot help concluding that what I am dealing with is something that never happened at all but has been unjustifiably smuggled in among my childhood memories. (Freud 1899a, 318)

This allows the official Freud to take up once again the claims of the prehistoric and the infantile:

> I see that I must take up again the defence of its genuineness. You are going too far . . . suppose now that this [the slipping away into childhood scenes—JF] cannot occur unless there is a memory-trace the content of which offers the phantasy a point of contact—comes, as it were, half way to meet it. Once a point of contact of this kind has been found—in the present instance it was the deflowering, the taking away of the flowers—the remaining content of the fantasy is remodelled with the help of every legitimate intermediate idea—take the bread as an example—till it can find points of contact with the childhood scene. (Freud 1899a, 318)

Freud's defense of the genuineness of the childhood scene points to both the potentials within it for meeting the adult fantasy halfway, as well as to its resistance to being simply made over by the later fantasy. Certain details of the scene do not fit in with the logic of the fantasy: the participation of the boy cousin in the scene or the presence of the peasant woman and the nurse, while the hallucinatory intensity of the yellow flowers and the delicious taste of the bread signal the overdetermined presence of fantasmatic pleasure.

What is striking about this account is that, despite the parallel of the screen memory with the dream as a form of wish fulfillment, Freud's defense of the genuineness of the childhood scene actually *reverses* his model of the dream. With the latter he writes to Fliess, "A recent wish only leads to a dream if it . . . is a derivative of the prehistoric one or can get itself adopted by one" (March 10, 1898, Masson 1895a, 302). With the screen memory, the childhood scene is merely the delegate of the organizing fantasy that comes from the later period. Despite its genuineness, it is merely "raw material" that was "utilizable," otherwise "it would not have been possible for this particular memory, rather than any others, to make its way forward into consciousness" (1899a, 318). Freud's assumption here seems to be both that the childhood experience—all childhood experience?—is inscribed somewhere (in a vast internal *poste restante*) and that it contributes nothing in the way of meaning or wishful fantasy to the formation of the screen memory. To take his example of the point of contact, the taking of the flowers existed only as a brutally literal gesture waiting for its figurative meaning to be conferred on it in retrospect by its metaphorical assumption into the order of signifiers and symbolic acts by the adult fantasy. However, if it had no preexisting *personal* significance for the small flower thief, then why was it recorded at all and in the form of a scene and a narrative with its own *dramatis personae* in excess of the requirements of the colonizing adult fantasy, as Freud himself points out? For the scene to have been available for retranscription and rewriting in the way Freud describes, a prior process of selection would had to have taken place. In order for it to be organized and encoded in the form of a scene and a narrative, however partial and enigmatic, a prior selection would have been necessary, not just of *this scene* out of the countless other moments of the child's life but also of *these sensory elements*—the yellow of the flowers, the taste of the bread—out of the manifold of sensory data that constituted *this moment* of experience. By ignoring this prior selection and the reasons for it, Freud's defense of its genuineness takes place at the expense of its meaningfulness and its afterlife in the psychic life of the young boy, prior to any appropriation as useful raw material by later adult fantasy.

One of the puzzling things about the "Screen Memories" essay is the partial disconnection between the schematic model of the screen memory set out at the beginning, on the one hand, in which, as I have already remarked, the displacement from experience to screen takes place metonymically between two adjacent elements within a simultaneous ensemble, and, on the other, the single example Freud offers for extended analysis. In the former, there is no question of early and later moments as the memorial elements are contemporary with each other, while in the latter a temporal structure emerges whose problems we have been tracing throughout this chapter. Indeed, 'Freud'-the-analysand offers his memory precisely as an *exception* to the model of the incomplete 'torso'-memory formed by displacement from the emotionally significant to the insignificant but simultaneous elements of an experience, which Freud-the-theorist had set out at the beginning. He then subjects his memory to a metaphoric interpretation (by appeal to relations of likeness and analogy—the flowers and the bread)—rather than to a metonymic one (the substitution of insignificant for significant parts within a larger whole, which is what his initial schema would require).

What also distinguishes 'Freud's' exceptional screen memory is that the question of temporal structure returns again, a question that had been preoccupying him since at least 1894, with Miss Lucy R. and other cases in *Studies on Hysteria* (1895d). However, insofar as he does address the temporal structure of screen memories, he proposes a purely formal solution to its problems: there are *retrogressive* screen memories in which recent experiences are displaced backward and screened off by childhood scenes (as in the present example), and there are *progressive* screen memories in which the disturbing experience is displaced forward and screened off by a later scene. This categorization solves nothing, however, because it says nothing about the relations *between* these different moments and the forms of their interaction. It appears to accommodate both earlier and later moments as the impelling and organizing forces in the production of the 'memory,' but neither here nor in his return to the same topic soon after in Chapter 4 of *The Psychopathology of Everyday Life* (1901b) does Freud analyze the crucial case of the "progressive" or forward-displaced memory (even though he acknowledges that it is the most common form of screen memory). It is the progressive screen memory that would approximate more closely than the others to the structure of trauma and afterwardsness that had most concerned him throughout the 1890s. It is true that, with this reverse scenario of the retrogressive screen memory, Freud dramatizes in his clinical dialogue something of the memory–fantasy oscillation that had beset him, and he attempts to stabilize it through his defense of the genuineness of the childhood scene and its resistant particularity, but he does so only insofar as the childhood memory is entirely subordinated to the power of retrogressive fantasy. The *Standard Edition* editors of *The Psychopathology of Everyday Life* tell us that in Freud's copy he noted the remark of a colleague in the Vienna Psycho-Analytical Society that "fairy tales can be made use of as screen memories in the same way that empty shells are used as a home by the hermit crab."[13] In Freud's account the childhood scene of the lush green meadow and the "deflowering" of the little girl by Freud and his male cousin, with its happy ending of the delicious bread, is just such an empty shell, waiting inexplicably to be given meaning and force from outside it.

What is striking, given the immediate context of Freud's theoretical development in the 1890s as traced here and in the previous chapters, is the apparent *theoretical amnesia* that marks the "Screen Memories" essay with regard to the temporal dynamics of trauma and the *nachträglich* interplay between its scenes. The complex double logic of afterwardsness, involving both deferral and retrospection, has here fallen apart into two formally separate alternatives to each other: a progressive determination of later 'memories' by earlier (of which Freud offers no example) and the retrogressive rewriting of earlier scenes as screens for later fantasies. Jean Laplanche has argued that what had held these opposed temporal dimensions together was the problematic of seduction and the figure of the other—"the unforgettable, prehistoric other person who is never equalled by anyone later" (December 6, 1896), the "prime originator" (October 3, 1897)—and the traumatizing transmissions and implantations from that other that provoke and awaken the "germs of sexuality" in the infant.[14] Due to Freud's failure to move from a pathological model of abuse to a generalized model of *primal* seduction within the relations of care and nurture between adult and infant, the traumatizing figure of the other, and the other's sexuality, recedes. Consequently, the theory of a distinctively infantile sexuality as an innate, biologically determined developmental program is elaborated in the *Three Essays* of 1905, without any more than a passing reference to that fun-

13. *The Psychopathology of Everyday Life* (1901b), *SE* 6, 49.
14. Jean Laplanche, "Notes on Afterwardsness" (1999b), in *Essays on Otherness*: 260–65. So much has seduction been forgotten that when Freud proposes an interpretation of seduction for one of the screen memories given by the Henris, he treats it as a purely factual circumstance with no recourse to the model of trauma or the conceptual arsenal of the seduction theory, as if the previous five years had never happened!

damental relation to the other that had been so persistent an element of the seduction theory.

Freud's essay concludes with a generalization of the model of the screen memory to call into question the commonsense understanding of childhood memories in general. The latter holds "that they arise simultaneously with an experience as an immediate consequence of the impression it makes and that thereafter they recur from time to time." Freud appeals to a characteristic of many such early memories, that "the subject sees himself in the recollection as a child . . . he sees this child, however, as an observer from outside the scene would see him" (Freud 1899a, 321). This spectator's relation to the scene, and to the figure of himself within the scene, Freud argues, contradicts the view that the scene is the immediate return of the original experience, for "the subject was then in the middle of the situation and was attending not to himself but to the external world" (ibid.). The taking up of an outsider or a spectatorial position vis-à-vis the past scene and the consequent contrast between "the acting and the recollecting ego" (ibid.) both indicate the work of revision at a later stage.

This skepticism about the authenticity of apparently spontaneous early memories leads to the further claim that immediate or unprocessed registrations of (at least early) experience are simply not available to retrospective consciousness. The pervasive falsification of memories—the displacement of events into different scenes, the merging or substituting of persons involved, the condensation of different experiences into one scene, in fact, the whole arsenal of condensation and displacement that Freud had first analyzed in the dream-work (which might justify the analogous term 'memory-work')—is a sign of the tendentious operation of repression and defense at a later stage of development. Consequently, "the falsified memory is the first that we become aware of: the raw material of memory traces out of which it was forged remains unknown to us in its original form" (322). Paradoxically, this leads the essay on "Screen Memories" to call into question the very distinction it set out to introduce, between screen memories, those puzzlingly clear and vivid but indifferent or enigmatic memory fragments of no apparent significance, and the rest of our childhood memories, especially those whose significance seems obvious to us and unquestionable. "It may indeed be questioned whether we have any memories at all *from* our childhood: memories *relating to* our childhood may be all that we possess" (322). With this final emphasis on the spectatorial conscious-ness and distance of so many memories, and on the constructedness of all memory formations as the outcome of the 'memory-work,' Freud has come down strongly on the side of the later moments' power to appropriate and back project their fantasies and concerns into the 'empty shells' of infantile memories. The priority of the prehistoric as in the model of the dream is completely reversed in the model of the retrogressive screen memory. By contrast, the *progressive* screen memory, which serves to cover over and re-press the disturbing and compelling infantile experience for which it stands in, remains unanalyzed and unexplored.

It is clear that the predominance of the retrogressive dimension is what leads to this generalized skepticism, not only about the authenticity of childhood memories but also the very capacity of the early experience they encode to mobilize their own resources of longing and fantasy, to act as drivers for the formation of later fantasies and representations. Conse-quently, I want to develop the previous criticisms of the dominance of the retrogressive dimension in Freud's deployment of the model of the screen memory by interrogating further the materials of memory that 'Freud'-the-analysand has produced. This will bear not on the central scene itself, with its lush meadow, the children, the flowers, and the bread, but, rather, on the highly charged memories of early childhood and adolescence that provide a *mise-en-scène* of desire. They are part of the associations that 'Freud' provides centering on the rural scenes of his infancy and his adoles-cent return to them. These constitute a scenography in two scenes and three moments: the most recent replicates the earlier scene, which itself is the cherished product of a nostalgic, backward glance toward a lost child-hood paradise from which the subject has been expelled. Expulsion was followed by "long and difficult years" of which "nothing was worth remem-bering" (ibid., 312), and across this exile the memory of infancy beckons: "I was never free from a longing for the beautiful woods near our home, in which . . . I used to run off from my father, almost before I had learnt to walk" (313)—an enigmatic and unelaborated scene in which only the out-line of a family drama is detectable: "beautiful woods near our home"; flight from the father; the earliest years "almost before" the age of walking; a permanent element of longing from which he is "never free." There fol-lows a return to the childhood scenes at the emotionally volatile age of seventeen, the prosperity and comfort of the old family friends with whom he is staying, whose fifteen-year-old daughter he promptly falls in love with. His "first calf love," he tells us. But this is also a repetition for which she is the occasion and agent provocateur (to use Charcot's metaphor, for she disappears soon afterward), and it is precisely her absence as much as her presence that "brought my longings to a really high pitch" (ibid.). The repetition of an old love is indicated quite clearly by the return to the *mise-en-scène* of his early longing: "I passed many hours in solitary walks through the lovely woods that I had found once more and spent my time building castles in the air" (ibid.). His adolescent fantasies, however, bear not on the future but on rewriting the past, an alternative past that would have happened had his father not finally succeeded in separating him from "the beautiful woods" and all that they enigmatically represent. The young girl–lovely woods connection seems to represent a new edition of a childhood fantasy, which might help explain why she lent herself to being represented by another childhood scene, of the meadow and the flowers. The fantasies are only sketched in outline—the connections between the fifteen-year-old daughter of the house, his three-year-old cousin, and the beautiful woods, apart from the color yellow, is not spelled out. What one can say, however, is that if his adolescent calf love is the driver of the deflowering scene, then his exiled longing for the beautiful woods and before that his original running away to them from his father are the drivers of that adolescent passion. The theoretical implications of this might be that the very availability of an infantile scene to the colonizing tendencies of later experience and the selective processes that led to its preservation, like the formation of the dream, are the result of the presence of early, unfulfilled wishes, fantasies, losses—'longings' seeking representation and ready for reactivation and retranslation. The very condition of possibility for the formation of a retrogressive screen memory, and its reverse side, would be such an unrecognized *nachträglich* repetition.

With Freud's generalized skepticism about the claims of memory, combined with the missing figure of the unanalyzed progressive screen memory, we are a long way from that other form of scenic reproduction with which this book began. The scenography of conscious memory and its critique, elaborated in 1899, pays a finely grained attention to the scenic organization and details of conscious memory. However, the very grounds of its critique of the naïve claims of memory indicate that the object of this scenography is a very different one from, for example, the compulsive repetition of the hysterical attack, with its decentering of the retrospective and recollecting ego that watches itself as actor in the screen memory. It is this adult ego that then fails to recognize as *its* memory the 'scenes of passionate movement' into which it is violently conscripted in the hysterical attack (or, as we shall later see, in the analytic transference). This is the action of a scene in the present that the ego cannot recollect but that seizes it, not in a transparent moment of revelation (beloved of the flashback melodrama, such as Hitchcock's notoriously 'Freudian' *Marnie*) but through a variety of *screens*—hysteria's auxiliary scenes, the day's residues of the dream, the analytic situation itself—that are as epistemologically unreliable as they are psychically compelling. As against the commonsense understanding of memory—"my memory *now* of that event *then*"—or the spectatorial structure of the screen memory—"I *now* see myself as I was *then*"—we have what still eludes Freud's metapsychology at the end of the 1890s and continues to disappoint and haunt his clinical practice: "a scene is being replayed through me, a scene remembers me, but it's not *my* scene, *I* don't recall it."

## FIVE

## The Scenography of Trauma: Oedipus as Tragedy and Complex

"If Freud is his own Copernicus, he is also his own Ptolemy."
—JEAN LAPLANCHE[1]

Jean Laplanche's terse but suggestive epigram summarizes an insight that has directed his systematic and critical archaeology of the Freudian conceptual field and the contradictory dynamics that have shaped it. It picks up on Freud's identification with the Copernican revolution as a paradigm of scientific thought and his alignment of psychoanalysis with the discoveries of both Copernicus and Darwin, as the third in a series of three major blows to human narcissism dealt by modern science.[2] Where Copernicus's heliocentrism had opened up the possibility beyond our solar system of an infinite universe without a single center, thus decentering the old geocentric Ptolemaic synthesis that positioned the earth as the central point around which the sun, moon, and stars moved, Darwin's theory of evolution

1. Jean Laplanche, "The Unfinished Copernican Revolution," in *Essays on Otherness*, ed. John Fletcher (London: Routledge, 1999), 60.
2. Sigmund Freud, "A Difficulty in the Path of Psycho-Analysis" (1917a), *SE* 17.

had decentered 'Man' in relation to the animal world, challenging traditional creationist myths of human origins. By analogy Freud saw the postulation of both the unconscious and the sexual drives by psychoanalysis as a decentering of the human subject in relation to himself, a recognition that *"the ego is not master in its own house"* (Freud 1917a, 143).

Laplanche rewrites Freud's analogy between the Copernican and psychoanalytic revolutions to foreground the contrary gravitational pulls at work on the Freudian field, especially in its foundational moment of crisis in 1897, which we have considered in Chapters 3 and 4, in which Freud elaborates and then abandons a theory of traumatic seduction for the first elements of a theory of infantile sexuality that was to come to fruition in the *Three Essays on the Theory of Sexuality* (1905d). Freud moved in the middle to late 1890s away from a trauma-based theory of psychopathology (primarily hysteria and obsessional neurosis) toward a drive-based theory of infantile sexuality in general, in which neurosis is but one of its vicissitudes and the Oedipus complex its major form. This is conventionally hailed as the establishment of psychoanalysis proper.[3] Laplanche has argued that despite the great gains made with the theory of infantile sexuality and of the drives, crucial elements had, however, been lost. In particular, what Freud encountered but failed to recognize as such, in the restricted and grotesque form of the pathological cases of infantile sexual abuse with which he worked, was the universal role of the adult other, with an unconscious and a fully formed sexuality, in the formation of an infantile subjectivity as yet lacking in both.[4] With the abandonment of the seduction theory this other-centered, 'Copernican' dimension is replaced by a 'Ptolemaic' movement of

3. For an orthodox critique and dismissal of Freud's seduction theory, see K. R. Eissler, *Freud and the Seduction Theory: A Brief Love Affair* (New York: International Universities Press, 2001). For a more thoughtful critique, see Jean G. Schimek, "Fact and Fantasy in the Seduction Theory: A Historical Review," *Journal of the American Psychoanalytic Association* 35 (1987): 937–65.

4. For Laplanche's theory of primal seduction as constituting the fundamental anthropological situation of the human being, see *New Foundations for Psychoanalysis* (1987), trans. David Macey (Oxford: Basil Blackwell, 1989): esp. Chapter 3, 89–151; *Essays on Otherness*: esp. 52–196, 260–65; Jacqueline Lanouzière, "Breast-feeding as Original Seduction and Primal Scene of Seduction" *New Formations* 48 (Winter 2002–3): 52–68. Dominique Scarfone, "'It was *not* my mother': From Seduction to Negation," *New Formations* 48 (Winter 2002–3): 69–76.

recentering on the subject, in which, according to Freud, the infant becomes the subject of his own developmental progression through the endogenously determined series of oral, anal, phallic, and genital stages. However, Laplanche proposes that "in Freud, one should speak, at almost every period, of an alternation between relapses into Ptolemaism and resurgences of the Copernican, other-centred vision."[5]

## Trauma and Its Scenes

In Freud's theory of traumatic seduction, as we have seen, there is a primacy of the other, a figure whom Freud called in a letter to Fliess "the prehistoric, unforgettable, other person who is never equalled by anyone later" (December 6, 1896).[6] This seductive and traumatizing other, as we have seen in previous chapters, is registered in a series of scenes marked by a distinctive temporal logic, which Freud wrestled with under the name *Nachträglichkeit* and its adjectival and adverbial cognates. Strachey's translation of it in the *Standard Edition* as 'deferred action' entailed a considerable narrowing of meaning, a reduction to a progressive linear movement in time, while Laplanche's more literal translation as 'afterwardsness' attempts to capture its double temporal dimension of progression and regression (an absolutely literal transposition of the German would be 'carrying-afterness'; the French translation is *après coup*).[7] Freud's grasp of it developed rapidly in the period 1895–97, as elaborated in Chapters 3 and 4, as the model of traumatic hysteria he inherited from Charcot was transformed by the difficulties of his clinical practice. As Laplanche and Pontalis point out, the word 'trauma' comes from the Greek word for wound, which itself derives from the verb 'to pierce.' In medicine it generally refers to the breaking of the skin surface due to external violence and its aftereffects on the organism as a whole. "In adopting the term, psychoanalysis carries the three ideas implicit in it over on to the psychical level: the idea of a violent

5. Laplanche, "The Unfinished Copernican Revolution," in *Essays on Otherness*, 60.
6. *The Complete Letters of Sigmund Freud to Wilhelm Fliess 1887–1904*, trans. and ed. Jeffrey Moussaieff Masson (Cambridge, Mass.: Harvard University Press, 1985), 213.
7. Jean Laplanche, "Notes on Afterwardsness," in *Essays on Otherness*, ed. John Fletcher (London: Routledge, 1999): 260–65.

shock, the idea of a wound and the idea of consequences affecting the whole organization."[8] A relatively simple cause-effect model in the "Preliminary Communication" (1893a), which traced each hysterical symptom back to the repressed memory of a traumatic event, gives way in the course of writing *Studies on Hysteria* (1895d) and the unpublished "Project for a Scientific Psychology" (1950a, [1895]) to a more complex temporal structure in which the initial traumatic scene is supplemented by a series of later auxiliary scenes that orchestrate the production of symptoms. In this account, as we have seen, it takes at least two scenes to make a trauma and the time lag between them (rather than being simply the overwhelming impact of a single event). The configuration of later scenes rhymes with the early traumatic scene, acting selectively back on certain features of the earlier scene that have remained unassimilated and unprocessed. What had been inscribed or deposited as excessive and unassimilable in a first scene is traumatically repeated, repressed and symptomatically symbolized, or revived and translated into the terms of a new scene and stage of development.

As we have seen in the cases of Katharina and Miss Lucy R. in *Studies on Hysteria* and of Emma in the "Project," the hysterical symptoms are then understood as the overdetermined end result of a palimpsestic superimposition of scenes. Freud formulated a stratified scenography of trauma in which the earlier scene, rather than acting "like an *agent provocateur* in releasing the symptom, which thereafter leads an independent existence . . . acts like a foreign body which long after its entry must continue to be regarded as an agent that is still at work" (1895d, 6). The figure of the agent provocateur was one of Charcot's favorite metaphors to indicate the merely secondary role of experiences of shock or trauma in precipitating an inherited predisposition to hysteria. Freud broke from Charcot's hereditarian framework, in which the traumatic event or accident had merely a mechanical and extrinsic connection to a symptom that is sustained by a hysterical constitution. He proposed instead a mode of direct causation in which the memory traces and associated excitations of the traumatic event continue to work in the present like a still-potent foreign body. We have

8. Jean Laplanche and J.-B. Pontalis, *The Language of Psychoanalysis* (1967) (London: The Hogarth Press, 1973), 465.

seen this action of past traumatic scenes coming alive again in the present moment in the report to Fliess, with which this book begins, in which Freud writes of an early scene of infantile seduction, traced back from an adult hysterical attack of "epileptiform convulsions": "I could hear again the words that were exchanged between two adults at that time! It is as though it comes from a phonograph" (Masson 1985a, 226).

In this exogenous model of trauma, an excitation that has been brought from the outside by the intrusive actions of the adult other breaches the boundaries and defenses of the infant or child subject. It remains unassimilable, an alien or foreign body in the first moment of its inscription, waiting to be revived and translated into the 'language' of later moments. It is in these later moments that either repression with the production of hysterical or obsessional symptoms takes place, or a relatively (always partial) successful binding and articulation of the original excessive and wounding inscription. Laplanche's critique of Freud's model of trauma argues that he failed to move beyond the instances of sexual abuse and its pathological aftereffects to a general model of *primal* seduction, which he had encountered in its extreme and pathological form but failed to recognize as such. What is at stake in Freud's other-centered theory of traumatic seduction is the infant's encounter with the unconscious and sexuality of the adult other, transmitted in the form of enigmatic signifiers, messages in verbal or nonverbal form, which are implanted through the ordinary ministrations of child care and nurture. It is this seductive but 'wounding' encounter with the enigmatic desire of the other, on whom the subject depends, that is lost in Freud's so-called abandonment of the seduction theory and in his move to a general theory of infantile sexuality in which the subject is recentered on his own spontaneous, endogenous sexual development.

*Oedipal Tragedies and 'Ptolemaic' Readings*

On September 21, 1897, Freud wrote to Wilhelm Fliess his letter of repudiation of his seduction theory, citing four reasons for his change of mind, which we have looked at in detail in Chapter 4. The repudiation was temporary, for within two weeks in the letters of October 3 and 4 Freud pursues the analysis of two of his own dreams as part of his self-analysis, in which he locates the "prime originator" of his own hysteria in the figure of his nurse: "She was my teacher in sexual matters" (Masson 1985a, 269). He affirms his conviction that the coming to light of "the scenes themselves" will lead to the therapeutic resolution of his hysteria. However, in the letter of October 15, Freud first formulated the germ of what he was only later in 1910 to call the "Oedipus complex,"[9] and which was to emerge as the replacement for the seduction theory:

> A single idea of general value dawned on me. I have found, in my own case too, [the phenomenon of] being in love with my mother and jealous of my father, and I now consider it a universal event in early childhood. . . . If this is so we can understand the gripping power of *Oedipus Rex* . . . the Greek legend seizes upon a compulsion which everyone recognizes because he senses its existence in himself. Everyone in the audience was once a budding Oedipus in fantasy and each recoils in horror from the dream fulfilment here transplanted into reality. (Masson 1985a, 272)

Here Freud sets up a relation between each former "budding Oedipus" in the audience, on the one hand, and both the Oedipus of legend and the Oedipus who walks the tragic stage, on the other. The latter two figures, the legendary Oedipus and the tragic Oedipus, are assumed by Freud to be identical (although they are not) because the ancient legend, he claims, seizes on the universal compulsion "which everyone recognizes because he senses its existence within himself." The play gives expression to this compulsion in the form of a "dream fulfilment here transplanted into reality." In a more elaborated reading of *Oedipus* three years later in *The Interpretation of Dreams*, Freud states: "King Oedipus . . . merely shows us the fulfilment of our own childhood wishes" (1900a, 262).

Freud also makes a parallel case about Shakespeare's *Hamlet*, that other great tragedy which, according to Freud, "has its roots in the same soil as *Oedipus Rex*," the soil of "primaeval dream-material" (ibid., 263). At first glance, a parallel between Hamlet and Orestes, the son bound to revenge the murder of his father Agamemnon by his mother Clytemnestra and her lover Aegisthus in Aeschylus's *Oresteia*, might seem the more appro-

9. Sigmund Freud, "A Special Type of Choice of Object Made by Men (Contributions to the Psychology of Love I)" (1910h), *SE* 11, 171.

priate comparison. However, despite their surface differences, there is a striking structural parallel between *Oedipus* and *Hamlet*. In both Sophocles' and Shakespeare's tragedies the definitive tragic crime, the killing of the King, has already happened and the drama constitutes a kind of post-tragic aftermath in which after effects and post traumatic repetitions occur. Hamlet like Oedipus is commissioned by a supernatural agent (his father's ghost, the Delphic Oracle) to bring to light and to redress a past traumatic event (the murder of the King, the father of each protagonist), and to bring to justice a criminal who turns out to be the reigning King (Claudius, Oedipus himself). In both cases, though differently, this involves the figure of an incestuously compromised Queen (Gertrude, Jocasta).

Despite the absence of a literal acting out and fulfillment of oedipal wishes in *Hamlet*, Freud claims that Hamlet's inability to take revenge on his uncle Claudius for his father's murder is due to the fact that Claudius is "the man who did away with his father and took that father's place with his mother, the man who shows him the repressed wishes of his own childhood realized" (265). The actions of the two tragedies, then, perform a similar but far from identical 'showing': where King Oedipus's actions show the post-oedipal subjects in the audience the "fulfilment of our own childhood wishes," Claudius's actions show Hamlet "the repressed wishes of his own childhood realized." The former "budding Oedipus" here is not so much in the audience of *Hamlet* as onstage in the person of the Prince. It is Hamlet the Prince, like the audience of Sophocles's play but not his own, who is imagined by Freud as the oedipal spectator watching the fulfillment by proxy of his now repressed infantile wishes.

However, the actions that perform this theatrical showing are different in each play, just as the relation of the play's actions to the wishes they are supposed to realize or fulfill is different in each case. In each play there is a *dislocation* between the oedipal wishes and their supposed realization, just as there is in each tragedy a different arrangement of the relations of action, showing, and watching. The 'oedipality,' so to speak, of each play's action is to be located differently. In Sophocles's play it resides in the objective character of the actions, for the protagonist does indeed kill his father and sleep with his mother. However, Oedipus, as the play makes clear, performed these actions unwittingly and against his will, and the play insists on this dislocation between the protagonist's conscious wish or will and the actions he turns out to have already performed. As the Chorus tell Oedipus: "Time, all-seeing, surprised you living an unwilled life" (l. 1213).[10] Critics opposed to Freud's reading of Sophocles have argued that because of this dislocation Oedipus cannot be said to have an 'Oedipus complex' in Freud's sense, that the play gives us, in Jean-Pierre Vernant's words, "Oedipus without the complex."[11] In an eloquent response to such a position, Jean Starobinski has argued that "Oedipus has no unconscious because he is our unconscious . . . one of the principal roles assumed by desire. He does not need any depth of his own because he is our depth. . . . To attribute a psychology to him would be foolish: he is already an instantiation of psychology. Far from being a possible object of psychological study, he has become a functional element in the creation of a psychological science. . . . In modern terms, Oedipus is instinct or, rather, its figurative counterpart."[12] Following Freud, Starobinski contrasts Oedipus with a Hamlet, "who has the three-dimensional character of a living person rather than the opaque, residueless plenitude of a psychic image" (Starobinski 1989, 160).

Now it is certainly true that Hamlet's presence in his play is characterized by the posture of a publicly proclaimed inwardness:

'Seems,', madam? Nay, it is, I know not 'seems.'
'Tis not alone my inky cloak, good mother,
Nor customary suits of solemn black,
Nor windy suspiration of forced breath,
No, nor the fruitful river in the eye,
Nor the dejected 'haviour of the visage,
Together with all forms, moods, shapes of grief,
That can denote me truly. These indeed 'seem';
For they are actions that a man might play,

10. Sophocles, *Oedipus the King: A Translation with Commentary*, trans. Thomas Gould (Englewood Cliffs, N.J.: Prentice Hall, 1970). All quotations from the play are taken from this edition.

11. Jean-Pierre Vernant, "Oedipus without the Complex," in *Myth and Tragedy in Ancient Greece*, ed. J.-P. Vernant and P. Vidal-Nacquet, trans. Janet Lloyd (Cambridge, Mass.: M.I.T. Press, 1988): 85–111.

12. Jean Starobinski, "Hamlet and Oedipus," in *The Living Eye*, trans. Arthur Goldhammer (Cambridge, Mass.: Harvard University Press, 1989), 156, 160.

But I have that within which passes show—
These but the trappings and the suits of woe.

(1.2. 76–86.)[13]

Hamlet's famous manifesto of interiority proclaims an inwardness "that passes show," but an inwardness that is at once proclaimed and withheld in the same gesture, just as he later rebuffs the clumsy probings of Rosencrantz and Guildenstern: "Why, look you now, how unworthy a thing you make of me. . . . Look you now, you would pluck out the heart of my mystery" (III. ii. 371–74). While it is indeed true that Sophocles's Oedipus does not exhibit Hamlet's self-conscious subjectivity, nevertheless I remain unpersuaded by Starobinski's response, for like Freud he seems to conflate the mythic or legendary Oedipus, who might well be seen as a figure for the trajectory of an impulse or a drive, with the tragic Oedipus, who has the layered nature of a palimpsest or an archaeological site (to use a favorite Freudian metaphor), a kind of depth therefore, but not a depth that can be enfolded into the circle of a single consciousness or lonely subjectivity.

In an almost geometrical antithesis to Sophocles's play, the 'oedipality' of the action in *Hamlet* does not reside in the objective character of the actions of regicide and incest, for after all, while Claudius is the murderer of the King, the King is his brother not his father, and while he marries the Queen, she is his sister-in-law not his mother. Nothing oedipal here, you might think, except in the eye of Hamlet the beholder. His is the one subject-position from which Claudius's actions can be responded to oedipally. It is only because the murdered Hamlet senior is Hamlet's father and the adulterous Gertrude is his mother that Claudius's actions might plausibly be claimed to resonate with Hamlet's repressed oedipal wishes. For the rest of us in the audience, our withers are unwrung. So there is a good reason Freud should invoke the protagonist rather than the audience of *Hamlet* as a former budding Oedipus, who is now interpellated by proxy through Claudius's actions.

In each play the psychodynamics of showing and seeing are different. Freud observes that the "child's wishful phantasy" in Sophocles's play is

---

13. William Shakespeare, *The Tragedy of Hamlet, Prince of Denmark* (1600), ed. T. J. B. Spencer (London: Penguin Books, 2005).

"brought into the open and realized as it would be in a dream," while in *Hamlet* "it remains repressed . . . we only learn of its existence from its inhibiting consequences" (1900a, 264). Freud's dream analogy, however, has its complications, not least because in Freud's model of the dream, with its distinction between latent dream-thoughts and manifest dream-scene, the fundamental wishful fantasy is only ever acted out by proxy or in disguise (at least for the post-oedipal subject). In Freud's account of *Hamlet* the oedipal fantasy is not realized in the actions onstage or in the events leading to the play's action but exists only in Hamlet's inferred unconscious mind, underlying his response to those actions and events. It is to be inferred from Hamlet's inhibition, expressed in his famous delay in killing Claudius, even when given the perfect opportunity to do so in the prayer scene, where the unguarded Claudius is unable to pray, and from what Freud calls his hysterical repudiation of his sexual feelings for Ophelia (though surprisingly Freud has nothing to say about his feelings for his mother). Freud forgets, perhaps, the play within the play, *The Murder of Gonzago*, which Hamlet himself stages, where the scene of oedipal usurpation is presented in thin disguise between a murderous nephew, Lucianus, and a murdered uncle, the Player-King, thus explicitly inscribing Hamlet himself as revenging nephew within the scene. It also repeats Claudius's fratricidal act of poisoning through the ear (the murdered King thus taking on the composite character of uncle, brother, and father). A similar argument can be made about the player's performance of the speech about Pyrrhus's killing of the aged King Priam of Troy and the grief of Queen Hecuba. The *singularity* of Hamlet's oedipal response to Claudius's actions, and its indirect or repressed presence in the play, has meant that, hitherto, Freud suggests, no one has been able to solve the mystery of Hamlet's psychology and his unaccountable delay. Claudius's actions of murdering his brother and marrying his sister-in-law do not represent the realization of his repressed infantile wishes to the hypothetically male spectator of *Hamlet* but only to Hamlet himself, who is the one person whose parents are the objects of Claudius's actions. The spectator's repressed oedipal wishes find representation, if at all, only in the figure of Hamlet, and there only negatively and indirectly, in his inhibition and delay in the killing of his father's killer and his mother's new husband, in his obsessive hatred for the latter, and in his denunciation of women's sexuality in the figures of his mother and Ophelia.

By contrast with *Hamlet*, Freud argues, with *Oedipus* the parricidal and incestuous fantasy is "brought into the open and realized" (1900a, 264). We have in the Greek play not a negative and indirect but a positive and direct representation of parricide and incest. However, this simple contrast of the two plays, between the indirect, repressed "more modern tragedy" (ibid.) and the "open and realized" fantasy of the ancient tragedy, ignores what I have called the *dislocation* between wish and its fulfillment in *Oedipus*, between the wishful protagonist and the action that shows us, the audience, "the fulfilment of our own childhood wishes" (ibid., 262) but not Oedipus his. For fleeing from Polybus and Merope, his adoptive parents, and from Corinth, his home city, upon receiving the Delphic Oracle's prophecy of his fate, Oedipus seeks desperately to avoid the transgressions it predicts. In fleeing the Oracle's predictions he meets a man who attacks him and whom he only then kills. On triumphing over the Sphinx, he is offered the kingship of Thebes and the hand of its widowed queen in marriage, which he only then accepts. The man he has killed turns out to have been the father he has never known and the woman he has married his unknown mother, but Oedipus himself is strangely absent from both these actions of which he is the ostensible protagonist. In the gap created by this dislocation between protagonist and the tragic actions, he turns out, only in retrospect, to have performed, the question of the Oracle insists with its brutal announcement in advance of Oedipus's fate.

In both his epistolary first thoughts sent to Fliess in 1897 and his later published account, Freud is concerned to displace the question of the Oracle and to dispute the play's status as a tragedy of fate or destiny. Its tragic power to move a modern audience is not to be explained, he argues, by the traditional contrast of the will of the gods or destiny and the struggle of the human protagonists to escape their fate but, rather, by "the particular nature of the material on which the contrast is exemplified" (ibid.). It is the material of parricide and incest, not their oracular form as a fate desperately resisted by the protagonist, which is crucial for Freud. Modern attempts to imitate the Greek tragedy of destiny have not worked, Freud argued, because we reject any "arbitrary individual compulsion," such as that contrived by Grillparzer in *Die Ahnfrau*, which turns instead on brother-sister incest. Oedipus's destiny "moves us because it might have been ours—because the Oracle laid the same curse upon us before our birth as upon him. It is the fate of all of us" (ibid.). The nature of this secular fate is further indicated as Freud develops his conception of Oedipus as everyman: "Like Oedipus, we live in ignorance of these wishes repugnant to morality, which have been forced on us by Nature" (ibid., 263). This ignorance, Oedipus's and ours as audience, Freud argues, in a return to Sophocles's tragedy in 1938 at the end of his life, "is a legitimate representation of the unconscious state into which, for adults, the whole experience has fallen."[14]

The reverse side of Oedipus's ignorance of what he has done is the foreknowledge of the Oracle of Apollo at Delphi, and its double warning of his fate, first to his father, Laius, before his birth, and later to Oedipus himself. Freud's reading performs a translation or reduction of the Oracle and its prophetic function: "The coercive power of the Oracle, which makes or should make the hero innocent, is a recognition of the inevitability of the fate which has condemned every son to live through the Oedipus complex" (ibid., 192). In an earlier retrospect, in 1924, Freud had commented, "Fate and the Oracle were no more than materialisations of an internal necessity."[15]

So an "internal necessity" with the inevitability of fate, one "forced on us by Nature," is what Freud translates Apollo's Oracle into. This reversal of an external agency, the Oracle, into an internal necessity, as merely the projection outward of that necessity, exactly repeats the logic that had characterized Freud's thinking in the moment of crisis and transition in 1897 in which *Oedipus*, as both tragedy and complex, had become the object of his thought. It is in the immediate wake of Freud's famous abandonment of the theory of traumatic seduction that he turns to the theme of *Oedipus*. The letter to Fliess, in which he announces his discovery of being in love with the mother and jealous of the father as "a universal event in early childhood," was written only three weeks after his previous announcement to Fliess of his repudiation of the paradigm of paternal seduction. In the earlier letter of September 21, 1897, the letter of the equinox, as Laplanche calls it, Freud had argued that, because "there are no indications of reality in the unconscious," one cannot distinguish "between truth and fiction cathected with affect." As a result, there is no way of telling whether the scenes reproduced in the analytic treatment are in fact memories, bearing the record of the

---

14. Sigmund Freud, *An Outline of Psycho-Analysis* (1940a), *SE* 23, 191–92.
15. Sigmund Freud, *Autobiographical Study* (1925d), *SE* 20, 63.

real event of seduction, as "there would always remain the solution that the sexual fantasy invariably seizes upon the theme of the parents" (Masson 1985a, 264–65). Freud presents here a choice between truth and "fiction cathected with affect," an opposition that has unfortunately dominated and misled the subsequent discussion, and especially the contemporary controversy over the seduction theory and the question of recovered memory.

However, the truth/fiction binary obscures a number of important issues. First, far from their being opposed alternatives, Freud had already assigned an increasingly important role to fantasy in the more complex late developments of his theory of traumatic seduction, where it functions as a 'psychic facade' that is meant to manage and process, through the work of condensation and displacement, the distressing affects and memories of traumatic primal scenes, as the letters to Fliess testify;[16] second, Freud's replacement theory of infantile sexuality, elaborated in the *Three Essays on the Theory of Sexuality* (1905d), grounded oedipal wishes precisely *in reality*, not in the reality of the event of seduction but in the reality of a biologically based, endogenous sexuality, unfolding through pregiven stages, as its inevitable expression (whereas fantasy as a concept virtually drops out of the *Three Essays*); third, and most pertinent for us, is that the misleading opposition between truth and fiction obscures a more fundamental shift in Freud's thought. This is a fundamental shift *away from* memory as the scene of the other's seductive and/or traumatizing intervention, an intervention by "the prehistoric, unforgettable, other person who is never equaled by anyone later" (December 6, 1896; Masson 1985a, 213), whom Freud had called, in the case of his own self-analysis, "the prime originator" (October 3, 1897; ibid., 268). Although he invokes fantasy as an alternative explanation to the real event of seduction, it is fantasy inevitably seizing on the theme of the parents but doing so as the expression of an "internal necessity," an endogenously unfolding psycho-biological reality, a "universal event" that is "forced on us by Nature." In this latter binary opposition of fantasy and the real event, the agency of the other is foreclosed,

---

16. In fact, the term 'primal scene' (*Urszene*), unlike its later narrow usage to refer to the scene of parental intercourse, is first formulated in this context to designate the originary moment of an excessive implantation or inscription regardless of the protagonists involved. For the role of fantasy, see Drafts L, M, and N, all written in May 1897 (Masson 1985a, 239–52) and discussed previously in Chapter 4.

while parental figures are reduced to being merely objects or projections of the fantasist's own wishes. In this movement of Freud's thought we have what Laplanche has called Freud's fundamental *fourvoiement*, or going astray, a movement from a Copernican, other-centered, exogenous model of traumatic seduction (albeit one confined to actual sexual abuse and its pathological aftereffects) to a generalized Ptolemaic model of endogenous development, that is, a recentering of the human subject as the protagonist of his own developmental *Bildungsroman*.

This foreclosure of the figure of the seductive and traumatizing other in Freud's metapsychology repeats itself in his interpretation of Sophocles's *Oedipus* in which Apollo and the Delphic Oracle are treated merely as materializations of Oedipus's own wishes and their inevitability. However, as we have seen, the action of Sophocles's play, its dramatic shape, cannot be described simply as the expression or fulfillment of Oedipus's wish, whether immediately or in delayed form. Indeed, Freud himself had described the play's action, with its "cunning delays and ever-mounting excitement," as "a process that can be likened to the work of a psycho-analysis," precisely because it reveals Oedipus as the author of actions that have already taken place in the past, before the play begins (1900a, 261–62). The action of the play takes the form not of a realization or fulfillment of wishes in the future but of an uncovering of past scenes and of Oedipus's implication in them. In particular, the scene at the forefront of the play's investigation is the murder of the former King Laius, for the identification of the regicide is a priority set by Apollo's Oracle for Oedipus as King of a devastated Thebes, when he sends to Delphi for advice and help over the plague that is destroying the city.

### Sophocles's Scenic Palimpsest

The killing of Laius is located within a specific place and scene, in the land of Phocis, *at a place where three roads meet.* Jocasta's first description of this bare but resonant topography provokes in Oedipus an intense response— "what a profound distraction has seized my mind" (l. 727)—a response that immediately alerts him to the possibility of his own implication in the scene acted there: "O, Zeus, what have you willed to do to me?" (l. 738), he cries out in reaction to Jocasta's summary narrative. The place where three roads meet is returned to in the play on a number of occasions, both before and after it is identified as the place of parricide. Gradually it is twinned with another scene, that of Oedipus's encounter with Jocasta in the marital bed. This scene is also revisited, both in lyrical evocations and finally in action, as Jocasta, crying out to her long-dead husband, Laius, locks herself in her bedchamber to kill herself and Oedipus breaks in to seek her there. It is in his return to the marital chamber, now conscious of his past actions and where he once again encounters the body of Jocasta, that Oedipus completes the tragedy's sequence of traumatic scenes, by blinding himself with the golden brooches taken from his wife-mother's dress.

This sequence of traumatic scenes, which rhyme with, pick up, and answer one another, has been the object of an illuminating commentary by the classical scholar Thomas Gould in his translation of *Oedipus the King*. Gould spells out the connections that are woven between these traumatic scenes by the play's poetic language. Following in Gould's footsteps, Cynthia Chase has invoked both Freud's model of trauma, as well as Laplanche's commentary on it, as a way of mapping the traumatic model of sexuality onto the textuality of Sophocles's play.[17] Chase's argument leads to a number of suggestive and striking formulations, but it also conflates different and antithetical moments in Freud's thinking of sexuality and his reading of *Oedipus*. In contrast with Chase, I have positioned Freud's reading of *Oedipus* at a particular turning point in his thought, at which, to invoke again Laplanche's recent distinction, a new Ptolemaic theory of an endogenous infantile sexuality is exemplified in an equally Ptolemaic reading of *Oedipus*. Freud's first formulation of what was later to become the 'Oedipus complex' functions not *in conjunction with*—as Chase would have it—but precisely *as a replacement of* the Copernican other-centered model of trauma, and its associated concepts in the form of the seduction theory. Furthermore, this foreclosure of the other has its effects precisely in Freud's erasure of the *daimonic* dimension of the Oracle, and the reduction of its pattern of agency, that binds the traumatic sequence of scenes into a compelling, indeed compulsive, unity.

17. Cynthia Chase, "Oedipal Textuality: Reading Freud's Reading of *Oedipus*," in *Psychoanalytic Literary Criticism*, ed. Maud Ellmann (London: Longman, 1994): 56–75.

As we have seen, Freud's 'oedipal' reading of *Oedipus* takes the protagonist's ignorance of what he has done as merely the figurative representation of the unconscious nature of his wishes to perform precisely those actions of parricide and incest, and Freud's Ptolemaic reading of the Oracle's prophecy takes it as merely the "materialisation of an internal necessity" (Freud 1925d, 63). However, a return to Freud's repudiated problematic of seduction and its scenography of trauma, in light of Laplanche's reformulation of its Copernican other-centered potential, will help us recapture the foreclosed dimension of otherness in Sophocles's tragedy, in both its forms, the parental (Laius and Jocasta) and the numinous-*daimonic* (Apollo and the Delphic Oracle). Chase suggests a homology between the two-scene model of trauma in the case of Emma from "Project for a Scientific Psychology" and the structure of *Oedipus*. The 'Phocal crime,' the murder of Laius at Phocis, constitutes the first 'primal scene' and the play's present scene of investigation the *second* scene. She later revises this to expand the first scene to include the entire oedipal drama that precedes the play's action, while the second scene includes all that is represented on the stage in the present time of the drama (Chase 1994, 62, 64), so Scene I, Oedipus's past actions, Scene II, Oedipus's current investigation of the killing of Laius in the present time of the play. This seems to me rather too formulaic in its neatness, deploying the two-scene model of deferred action or afterwardsness without the alterity, the relation to the other that Laplanche's revisionary critique of Freud has located in it. For the play's presenting symptom, as it were, the traumatic crisis whose eruption provokes the opening scene of civic emergency, in the present time of the play and its subsequent investigative action, is the plague that smites the city of Thebes: the city "dies in the fruitful flowers of the soil, / . . . in its pastured herds, and in its women's / barren pangs" (ll. 25–27). This curse on the city's fertility constitutes the present emergency that motivates the turn to the past, and it is presented as the result of precisely the daimonic activity that Freud's Ptolemaic reading forecloses: "The fire-bearing god [*daimon*] has swooped upon the city, hateful plague" (ll. 27–28).

The Delphic Oracle's recommended cure for the plague is for the city to take up again the interrupted search for the killer of Laius, long since abandoned due to the visitation of the Sphinx and the drama of Oedipus's triumph over her. King Oedipus's investigation, thus directed, takes as its prescribed target the killing of his predecessor, King Laius, at Phocis, the place where three roads meet. Rather than being a hidden 'primal' scene, as Chase suggests, the Phocal scene in its first manifestation in the play is the most recent, uppermost scenic layer of the memorial palimpsest that confronts Oedipus. His rehearsal for Jocasta of his memory of the events enacted there fills out her bare secondhand report of the killing of Laius with the drama of a murderous encounter, an encounter that condenses many of the play's other traumatic scenes. Oedipus's narration presents him as arriving at the "exact location" in what is virtually a single movement of rebound from Apollo's prophecy:

> But Phoebus sent me away
> dishonouring my demand. Instead, other
> wretched horrors he flashed forth in speech.
> He said I would be my mother's lover,
> show offspring to mankind they could not look at,
> and be his murderer whose seed I am.
> When I heard this, and ever since, I gauged
> the way to Corinth by the stars alone,
> running to a place where I could never see
> the disgrace in the Oracle's words come true.
> But I soon came to the exact location
> where as you tell of it the king was killed.
> Lady, here is the truth. As I went on,
> when I was just approaching those three roads,
> a herald and a man like him you spoke of
> came on, riding a carriage drawn by colts.
> Both the man out front and the old man himself
> tried violently to force me off the road.
> The driver, when he tried to push me off,
> I struck in anger. The old man saw this, watched
> me approach, then leaned out and lunged down
> with twin prongs at the middle of my head!
> He got more than he gave. Abruptly—struck
> once by the staff in this my hand—he tumbled
> out, head first, from the middle of the carriage.
> And then I killed them all.

> (ll. 788–813)

Oedipus's ambiguously phrased narration presents himself, in recoil from the prophecy, as running to a place which he intends as a place where the prophecy will not be fulfilled but which he actually describes as a place of ignorance or unconsciousness, "a place where I could never see the disgrace in the Oracle's words come true." Running to this place of not seeing, he soon comes to the "exact location" where the three roads meet and someone, perhaps the king, Laius, was killed. In this overdetermined place, the narration orchestrates an escalating sequence of violent acts, which take the form of a double exchange of blows that climax in Oedipus's killing of Laius and his retinue. The killing is a violent response to the violence offered to Oedipus and, significantly, it begins with the attempt by both Laius and his herald to force Oedipus off the road: "Both the man out front and the old man himself / tried violently to force me off the road." Oedipus, a single traveler, just approaching the place where three roads meet, becomes an obstacle to the passage through it of an unknown figure of some consequence, riding in a carriage and preceded by a herald. The first exchange of blows takes place between the herald/driver and Oedipus: "The driver, when he tried to push me off / I struck in anger." The second exchange of blows frames in close up "the old man," as he is twice called, caught in a sequence of actions that are premeditated and have an intentional quality, beyond the spontaneous and reactive aggression that preceded it.

> The old man saw this, watched
> me approach, then leaned out and lunged down
> with twin prongs at the middle of my head!
>
> (ll. 807–9)

Gould's commentary enables the English language reader to hear the resonance of Laius's gesture, carefully aimed and targeted as it is, that both repeats earlier and prefigures later moments in the play. In particular, the verb 'lunges' repeats and reverses the previous remark of Oedipus about his predecessor on the throne of Thebes and in Jocasta's bed:

> It's I who have the power that he had once,
> and have his bed, and a wife who shares our seed,
> and common bond had we had common children
> (had not his hope of offspring had bad luck—
> but as it happened, luck lunged at his head).
>
> (ll. 259–63)

Where luck, chance—*tuche*—had lunged at Laius's head, Laius in turn "lunged down with twin prongs at the middle of my head." The same verb to lunge—*enallesthai*—is used again here, to describe Laius's action, now aimed at Oedipus's head, that provokes in turn Oedipus's parricidal lunge, a blow by which "struck / once by the staff in this my hand / he tumbled out head first, from the middle of the carriage" (ll. 810–12). So it is now revealed that it was Oedipus's blow that was the bad luck that had lunged at Laius's head, but that it came in reply to Laius's lunge at Oedipus's head, and that both are the lunge of *tuche*. *Tuche* can mean chance, contingency, or, in this case, bad luck, but as Gould points out, it comes increasingly in the course of the play to be seen as a pattern, and to testify to the unseen action of a divinity, or *daimon*.

The weapon Laius uses—"the two prongs"—is a double-pointed goad used on horses and cattle. This both repeats and prefigures the motif of a dual attack or double violence directed at Oedipus's body that is found throughout the tragedy. Tiresias had already predicted that Oedipus will feel "a mother's and a father's double-lashing, terrible-footed curse" that "will drive you out" (ll. 417–18). As Gould notes, the word *diplos*, meaning double, is used throughout the play, and in Tiresias's prediction it references a violence coming from the parental couple or double. Both the "lunge" and the "twin prongs," as well as the "double-lashing curse," all point forward to the other scene that matches Oedipus's narration of the Phocal scene, to Oedipus's reencounter with Jocasta, reported by the messenger as having just taken place offstage, but within the time of the play.

> She came in anger through the outer hall,
> and then she ran straight to her marriage bed,
> tearing her hair with fingers of both hands.
> Then, slamming shut the doors when she was in,
> she called to Laius, dead so many years,
> remembering the ancient seed which caused
> his death, leaving the mother to the son
> to breed again an ill-born progeny.
> She mourned the bed where she, alas, bred double—
> husband by husband, children by her child.
> From this point on I don't know how she died,
> for Oedipus then burst in with a cry,

and did not let us watch her final evil.
Our eyes were fixed on him. Wildly he ran
to each of us, asking for his spear
and for his wife—no wife: where he might find
the double mother-field, his and his children's.
He raved, and some divinity [*daimonon tis*][18] then showed him—
For none of us did so who stood close by.
With a dreadful shout—as if some guide were leading—
he lunged through the double doors; he bent the hollow
bolts from the sockets, burst into the room,
and there we saw her, hanging from above,
entangled in some twisted hanging strands.
He saw, was stricken, and with a wild roar
ripped down the dangling noose. When she, poor woman,
lay on the ground, there came a fearful sight:
he snatched the pins of worked gold from her dress,
with which her clothes were fastened: these he raised
and struck into the ball-joints of his eyes.
He shouted that they would no longer see
the evils he had suffered or had done,
see in the dark those he should not have seen,
and know no more those he once sought to know.
While chanting this, not once but many times
He raised his hand and struck into his eyes.
Blood from his wounded eyes poured down his chin,
not freed in moistening drops, but all at once
a stormy rain of black blood burst like hail.
These evils, coupling them, making them one,
have broken loose upon both man and wife.
The old prosperity that they had once
Was true prosperity, and yet today,
Mourning, ruin, death, disgrace, and every
Evil you could name—not one is absent.

(ll. 1241–85)

18. Sophocles, *Oedipus the King*, footnote to l. 1258, 143.

This extraordinary sequence is itself *diplos*, or double, in that it breaks down into two moments: first there is the moment of Jocasta's return to the marriage bed calling out to Laius, and then there is Oedipus's return to the same marriage bed seeking Jocasta. Jocasta in anger slams shut the doors of the marital chamber against Oedipus, locking him out, and crying out to Laius she invokes the memory of an earlier scene also enacted there, their sexual encounter—"the ancient seed"—which conceived Oedipus and killed Laius, formulated as one continuous action: "the ancient seed which caused / his death, leaving the mother to the son / to breed again an ill-born progeny." The conception, death, paternal absence "that leaves the mother to the son to breed again," and the consequent incest are all presented here as one telescoped and doubled up action *in the same place*: "the bed, where she, alas, bred double / husband by husband, children by her child." This doubled breeding, the second conception repeating and taking the place of the first, makes clear the way the play condenses or telescopes different moments together, such that one scene is operative within another in a way that confuses forward linear chronology. This strange temporal structure that condenses conception, death, and a second conception relocates the killing of Laius, which had hitherto been the exclusive focus of attention, within the larger gravitational field of maternal incest and its scene.

When the Oracle of Delphi specifies the pollution to be driven out of Thebes in order to cure the plague, it mentions only the presence of the killer of Laius in the city. Nothing is said by the Oracle about the double nature of Oedipus's crime, parricide and incest, and the double blood relation—father–son, mother–son—involved. When Oedipus as King pronounces a formal curse and warrant of expulsion on the killer, when he begins the investigation and when he responds to Jocasta's clue, her almost casual mention of the place where three roads meet, it is regicide and Phocis as the scene of regicide *only* that is intended. However, Oedipus's narration of what turns out to be the scene of parricide resonates with other moments and scenes. This becomes clearer when the self-blinded Oedipus, far from being a figure of repression, as Cynthia Chase suggests,[19]

19. She claims that "he 'represses' the scene of the crime by blinding himself" and proposes an "analogy between Emma's hysterical forgetting and Oedipus' self-blinding"; see Chase, "Oedipal Textuality," 63.

looks back on the Phocal scene from a position now of belated knowledge, *not* unconsciousness, and at last rehearses it in full recognition of its double—"diplos"—nature:

> You three roads, and you, secret ravine,
> you oak grove, narrow place of those three paths
> that drank my blood from these my hands, from him
> who fathered me, do you remember still
> the things I did to you? When I'd come here,
> what I then did once more? Oh marriages! Marriages!
>
> (ll. 1398–1403)

Behind the regicide is the parricide and behind that is the maternal incest. The parricide enables and makes way for the incest that is the fulfillment of its logic. The later scene of the incest acts back on the earlier scene of parricide, absorbing it into itself such that the scene of one was always already the scene of the other. This backward, *nachträglich* refiguration of the scene now becomes obvious here, as the bare topography of the crossroads is embellished and filled out as the "secret ravine, / oak grove, narrow place," the geography of sex and the maternal body, the place where the son's trespass provokes the father's murderous lunge and he replies with his own parricidal blow. As Gould comments: "This vivid picture . . . must be a return, at one and the same time, to the place where he assaulted his father and to the place—that is, the part of the body—where he assaulted his mother" (156, note to l. 1398). The implicit presence of the mother at the scene of parricide, the spilling of the father's blood in the *maternal* space of the "secret ravine" and the "narrow place," is established by a shift of rhetorical register in Oedipus's intimate address to and personification of that place: "you, secret ravine, / you oak grove, narrow place of those three paths / . . . do you remember still / the things I did to you?" The doubled nature of this spilling is made explicit by Oedipus's next question: "When I'd come here, / what I did once more? O marriages! Marriages!" The spilling of his father's blood and the spilling of the son's seed are one continuous and doubled action *in the same place*. The place where three roads meet and the mother-field of double sowing are the same doubled scene, and the three roads are the lifelines or fates of Laius, Jocasta, and Oedipus that meet and encounter each other in that overdetermined *mise-en-scène*. It is only now, in retrospect, that the full incestuous dimension is released of the scene of parricide, a scene that is chronologically first but that functions as a facade or screen memory, that covers over the doubled 'palimpcestuous,' as it were, scene of double sowing.

The second half of the diptych in the marital chamber stages Oedipus's attempt to confront his wife-mother who has shut herself away from him behind the locked doors of the marital chamber. Where Jocasta had called to "Laius, long dead" to rehearse their past sexual encounter that conceived Oedipus, Oedipus, now calling both for a spear and "the double mother-field, his and his children's," is possessed of a violence that is also presented as both a repetition of previous scenes and as impelled by a *daimon*: "He raved, and some divinity [*daimonon tis*] then showed him— . . . / With a dreadful shout—as if some guide were leading— / he *lunged* through the double doors; he bent the hollow bolts from the sockets, burst into the room" (ll. 1258–62, emphasis added). This *daimon*-led lunge through the double doors of the marital chamber recapitulates the lunge of Laius and that of *tuche* that was Oedipus's parricidal blow, while at the same time it repeats, now in the present time of the tragedy, like a transferential acting out, the incestuous primal scene between wife-mother and husband-son. Oedipus penetrates to the marriage bed, the most secret part of the house, to encounter once again Jocasta's body, only this time "hanging from above, / entangled in some twisted hanging strands." It is a shocking and enigmatic image. Jocasta's suicide has preempted Oedipus's violence and her self-violence seems to deflect or direct Oedipus's aggression back onto himself, and to prompt a similar self-violence in him. The strangeness of Oedipus's terrible act of self-blinding is that his gesture appears to reach out and to take or receive that violence from Jocasta:

> He snatched the pins of worked gold from her dress,
> with which her clothes were fastened: these he raised
> and struck into the ball-joints of his eyes.

> (ll. 1268–70)

Whatever Oedipus's explanation of his terrible act, either in the very performance of it or to the horrified Chorus that questions him afterward, whether as a punishment or an attempt to erase the forbidden sight of "those he should not have seen," it is the poetic formulation of it in Sophocles's dramatic verse that locates it as the climactic moment of a whole sequence of scenes.

## Traumatic Wounding and the Power of the Daimon

Jocasta's twin golden pins or brooches belong to the whole series of dual attacks on Oedipus's body, which I have invoked in commenting on the twin prongs of Laius's goad and on the double-lashing, terrible-footed parental curse predicted by Tiresias the prophet. Gould's invaluable commentary has enabled us to see a further repetition in the strange trope of "the ball-joints of his eyes." As Gould points out, the Greek term here is '*arthra*', meaning joints (as in arthritis), and it is a unique use of it to refer to the eyes. He refers us back to two earlier appearances of the word, each referring to Oedipus's feet. There is Jocasta's casual reference to the baby son that she and Laius had long ago abandoned in response to the prophecy of the Delphic Oracle:

> As for the child I bore him [Laius], not three days passed
> before he yoked the *ball-joints* of its feet,
> then cast it, by other's hands, on a trackless mountain.
>
> (ll. 717–19, emphasis added)

Later the Corinthian messenger who brings both the news of the death of Polybus, Oedipus's supposed father, and eventually the identity of Oedipus as the cast-out offspring of Laius and Jocasta, also refers to "the ball-joints of your feet," which Oedipus reluctantly acknowledges as "that ancient trouble" (ll. 1032–33). The piercing and yoking together of the infant's ankles, which Gould takes as the meaning of *arthra*, is the tragedy's moment of trauma as wounding, the first of the dual woundings of Oedipus brought to a final traumatic repetition via a tropological transfer from feet to eyes, with Oedipus's repeated double piercing of the arthra or "ball-joints" of his eyes. In the earlier exchange between Oedipus and the messenger, the piercing of the arthra or ball-joints of the feet are referred to as acts of signification; so the messenger says, "The ball-joints of your feet might testify" (l.1032), and Oedipus replies, "A fearful rebuke those tokens left me" (l.1035). These dual woundings, to the feet, to the head, and finally to the eyes, constitute the realization of Tiresias's prediction of "a mother's and a father's double-lashing, terrible-footed curse." However, paradoxically, it is an attack that had begun *before* the acts of parricide and incest that it both provokes and punishes.

These repeated double woundings are part of a larger pattern of *daimonic* repetition that is made quite explicit in the wake of this terrible scene, as the self-blinded Oedipus comes on stage singing: "Divinity [*daimon*], where has your lunge transported me?" (l. 1311)—that same word *enallesthai* once again. As Gould argues at length, the repeated 'lunges' by different agents in the play belong to a whole family of similar verbs—to lunge, to swoop, to leap on, to mount, to pierce—whose repeated pattern is only now acknowledged as the *daimonic* work of Apollo in and through the activity of human agents. When asked by the Chorus, who seem to regard the self-blinding to be as terrible as the parricide and incest, "What divinity [*daimon*] raised your hand?," Oedipus replies:

> It was Apollo there, Apollo, friends,
> who brought my sorrows, vile sorrows to their perfection,
> these evils that were done to me.
> But the one who struck them with his hand,
> That one was none but I, in wretchedness.
>
> (ll. 1329–33)

We have here a bifocal vision, characteristic of fifth-century Athenian tragedy, in which the human actor affirms his agency but simultaneously acknowledges the *daimonic* pattern of repetition, through which Apollo brings Oedipus's "vile sorrows to their perfection" in Oedipus's own act of self-blinding. A similar moment occurs in *The Oresteia* of Aeschylus, where Clytemnestra proclaims her ownership of the deed of murder of her husband, King Agamemnon: "And I stand where I struck, with the deed done. /And so I acted—and I will not deny it" (*Agamemnon*, ll. 1379–80). Only minutes later, however, she declares:

> You aver that this deed is mine.
> But do not consider
> that I am Agamemnon's consort!
> But in the likeness of this dead man's wife
> the ancient savage avenger

of Atreus, the cruel banqueter,
slew him in requital.

(ll. 1497–1503)[20]

Having claimed the murder of her husband, Agamemnon, as her own, Clytemnestra then invokes the *daimon* of the House of Atreus as the revenging
force that strikes down Agamemnon, the son of Atreus, cursed by his rival
and brother Thyestes, to whom he had served the flesh of his sons in a dish.
This bifocal vision of a simultaneously *daimonic* and human agency must
call into question Starobinski's account of a one-dimensional Oedipus who
simply is the exemplification of drive or desire, "the opaque residueless
plenitude of a psychic image," for Sophocles's Oedipus carries around with
him an unknown but still-active past, in both his name and wounded body,
a past that takes possession of his proud exercise of investigative reason,
diverts it and turns it into a maddened *daimon*-led repetition of the tragedy's founding trauma. In and through Oedipus's chosen act of self-blinding,
other forces are at work, and Oedipus laments their continuing double attack; using the same word, *kentra*, that denoted the twin prongs of Laius's
double-pointed goad, Oedipus sings: "Alas! / Again alas! Both enter me at
once: / the sting of the prongs [*kentra*], the memory of evils," while the Chorus comments, "You carry double griefs and double evils' (ll. 1316–20).

The investigation in the present moment of the play does not just neu-
trally interrogate the truth of actions that are past and done, determining
the accuracy of the various shepherds' and messenger's reports as evidence.
The play's tragic action, beginning with the eruption of the *daimonic*
'swooping down' of the plague-god, culminates in two acts, Jocasta's suicide and Oedipus's self-blinding, which are part of a pattern of repetition in
which past scenes and acts are reproduced, coming alive in new forms in
the present. These are not to be construed on a simple wish-fulfillment
model, as the inevitable wishes of the infant Oedipus "imposed by Nature"
in Freud's words and finding expression unconsciously, the figuration of
pure instinct or drive, as in Freud's and Starobinski's readings. Rather, the
tragedy's 'oedipal' actions of parricide and incest burst out of the Ptolemaic

20. Aeschylus, *Agamemnon*, trans. Hugh Lloyd-Jones (Englewood Cliffs, N.J.: Prentice
Hall, 1970), 91, 97–98.

framework of a single subject centered on his own wishes, being moments in a chain or sequence in which the initiative of the other, the precursor, is fundamental and originary. It is with this 'Copernican' perspective I want to end.

## Maiming and Naming

In the first instance the precursors are Laius and Jocasta, who are not just passive objects of Oedipus's wishes and actions but initiators. I am thinking here of that casually mentioned event long ago, the casting out to die of the royal couple's fatal offspring, the baby-son with the yoked and pierced *ar-thra* of his feet, a sign of rejection—or, as he calls it himself, a "token of rebuke." These are wounding acts of signification that both mark the body and deliver a violent and enigmatic signification that Oedipus is fated unknowingly to act out. One of the enigmatic significations they deliver is Oedipus's own name, as the messenger points out to Oedipus: "that [the wounded feet—JF] was the chance [*tuche*] that names you who you are" (l. 1036). This 'arthritic' primal wounding of the feet gives rise to one of the two competing derivations of Oedipus's name—from *oidein*, to swell, and *pous*, meaning foot—"swollen-footed," as its encrypted secret reference point; "Swellfoot the Tyrant," as Shelley translated the play's title. However, the derivation of his name that Oedipus himself explicitly plays on is from *oida*—I know. In his attack on the prophet Tiresisas, who failed to solve the Sphinx's riddle with augury and divination, Oedipus boasts:

> I came along, yes, I
> Oedipus the ignorant and stopped her—
> by using thought not augury from birds.

> (ll. 396–97)

Oedipus the ignorant—*ho meden eidos Oidipous*. In a much-quoted sentence, M. L. Earle states: "As 'Knowfoot' (*eidos tous podas*) he solves the riddle about feet" (*Sophocles*, 63). In the strange multiform, polymorphous creature described by the Sphinx's riddle, which changes shape from four feet to two feet to three feet and is at his weakest when supported by most feet, Oedipus recognizes the figure of 'Man' in his various stages of development, from infancy to old age. As such, his exercise of *gnome*, or reason, vanquishes the predatory female *daimon*, the Sphinx, reducing the numinous and enigmatic monster to 'Man,' its supposed human source. This wins him recognition from Hegel, Heidegger, and many other philosophers for his exemplary posture of demystifying philosophical reason, as a type of the fifth-century Athenian Enlightenment.[21] However, underpinning his ironically mock-modest boast to Tiresias of being *"ho meden eidos Oidipous"*— "Oedipus the ignorant", 'the nothing-knowing Knowfoot'—is the underlying connection between the Sphinx's riddle—*tetra-pous, di-pous, tri-pous* (four-footed, two-footed, three-footed) and his "ancient trouble" with his feet; he is *Oidipous*—"Knowfoot"—the one who knows about feet, only because he is, always already, marked and inscribed as "Swellfoot"; his identity and its capacities are determined in the trauma of that primal wounding, that is, as Chase observes (1994, 74, n. 16), both a maiming and a naming, the secret work of *tuche*, as the Corinthian messenger tells him.

If Oedipus's proud epistemic stance as "Knowfoot" is unwittingly grounded in his condition as "Swellfoot," as the effect of that "terrible-footed"—*deinopous*—parental curse, it is utterly undermined and subverted by that other dimension of the play's repetition-compulsion, not the human ancestral but the numinous-daimonic. The parental curse, in its "double-lashing"—*amphiplex*—bodily inscription and casting out, represents the struggle of Laius and Jocasta to *avoid* the Oracle's fate and to abort or turn aside the predicted actions of parricide and incest. However, the swooping, lunging, piercing 'daimonism' of the play, emanating from precisely Apollo and his Oracle, can only make sense if understood as the god or *daimon*'s enigmatic *desire for* the very double scene of parricide and incest that both Oedipus and his parents, in their different ways, recoiled from and struggled against. Aeschylus's great trilogy encloses the transgenerational *daimon* of the House of Atreus in a genealogical prehistory going back to the legendary Feast of Thyestes, and it completes itself in the purging of the matricide Orestes and the sublimatory transformation of the *Erinyes*, the avenging maternal Furies, into the Eumenides, the Kindly Ones, who will live be-

---

21. For a systematic consideration of Oedipus's relation to both the Athenian Enlightenment and the Western philosophical tradition, see Jean-Joseph Goux, *Oedipus Philosopher*, trans. Catherine Porter (Stanford, Calif.: Stanford University Press, 1993).

neath the city and sustain its fertility.[22] Aeschylus's trilogy appears to offer us this sublimation of the Erinyes into the Eumenides, as a translation without remainder or residue. By contrast, in this tragedy at least (as we do not have his other lost Oedipus plays), Sophocles makes little or nothing of the ancestral prehistory of the Labdacid dynasty or of the crimes of Laius. The ending of *Oedipus The King*, in contrast with *The Oresteia*, is bleakly devastating, without remedy or resolution, other than the final lunge of the *daimon* that transports Oedipus from self-blinding to exile. He exits from the stage as the self-cursed and self-blinded embodiment of the *miasma*, or pollution, with which Thebes is stricken, and who must be driven out as a *pharmakos*, or scapegoat, to ensure the cleansing of the city.

In the process of transgenerational trauma, there are two structural possibilities: there is the normal process of translation and binding of the traumatizing enigmatic signifiers, inscriptions, and implantations coming from the adult other, together with an accompanying repression and exclusion of what cannot be translated and incorporated into the ego and its archives; alternatively, there is the unbound and unbinding 'intromission,' as Laplanche calls it, of enigmatic signifiers with their wounding, scarifying acts of signification, messages inflicted with such violence that the recipient's processes of translation, binding, and sublimation are paralyzed and disabled. The outcome of the latter process is often psychosis, with its desperate attempts to expel such intolerable burdens, which psychoanalysis specifies in the various psychotic mechanisms of repudiation (Freud), foreclosure (Lacan), and projection (Klein).[23] A 'traumatological' or 'Copernican' reading of Sophocles's tragedy, which seeks to reclaim the *Wiederholungszwang* or traumatic repetition-compulsion foreclosed by Freud's 'instinctualist—Ptolemaic' reading of the play, comes up against something very like Laplanche's overriding structure of violent intromission. This *daimonic* agency preempts any binding or sublimation, converting all attempts at resistance or substitution, by Oedipus and his parents, into the very instruments of its own proliferation. By contrast, in *Oedipus at Colonus*,

---

22. For a compelling reading of Aeschylus's *Oresteia* in relation to the question of the *daimon*, see Robin Grove, "The *Oresteia* and the Furies," *The Critical Review* (Melbourne) 13 (1970): 2–33.

23. Jean Laplanche, "Implantation and Intromission," in *Essays on Otherness*, ed. John Fletcher (London: Routledge, 1999): 133–37.; Scarfone, " 'It was *not* my mother,': 69–76."

written twenty-five years later, Oedipus's final resting place is a sacred site associated with precisely the Eumenides, Aeschylus's sublimated Kindly Ones—but that is another play and another story.

The paradox of Freud's engagement with Sophocles's tragedy is that Freud takes as a prototype for the 'universal event in early childhood,' that is supposed to ground his developed theory of sexuality, a play whose very dramatic construction challenges his proposed model of a spontaneous emergence of incestuous and jealous impulses in infancy. Oedipus-Knowfoot, who knows about feet and so defeats the Sphinx by the exercise of reason, is exposed as Oedipus-Swellfoot, named for a wound, the ancestral marker of his possession by the *daimonic* fate that provokes the very impulses that he comes to name in Freud's theory. In order to exemplify his move from an exogenous model of trauma to an endogenous model of natural development, Freud is drawn to a text whose *nachträglich* sequence of scenes enacts the very traumatology he is seeking to replace. The same case can be made about *Hamlet* and its figuring of a spectral other in the ghost of Hamlet's father, who does not appear in Freud's 'oedipal' reading.[24] We will also find in Chapter 11 that, in that other turning point and moment of theoretical crisis of the death drive in 1919, Freud is similarly drawn to Hoffmann's novella, *The Sandman* (1816), only to elaborate a normalizing, 'oedipal-Ptolemaic' reading that attempts to contain the daimonic repetitions and traumatic scenography of Hoffmann's uncanny text within the singular subjectivity of the protagonist.

24. A compelling reading of both tragedies along 'Copernican' lines is elaborated by Nicholas Ray in *Tragedy and Otherness: Sophocles, Shakespeare and Psychoanalysis* (Bern: Peter Lang, 2009).

**Part III   Screen Memories and the Return of Seduction**

# Leonardo's Screen Memory

The concept of the screen memory, as it is elaborated in Freud's two texts of 1899 and 1901, both resumes and silences the theoretical perturbations that had agitated him in his struggles in the 1890s to understand and to treat the disturbing phenomena of child sexual abuse and their *sequellae*, the range of hysterical, obsessional, and paranoid symptoms that his writings of the mid-1890s describe and analyze. In my discussion of the screen memory in the final section of Chapter 4, I remarked on the theoretical amnesia that appears to characterize Freud's critique of the commonsense understanding of memory in the "Screen Memories" paper of 1899. The ghost of the seduction theory (only gradually and unevenly abandoned) stalks its pages, as Freud rehearses yet again the question of the relation between early infantile moments of experience, their residues and deposits, and later moments marked by the formation of neurotic symptoms, dreams, screen memories, fantasies. The 1899 essay presents a formal schema that allows for both *regressive* screen memories (where later experiences and fantasies borrow earlier 'innocent' memories as screens, just as, in Freud's borrowed metaphor,[1] hermit crabs hide themselves in abandoned empty shells), and *progressive* screen memories (where highly charged childhood scenes are encoded within and screened off by apparently anodyne later scenes, as in the Emma case from "Project for a Scientific Psychology" (1950a [1895]), discussed in Chapter 3).

The latter possibility of a *progressive* screen memory, however, despite being acknowledged as the most common form of screen memory, is proposed by Freud only to be ignored. This is the case both in the 1899 text and in Freud's return to the subject two years later in *The Psychopathology of Everyday Life* (1901b), where the memories analyzed involve either regressive borrowings of earlier scenes or displacements onto adjacent contemporary elements of the same situation. The absence of any analysis of the so-called *progressive* screen memory represents the temporary triumph of the retrogressive perspective voiced in the September letter of repudiation of 1897 to Fliess; it signals the marginalization of the problem of infantile trauma and the temporal logic of afterwardsness that characterized its repetition, and whose adventures we have traced in previous chapters. Assimilated in practice to the retrogressive dimension, the screen memory in these two texts is the very antithesis of the dream, despite the emphasis on what I have called the 'memory-work' of displacement and condensation modeled on the dream-work, for it is in the dream that the priority of the infantile and the 'prehistoric' is affirmed over the 'day's residues' of contemporary experience.

The question of the priority of the infantile in relation to memory, however, reasserts itself in Freud's texts on Leonardo and Goethe. Here the model of the screen memory is invoked again, but in a way that is ambiguous and marked by conceptual slippage. This is more obvious in the later essay "A Childhood Recollection from *Dichtung und Warheit*" (1917b), where the term 'screen memories' actually appears as such, rather than in the earlier, more substantial text *Leonardo da Vinci and a Memory of His Childhood* (1910c), where the term does not feature. The connection between the Leonardo and Goethe examples is made by Freud himself, who rehearses the Goethe paper in a footnote added in 1919 to the earlier Leon-

1. *The Psychopathology of Everyday Life* (1901b), *SE* 6, 49.

ardo study. The Goethe example is the simpler of the two. It involves a childhood incident of no apparent emotional significance that Freud sees as belonging to a class of similar memories: "Generally they seemed indifferent, worthless even, and it remained at first incomprehensible why just these memories should have resisted amnesia."[2] The memory in question is the single incident Goethe recalls from "the earliest years of childhood" (1917b, 147) in his autobiography. It involves the young Goethe playing with his small child-size crockery and utensils in the hall of the family house: "Since this seemed to lead to nothing, I threw a plate into the street, and was overjoyed to see it go to bits so merrily" (ibid.). Watched by his neighbors, the adult von Ochsenstein brothers, he is urged by them to do it again and again as he smashes in quick succession all his miniature pots and dishes, only then to proceed to plunder the dresser in the family kitchen of its large earthenware plates and to hurl them also into the street. Goethe concludes that after so much destruction "there was at least an amusing story, which the rascals who had been its instigators enjoyed to the end of their lives" (ibid., 148).

Freud interprets the apparent "utter innocence and irrelevance" of Goethe's memory by grouping it with childhood memories with a similar content—children hurling household objects, glasses, shoes, brushes, crockery, and even father's heavy mountaineering boots, out of windows and doors. In all these vignettes the child is angry and the anger can be related to the birth of a younger sibling. Goethe's incident is also dated by Freud in relation to the birth of a younger brother, Hermann Jakob, who is not mentioned in this main account of his childhood but who is referred to later in an account of childhood illnesses as dying young at the age of six when Goethe was ten, and when his indifference to his brother's death prompted a reproach from his mother. Freud suggests that "the throwing of crockery out of the window was a symbolic action, or, to put it more correctly, a *magic* action, by which the child (Goethe as well as my patient) gave violent expression to his wish to get rid of a disturbing intruder" (152). He adds persuasively: "A child who breaks crockery knows quite well that he is doing something naughty . . . he probably has a grudge against his parents

2. Sigmund Freud, "A Childhood Recollection from *Dichtung und Warheit*" (1917b), *SE* 17, 148.

that he wants to satisfy; he wants to show naughtiness." Rather than just a pleasure in destruction for its own sake—the satisfying shower and sound of fragments—it is the act of expulsion that is crucial: "this 'out' seems to be an essential part of the magic action and to arise directly from its hidden meaning. The new baby must be *got rid of*—through the window" (ibid.). Now this persuasive analysis is of the *content* of the memory, not of the memory process itself. The memory is taken by Freud as a transparent window onto the childhood scene *as a scene*, in which the child performs the symbolic action of expulsion of his hated rival. It is taken as the reliable record of a single real event, albeit one that has a hidden symbolic meaning. From Freud's explanation, we would deduce that it is not, strictly speaking, a *screen memory*, in which an indifferent memory is recalled or even constructed as a substitute for a repressed or excluded experience; rather, in the Goethe example, the symbolic displacement takes place in the child's action *in the past*, not in the adult's remembering *in the present* (which is assumed to be unproblematic). We have a contrast between a 'memory' as a screen for an unremembered experience and the memory of an action that had itself been symbolic.

This is also the case in the extended analysis of Freud's own memory of his missing mother and her sudden return that Freud performs in his second treatment of screen memories in *The Psychopathology of Everyday Life* (1901b). Here the symbolization is, first of all, the work of Freud's elder half brother, whose playful reference to young Sigmund's missing nurse, that she is "boxed up" ("*eingekastelt*," meaning she has been imprisoned for household thefts), leads the child, in the later moment of his mother's absence during a confinement, to demand that his elder brother open the wardrobe (*kasten*) or "box" to let his absent mother out. Freud's later reinterpretation of the scene, in which the box stands for the mother's body and the scene turns on the wish that no more babies come out of mother's "box," attributes to the young Sigmund the symbolic displacement from the mother's body to the wardrobe/box.[3] Once again there is a memory taken unproblematically at face value as the record of a real event, although one in which a symbolic displacement had taken place in the past (from the

3. Sigmund Freud, "Childhood Memories and Screen Memories," *The Psychopathology of Everyday Life* (1901b), *SE* 6, 50–52.

mother's body to the *kasten* or box). The memory process itself is assumed to be transparent (i.e., these events really were as Freud or Goethe remembered them).

Freud seems briefly to acknowledge the distinction between memory as content and memory as process when he observes that the work of interpretation of these enigmatic memory fragments and scenes "either showed that their content required to be replaced by some other content, or revealed that they were related to some other unmistakably important experiences and had appeared *in their place* as what are known as 'screen memories'" (ibid., 148, emphasis added). Given this distinction between symbolic displacement in the past and a screen memory based on substitution in the formation of the memory itself, Freud's interpretation based on the replacement of one content—throwing out household objects—by another—throwing out the new baby—would seem to imply that Goethe's memory belongs to the first category and is therefore *not*, in Freud's terms, a screen memory. Freud's interpretation does not discover another "unmistakably important experience" *with its own scene* that is being screened out by a later or earlier memory but, rather, "some other content" behind the single, accurately remembered scene.

On reflection, however, Freud's point from the 1899 "Screen Memories" paper, that a retrospective revision betrays itself as the recollecting ego watches itself from the outside and from a later moment, might lead one to notice that Goethe writes: "The von Ochsensteins, who saw how delighted I was and how joyfully I clapped my little hands, called out 'Do it again!'" (ibid., 147–48). The betraying detail here is, of course, the "little hands." This is not the child's perspective but the adult's, and together with the von Ochsensteins and their supposedly encouraging role in the whole scene, it betrays the activity of revision. Indeed, Goethe's narrative ends with the von Ochsensteins as "the rascals who had been the instigators" (ibid., 148), thus shifting the blame from himself onto the adults. However, as Freud himself had remarked, the child's activity of throwing out his pots and plates had begun *before* the adult encouragement; moreover, that adult neighbors should have urged on the wholesale destruction of the family crockery service seems highly implausible. The absence of any account of parental punishment is also striking. All these features would suggest the revised and reconstructed nature of Goethe's memory, which Freud ignores but which would be the basis for its identification as precisely a screen memory proper, in which the remembered retrospectively humorous scene replaces a different and more distressing one. This is not to deny the force of Freud's identification of the sibling rivalry being acted out symbolically in the throwing out and smashing of the crockery but instead to raise the question of the edited and idealized nature of the scene (Goethe's "little hands," the absence of parental punishment, the adults as rascals/instigators, the element of guilt suggested by the mother's later reproach to Goethe over his indifference to his brother's death, etc.). So Freud's account appears to place Goethe's childhood memory as akin but *not* identical to a screen memory. However, as a memory where the displacement belongs not just in the past to the memory-content (the clear-cut memory of a symbolic action) but to the memory-process itself (the memory acts as precisely a *screen* or cover for *another* scene), the very details of Freud's example from Goethe would seem to speak against him, and to suggest that Goethe's is indeed a screen memory.

### Early Scenes, Later Fantasies: A Reprise

In the second chapter of his study, *Leonardo da Vinci and a Memory of His Childhood* (1910c), Freud considers Leonardo's memory of his infantile encounter with a bird in his cradle and makes it the focal 'scene' for his analysis of Leonardo's personality, his sexual, intellectual, and artistic development, and some of his greatest paintings. Surprisingly, the term 'screen memory' is not used in the Leonardo study, although the concept is invoked and, in a footnote added in 1919, precisely in relation to his later analysis of Goethe's childhood memory. What is at work here, in Freud's discussion of both Goethe's and Leonardo's childhood memories, is the model of the *regressive* screen memory as elaborated in the 1899 essay. Given the fabulous nature of Leonardo's so-called 'memory'—"while I was in my cradle a vulture came down to me, and opened my mouth with its tail, and struck me many times with its tail against my lips"[4]—Freud's ini-

---

4. S. Freud, *Leonardo da Vinci and a Memory of His Childhood* (1910c), *SE* 11, 82. Notoriously, Freud relied on an incorrect German translation of the Italian term *'nibio'*, which

tial presentation proposes the view that "the scene with the vulture would not be a memory of Leonardo's but a phantasy, which he formed at a later date and transposed to his childhood" (1910c, 82). The back projection of a later fantasy into the time of childhood matches exactly Freud's analysis of the screen memory of the stolen flowers and the delicious bread from the 1899 paper. However, the emphasis falls slightly differently, as he goes on to mount a contrast between the formation of childhood memories and adult memories, which is part of a larger comparison between personal memory and collective memory.

As against the commonsense view of childhood memories as "fixed at the moment of being experienced and afterwards repeated," Freud proposes that they are "only elicited at a later stage when childhood is already past; in the process they are altered and falsified, and put into the service of later trends" (ibid., 83). Although as a result they are scarcely to be distinguished from fantasies, at least there is an acknowledgment of the part played by early memory traces, inscribed prior to the formation of the fantasy, which therefore has a memorial dimension of some kind. Are these memory traces to be mere vehicles, shells for the hermit crab of later fantasy, or do they make a significant contribution of their own, not only to the material but also to the *meaning* of the resultant 'screen memory'?

The schematic analogy that Freud sets out is, first, between an initial moment of history writing, the keeping of contemporary records of current events, and "a man's conscious memory of the events of his maturity" (84) which, as Laplanche points out, is assumed not to entail any serious distortion and hence is "an ideal model that the psychology of everyday life would correct."[5] The second moment of Freud's analogy claims that "the memories that he has of his childhood correspond, as far as their origins and reliability are concerned, to the history of a nation's earliest days, which was compiled later and for tendentious reasons" (84). Freud's conception of the latter stresses two things: first, the *memorial* material of "traditions and legends," "the traces of antiquity that survived in customs and

---

means 'kite,' and not 'vulture.' Also the final phrase should read "within [*dentro*] my lips," as the *SE* editor points out.

5. Jean Laplanche, "A Short Treatise on the Unconscious" [1993], in *Essays on Otherness*, ed. John Fletcher (London: Routledge, 1999), 96. Henceforth, Laplanche 1993.

usages"; second, the *rewriting* that this interpretation of past "traces" entails as "an expression of present beliefs and wishes rather than a true picture of the past," for "many things had been dropped from the nation's memory, while others were distorted and some remains of the past were given a wrong interpretation to fit in with contemporary ideas" (83).

Laplanche comments that this is a model not of unconscious elements or scenes but of conscious screen memories whose function is precisely to prevent the resurgence of the repressed, and he hails it as "a very exact resurfacing of the model of afterwardsness or the two-phase trauma" (Laplanche 1993, 96). However, as I have noted in my commentary on the 1899 "Screen Memories" essay in Chapter 4, there are *two* main models of the screen memory, each with its own temporal structure, of which the regressive screen memory is the only one Freud explores. This is what Freud invokes here to account for both personal and collective memory. What impels its formation is "a phantasy from a later period" (1910c, 84) that conscripts the infantile or historical pasts for its own contemporary purposes. *Pace* Laplanche, what is absent once again, unfortunately, is the unaddressed possibility of the *progressive* screen memory, which is the variant that would more precisely correspond to the traumatic model of afterwardsness, whose resurfacing is hailed somewhat prematurely by Laplanche's comment, just quoted. As with the "Screen Memories" essay, Freud resists the total dominance of the regressive perspective by insisting on the presence of the "raw material" of memory traces, albeit in distorted form. However, as I have argued in Chapter 4, with the regressive model the genuineness of, for example, the stolen flowers motif is defended at the expense of its meaningfulness, a meaningfulness that is imposed on it only by the fantasy of the later moment. It is the empty shell that the hermit crab of revisionary memory comes to occupy for its own purposes. Here the early memory traces become the screen for the later fantasy, which is repressed and returns in infantile disguise. In the 1899 example, these are Freud's adolescent sexual wishes for the daughter of the old family friends he was staying with, thus exemplifying "the slipping away of repressed thoughts and wishes into childhood memories."[6] As I have argued, this is the *reverse* of the models of both trauma and the dream (Freud's two key concerns in

6. Sigmund Freud, "Screen Memories" (1899a), *SE* 3, 317.

the 1890s), in which the priority of the infantile over postpuberty traumas or the recent 'day's residues' was repeatedly affirmed.

Even as he establishes the dominance of the regressive perspective, however, the emphases of Freud's argument begin to shift. In an echo of the oscillations of the mid-1890s, his critical agnosticism about the distorted revisions of the early past, which had led to his sense of impasse and failure in the letter to Fliess (September 21, 1897) announcing a *temporary* repudiation of his seduction theory, gives way to the claim that "if it were only possible, by a knowledge of all the forces at work, to undo these distortions, there would be no difficulty in disclosing the historical truth lying behind the legendary material" (1910c, 84). This goes with Freud's renewed confidence that the techniques of psychoanalysis can disclose the material concealed behind Leonardo's childhood fantasy. As an example in miniature of such a success Freud then interpolates, in a footnote added in 1919, a summary of his 1917 analysis of Goethe's childhood memory. The real significance of this for us, however, is the conceptual slippage it unwittingly demonstrates on the question of screen memories, for while he rehearses his persuasive analysis of the magical act of expulsion in Goethe's childhood, Freud seems to forget his previous distinction between events in which a past symbolic displacement has taken place (one scene with a hidden meaning, the latent content of a transparent memory) and memory processes that themselves screen what actually happened (two temporally separated scenes in which one covers or screens out the other), by virtue of which, according to Freud's own analysis, Goethe's memory *as he describes it* is not a screen memory. However, in the inserted footnote of 1919 Freud collapses this distinction by assimilating Goethe's memory to Leonardo's as examples of "the earliest memory of childhood, preserved in disguises such as these" (ibid., 85), without analyzing the distorting and screening processes that do indeed make it, as I have argued, a genuine screen memory (whereas in his short essay of 1917 on Goethe's memory, he had treated it as an *undisguised* memory of an act that had a hidden meaning).

In his tacit rewriting of his previous account of Goethe, Freud makes clear that the regressive model is still the operative one, as he ascribes the organizing motive of Goethe's memory's to a *later* moment of adult writing rather than to a resurgent infantile repetition: "at the place in the book where he describes the episode the intention is to triumph over the fact that a second son was not in the long run permitted to disturb Goethe's close relation with his mother" (ibid.). In this later account, what is disguised is the retrospective triumph, which could only have been felt *after* his brother's death, years later than the remembered episode of the three-year-old Goethe's plate smashing at his newborn rival's unwelcome appearance. This only apparently innocuous magical act is recalled by Goethe the writer, both to express and disguise the writing adult's *Schadenfreude* and accompanying guilt.[7]

There is, however, an elision in Freud's overall argument between the retrievability and knowability of these earliest scenes—"as a rule the residual memories . . . cloak priceless pieces of evidence about the most important features of his development" (84)—and the different question of the *motivating force* for the formation of screen memories. Despite Freud's renewed confidence in the techniques of psychoanalysis to undo later distortions and disclose "the historical truth behind the legendary material" (ibid.), the motivating force in all his analyses of screen memories has been *not* the traumatic kernel of an originary earliest moment but, rather, the wishful fantasy emanating from a later one (as in the case of Goethe's and Freud's own screen memories). Up to this point in Freud's argument, it is the *later* fantasy that organizes and mobilizes the childhood scene. As I have argued, what is missing in Freud's discussion of screen memories is the possibility of an infantile resurgence acting through later scenes and representatives, as we have seen in the case of Emma from "Project for a Scientific Psychology," where the earlier scene of molestation by the shopkeeper acts through the parallel details of the later 'innocent' scene to provoke both its postpuberty sexual excitation and Emma's subsequent hysterical reaction of phobic flight. The priority of the earliest scenes is also clear in the case of Miss Lucy R. in *Studies on Hysteria*, discussed extensively in Chapters 2 and 3.

---

7. According to Bettina Brentano, Goethe's mother was struck by his lack of grief at his little brother's death and his apparent annoyance over the grief of his family, and she reproached him for not being fond of his brother. Goethe responded by producing piles of paper on which he claimed were written stories and lessons, "saying that he had done all this to teach his brother" (Freud 1917b, 328). A note of guilty self-justification seems clear, although Freud does not comment on it.

## Leonardo's 'Primal Scene'

> "It seems at any rate . . . as if the key to all his achievements and misfortunes lay hidden in the childhood phantasy of the vulture."
> —(Freud 1910c, 136)

In Freud's actual analysis of Leonardo's famous bird memory,[8] we find an unannounced *reversal* of the temporal structure that had hitherto characterized his account of the screen memory and its retrogressive logic. The temporal dimensions are complex, and the details of the argument are not always clear. Freud's initial critical discussion of Leonardo's claims for this as a veridical memory of a real if marvelous event, when he had been visited in his cradle by a bird, proposes that it is in fact "a phantasy, which he formed at a later date and transposed to his childhood" (1910c, 82), that is, at this point the retrogressive model seems still in place. However, what is the motivating force for this retrogressive transfer?

Despite this back projection of a later fantasy into an earlier period in the form of a memory, Freud performs a series of 'translations' of the scene with the bird, decomposing it into a layered structure of scene upon scene, each with its own specific signification. In this scenic palimpsest, the later fantasy scene with the bird translates and stands in for earlier scenes, some of which Freud designates as memories and one a fantasy. The temporal complexity resides partly in the fact that *both* retrogressive and progressive logics are in play, although in a significant about-turn ultimately priority is accorded to the earliest scenes as sources for the impulsion that drives the formation of the fantasy. These scenes—or their condensation—have the

---

8. It has long been established that Freud had relied on a mistranslation of the text of Leonardo's original memorandum in which the Italian term *nibio*, or kite, is misconstrued as "vulture." However, I am as much concerned with the conceptual structure of Freud's vulture reading of Leonardo's 'memory' as with the important question of its adequacy as an interpretation. In response to the art-historical critique of Freud's interpretation by Meyer Schapiro and others, what one might call a psychoanalytically motivated 'kite reading' has been elaborated by K. R. Eissler, in *Leonardo da Vinci: Psychoanalytic Notes on the Enigma* (New York: International Universities Press, 1961), and Jean-Pierre Maïdani-Gerard, in *Léonard de Vinci: Mythologie ou théologie* (Paris: Presses Universitaires de France, 1994); also see R. Richard Wohl and Harry Trosman, "A Retrospect of Freud's *Leonardo*," *Psychiatry* 18 (1955): 36–37.

status of a "primal scene" (*Urszene*) in the sense in which Freud first uses the term in his letters to Fliess, as the originary scene of traumatic seduction/excitation, which in its tendency to recur requires management, and what Freud sometimes calls "sublimation," through its translation into "protective fictions" or fantasy.[9] Significantly, Freud returns to something like the fantasy-memory relation that he had formulated in the late unpublished stages of his seduction theory in the letters to Fliess, before they were polarized into mutually exclusive alternatives by the current of his thought that rejected the whole problematic of seduction.

The first translation that Freud performs on the "special language" of the fantasy focuses on the bird's tail: "a tail, '*coda*,' is one of the most familiar symbols and substitutive expressions for the male organ, in Italian no less than in other languages" (1910c, 85). The intrusive, even aggressive, activity of the bird's tail signifies a specific sexual act, Freud suggests: "The situation in the phantasy, of a vulture opening the child's mouth and beating about inside it vigorously with its tail, corresponds to the idea of an act of *fellatio*, a sexual act in which a penis is put into the mouth of the person involved" (86). Freud does not attempt to explore this fantasy in its own right, other than to remark that it is a "passive homosexual fantasy" (87). In order to preempt the anticipated disgust and indignation of his *bien-pensant* reader, Freud passes rapidly on to assert both the general incidence of a fantasy of fellatio in both women and passive homosexual men, and to diminish its offensiveness by tracing it back to "an origin of the most innocent kind": "It only repeats in a different form a situation in which we all once felt comfortable—when we were still in our suckling days . . . and took our mother's (or wet-nurse's) nipple into our mouth and sucked at it" (ibid.). In addition to transforming the "loathsome sexual fantasy" into an "innocent" and "comfortable" "scene of human beauty," one given artistic and religious sanction, as Freud remarks, by so many representations of the Madonna and Child, Freud has also given the fantasy a psycho-biological foundation: "The organic impression of this experience—the first source of pleasure in our life—doubtless remains indelibly imprinted on us" (ibid.).

9. Sigmund Freud, "Draft L," Letter to Fliess, May 2, 1897, *SE* 1, 248. I have used here Strachey's translation from the *Standard Edition* because it gives an accurate translation of Freud's German term *Urszene* and not an interpretation of it, as Masson's translation does.

Behind the fantasy of fellatio (Freud does not claim it to be an unconscious memory—but why not ?) lies its originary reminiscence: "What the phantasy conceals is merely a reminiscence of sucking—or being suckled—at his mother's breast" (ibid.), which is presumably why Leonardo's encounter with the bird takes place in the cradle and not (as its homosexual content might warrant) in a scene from later life. However, if the scene of intimate, even aggressive, intrusion conflates a later (adult or adolescent) fantasy with an indelible infantile reminiscence of oral pleasure, Freud's location of its infantile origins leaves certain questions postponed or unanswered. What is postponed is the general psychoanalytic account of how male homosexuality supposedly arises from a particular attachment or fixation to the mother, thus allowing Freud's reduction of the fantasy to its maternal origins; but what is unanswered, indeed, not even asked, is: "Whose penis is being sucked?" If the infant's partner in the original scene is his mother, even a phallic mother, then in what sense is it a *homosexual* fantasy? If it is a homosexual fantasy, then what elided male figure, bearer of the intrusive penis, is the active partner in the "passive *homosexual* fantasy" (emphasis added) that Freud identifies but does not explore? The possibility of a disguised memory trace of sexual abuse of the child Leonardo at whatever age is not considered, although the latter had featured prominently in the material Freud had reported in the 1890s in his letters to Fliess.

At this point in Freud's analysis it might look as if, once again, the temporal structure of the fantasy is the familiar one of a retrogressive screen memory, in which a later homosexual fantasy, a scene of oral sex between Leonardo and a male partner, is being disguised in an innocent if enigmatic childhood scene. Is Leonardo's 'memory' merely a homosexual variant of Freud's 1899 fantasmatic memory of 'deflowering' disguised as a childish scene? The difference between Freud's two analyses lies in the weight he gives to Leonardo's infantile scene as a *universal* scene of origins, whose ontological and mythological importance centers on the figure of the mother. In identifying the bird as a representative of the mother, Freud in effect *reverses* the regressive logic of the screen memory by revealing behind the later homosexual fantasy an earlier archaic memory of being suckled at the breast, acclaiming it as an indelible trace of originary pleasure. This is the earliest organizing scene, Freud claims, disguised behind Leonardo's bird memory.

But why should this infantile experience be represented *in disguise* in the form of Leonardo's bird memory? At this point Freud's mistranslation of Leonardo's Italian term *nibio*, or kite, as a vulture becomes crucial.[10] Freud asks the pertinent question: "We find his mother replaced by—a vulture. Where does this vulture come from and how does it happen to be found in its present place?" (ibid., 88). The answer to Freud's first question leads to an excursus through the ancient Egyptian mythology of Mother goddesses. He notes that the Egyptian hieroglyph for the mother is a picture of a vulture and that the Egyptians worshipped a Mother goddess called *Mut* with the head of a vulture. Conceding that Leonardo could not have known this as Egyptian hieroglyphs were only decoded by the French scholar Champollion in the early nineteenth century, Freud turns to various ancient Greek and Latin treatises that report that the vulture was regarded as a symbol of motherhood because of the belief in Antiquity that only female vultures existed; there were no males of the species. They reproduced through impregnation by the wind. According to the modern editor of the treatise on hieroglyphs by Horapallo Nilous, from which Freud quotes, this fact led to the fable of the vulture's single-sex reproduction being cited widely by the Church Fathers as a proof taken from natural history of the possibility of the Virgin Conception and Birth of Christ by his mother Mary. Through this connection Freud postulates that the widely read and learned Leonardo would have been familiar with the fable of the vulture, and he attributes its interest for Leonardo to the two facts about his childhood established by scholars at the time Freud was writing. These are that, first, he was born as the illegitimate son of a certain Caterina, a peasant woman, and a distinguished notary, Ser Piero da Vinci, who married a woman of his own class, Donna Albiera, in the year of Leonardo's birth,

10. The *SE* editor in noting Freud's error attributes it to the German translations of Leonardo's text (or Merezhkovsky's fictionalized biography of Leonardo) that Freud was using. Maïdani-Gerard argues, following Laplanche's suggestion (Jean Laplanche, *Problématiques III: La sublimation* [Paris: Presses Universitaires de France 1980], 74–78), that Freud spoke and read Italian, quoting Italian sources in the original in his text, and that he had made his *own* translation of Leonardo's memorial note. Consequently, the mistranslation is a *lapsus*, or parapraxis, of Freud's, motivated by his wish to substitute an Egyptian mythology of the virgin-mother goddess, Mout, for the more pertinent Catholic theology of the Virgin Mary, for which Freud had a distaste (substituting a "Moutology" for a "Mariology," as Maïdani-Gerard puts it).

1452; and, second, that Leonardo's name appears on a tax register at the age of five, as an illegitimate son dwelling in his grandfather's house in the town of Vinci.

It is in this context that Freud answers his second question—"Why a vulture?"—and reconstructs the origin of Leonardo's vulture fantasy. Reading in one of the Church Fathers or a work of natural history, Leonardo comes across the fable of the female vulture's reproduction without the male, which rhymes with his situation as the offspring of a single mother: "a memory sprang to his mind, which was transformed into the phantasy that we have been discussing, but which meant to signify that he also had been such a vulture-child—he had had a mother but no father" (ibid., 90). Freud does not consider the implication of the legend that as a "vulture-child" Leonardo would not himself have been male. Freud's aim, he tells us, is to separate out the "real memory" that is the "real content" of the fantasy: "the replacement of his mother by the vulture indicates that the child was aware of his father's absence and found himself alone with his mother" (91). While there is no record of Leonardo's circumstances between his birth and his recorded presence at the age of five in his grandfather's house, Freud draws the following implication from the vulture fantasy: "Leonardo, it seems to tell us, spent the critical first years of his life not by the side of his father and stepmother, but with his poor, forsaken, real mother, so that he had time to feel the absence of his father" (ibid.). Freud appeals plausibly enough to the unlikelihood of the husband's illegitimate offspring being presented to a new bride at the start of the marriage (and it would be standard practice for Caterina to have acted as wet-nurse before surrendering him later on to his father). He speculates that it was only when the childlessness of Ser Piero's marriage had become apparent that little Leonardo would have been received, between the ages of three and five, into his father's and stepmother's care.

Freud's speculative construction, harmonizing the vulture fable with the bare minimum knowledge of Leonardo's early years, has a certain plausibility. It is, however, undermined by the fact that Leonardo symbolized the 'prime originator' of his early years as a kite and not as a single mother-vulture. Furthermore, the vulture fable, in which there are no male vultures, signifies not an absent father ("he had time to feel the absence of his father"), a father-shaped absence, but the absence of *all* fathers, that is, there were no fathers to be absent. Contemporary Leonardo scholarship has also established that Caterina was herself married in the same year as Leonardo's birth and his father, Ser Piero's, marriage. So the picture of the "poor, forsaken real mother" with whom Leonardo found himself alone as a husband-substitute for his first three to five years is also thrown into question by Caterina's rapid marriage to another man and birth of a daughter. Of course the psychological significance of the recorded facts cannot be inferred from their bare record, and it might well be the case that Caterina's relation to the distinguished and wealthy Ser Piero was a precious one whose loss was much regretted, and that her relation to their son was an intensely invested one, despite her new husband and baby daughter. We know nothing about Caterina's state of mind. Leonardo's fantasmatic memory of the *kite* throws no obvious light on these questions. However, as psychoanalytic commentators both before and after Meyer Schapiro's critique of Freud have pointed out, a fable of the kite does appear in Leonardo's *Notebooks*, in which it is an emblem of Envy, who "when it sees its young ones growing too big in the nest, out of envy, it pecks their sides, and keeps them without food."[11] While this negative image of the mother is only one element in Leonardo's quite extensive writing about kites, with whose habits and abilities he was fascinated (and it is a recorded piece of folklore rather than part of Leonardo's scientific discourse), nevertheless, this negative image of the kite as jealous parent is part of the associational field around his choice of bird as the figure in his screen memory.

What is significant for our purposes is the psychological process that Freud proposes, in which the supposed encounter with the fable of the vulture in adulthood (or late adolescence at least) elicits a memory that is then turned into a fantasy. He does not specify the content of the memory other than to say that with it "was associated, in the only way that impressions of so great an age can find expression, an echo of the pleasure he had at his mother's breast" (ibid., 90). It is not at all clear from this bare account, however, *why* the echo of this early oral pleasure required translation into the vulture fantasy. The memory-fantasy model from the seduction theory assumes that the memory traces in question are in some way disturbing, excessive, unworked through and traumatic, and consequently the work of

11. See Wohl and Trosman 1955, 36; Eissler 1961.

fantasy as a protective fiction is required to bind and manage them. It is not clear how the vulture—even supposing it had been a vulture—does this. As a signifier of paternal absence, an absence that was provoking, even distressing (Freud infers that "the child . . . began to brood on this riddle with special intensity" [ibid., 92]), it is surprising to see it survive into the manifest content, as it were, of the memory. One might have expected the bird that supposedly substituted for the lonely mother in her abandoned state to have a compensatory if not affirmative signification for Leonardo rather than the distressing reference to his fatherless state that Freud attributes to it; otherwise the substitution would not have accomplished its protective-defensive purpose.

## Vulture into Kite

In fact, if we substitute the kite for the erroneous vulture, that is what we do find. Leonardo himself jots down the 'memory' of the kite in the upper margin of the verso of a sheet that is the last of a run of four sheets in Leonardo's unpublished *Codex Atlanticus* dealing both with the flight of birds and in particular the kite, and with the fall of homogenous bodies in an atmosphere of uniform density, all closely written and illustrated with sketches.[12] The highly personal childhood memory is a striking break in the register and continuity of his scientific discourse, for which, nevertheless, its bridging passage offers it as a personal myth of origins:

> *To write thus clearly of the kite would seem to be my destiny,* because in the earliest recollections of my infancy it seemed to me when I was in the cradle that a kite came and opened my mouth with its tail, and struck me within upon the lips with its tail many times.[13]

12. Maïdani-Gerard reproduces the four pages in their original layout with marginal glosses and sketches of birds in flight, and he gives a detailed summary of their contents so as to reproduce the precise context in which Leonardo's memory occurs and to give an interpretation of its irruption into his densely argued scientific text. See Maïdani-Gerard 1994, 23–36.
13. *The Notebooks of Leonardo da Vinci*, ed. E. MacCurdy (London: Jonathan Cape, 1938), vol. 2, 521, emphasis added.

Questo scriver si distintamente del nibio par che sia mio destino, perchè
nella mia prima recordatione della mia infantia e' mi parea che, essendo io in
cullo, che un nibio venissi a me e mi apprisse la bocca colla sua coda e molte
volte mi percuotesse con tal coda dentro alle labbra.[14]

As Eissler helpfully points out (1961, 13) the Italian "parea" is stronger than
"it seemed" and should be "appeared" or "became visible" (Maïdani-Gerard
makes much of this point which, he argues, gives the memory the status of
a vision or hallucination). Leonardo himself grounds his scientific interest
in the kite and more generally the flight of birds (to which we can add his
long-term ambition to build a flying machine, to achieve flight himself) in
this memory that has something of the force of an initiation leading to a
destiny.

Meyer Schapiro's art-historical critique of Freud's interpretation of
Leonardo's memory gives a persuasive account of the *explicit* significations
attached to the motif of the initiation of an infant in its cradle, especially
through the mouth, by symbolically significant animals. He points to an
established literary pattern or topos that is an omen of future genius and
success. While the infant Midas slept, ants filled his mouth with grains of
wheat signifying his future fabulous wealth; with the infant Plato, bees
settled on his lips signifying his future sweetness of speech and eloquence;
with the great lyric poet Stesichorus, a nightingale alighted on the sleeping
infant's mouth; with Pindar—and, later, St. Ambrose of Milan—swarms of
bees were said to have deposited wax on his lips or entered his mouth as a
hive. Schapiro persuasively establishes this as a topos of inspiration and
predicted greatness.[15] Leonardo's screen memory seems to fit this legendary and celebratory formula, with the role of initiator played by the kite,
the bird whose prowess in flight was the object of his fascination and extended study. It was inevitable for Leonardo that the kite as initiator and
inspiration would be his model in his ambition to imitate the flight of birds.
Consequently he boasts in a lyrical anticipation of success that transforms

14. Leonardo da Vinci, *Codex Atlanticus*, F.65v. Quoted in Freud 1910c, 82.
15. Meyer Schapiro, "Freud and Leonardo: An Art Historical Study," *Journal of the History of Ideas* 17, no. 2 (1956): 147–78,, reprinted in Meyer Schapiro, *Theory and Philosophy
of Art: Style, Artist and Society* (New York: George Braziller, 1994), esp. 160–64.

the infantile scene of passivity and aggressive intrusion into an apotheosis in which Leonardo will achieve flight and assume the heavens:

> The great bird will take its first flight upon the back of its Great Swan; it will fill the universe with stupefaction and all writings with renown, and be the eternal glory of the nest where it was born.[16]

Maïdani-Gerard devotes a valedictory Coda to Leonardo's fantasy of apotheosis, locating it in the shorter Codex on the Flight of Birds, where it appears in two forms: first a prose announcement of the proposed flight on the final page, and then on the opposing inside cover a more riddling and poetic proclamation, made up of rhythmically repeated phrases, half-rhymes and internal echoes.[17] The "great bird" is Leonardo's flying machine and the "Great Swan" is Monte Ceceri (*'cecero'* is the Italian for swan), the hill outside Florence where he made his attempts at flight. The kite's initiatory visitation to Leonardo in his cradle, understood as an omen of success, is a fitting fantasmatic prelude to the magnitude of Leonardo's later ambition—to be the first man to achieve the power of flight.

Schapiro has established what he called, after Freud's dream theory, the "manifest content" of Leonardo's kite memory as a fantasy of initiation and empowerment, while he declined to consider its *unconscious* meanings and resonances. To explain the need for the formation of a screen memory, however, some account needs to be given of the disturbing unconscious processes that formed it, the memory traces, emotional complexes that needed to be translated, whether repressed or transformed by the compensatory fantasy of empowerment in the form of a memory. Freud's translation of the manifest scene or 'screen' of the bird's visitation into the universal infantile situation of suckling, for all the indelibility of its pleasures, does *not* provide this motivation. However, in addition to the scene of suckling, he adds a second infantile scene, which is derived not from the identity of the bird as 'vulture' but from its aggressive and intrusive actions toward the child: ". . . and opened my mouth with its tail, and struck me within upon the lips many times" (da Vinci, 521). The Italian phrase, here

16. Freud (1910c) *SE* 11, 125.
17. Maïdani-Gerard prints both versions as part of his persuasive analysis of Leonardo's animating fantasy and its multiple identifications (1994, 277–81).

somewhat awkwardly translated by MacCurdy as "within upon the lips," is *"dentro alle labbra."* Renato Almansi, cited by Eissler, gives the literal translation as "and struck me with such a tail inside of the lips many times" (Eissler 1961, 13). Herzfeld's German translation quoted by Freud has *"gegen meine Lippen,"* translated by the *Standard Edition,* as "against my lips."[18] What is at stake here is the insistence in Leonardo's original Italian on the penetration of the mouth, the breaking in of the infant's bodily boundaries and, unlike the legendary gifts of grain, wax, or honey, the aggressive occupation of its inner body space: "struck me . . . inside of the lips many times." Leonardo's 'memory' registers verbally the note of aggression and excess— *"me percuotesse,"* "struck me"—even as it frames it within the legendary formula of inspiration and predicted greatness.

## The Return of Seduction

In the framework of his vulture translation, Freud infers from the vulture's actions "the intensity of the erotic relations between mother and child" (1910c, 107). From the combination of maternal activity and "the prominence of the mouth zone," he infers that "a second memory is contained in the phantasy." Given his starting point in the mother-vulture equation, he reconstructs this second scene thus:

> This may be translated: 'My mother pressed innumerable passionate kisses on my mouth.' The phantasy is compounded from the memory of being suckled and being kissed by his mother. (1910c, 107)

After his analysis of two of Leonardo's greatest paintings (which will be considered in the next chapter), Freud returns to this inferred scene of maternal seduction, the excessive maternal sexualization of the child: "the violence of the caresses" that was "fateful for him; it determined his destiny and the privations that were in store for him" (1910c, 115–16). This seductive excess is contextualized by Freud in terms of his inferred narrative of

18. Maïdani-Gerard (1994, 3–19) gives a detailed presentation and examination of both the Italian and the German translations of the phrase, including Herzfeld's two variant translations.

maternal abandonment: "Like all unsatisfied mothers, she took her little son in place of her husband, and by the too early maturing of his erotism robbed him of a part of his masculinity" (ibid., 117). This somewhat cryptic formulation with its combination of premature ripening and virtual castration ("robbed him of a part of his masculinity") refers to the thesis of Leonardo's maternal fixation, and the consequent absence of an actual sex life that supposedly resulted from the repression of his intense maternal attachment. This is central to Freud's account of the adult Leonardo's sexuality.

This picture of an excessive, even traumatizing, maternal seduction certainly provides a possible motivation for the defensive formation of a screen memory. The latter's function would be to harness and sublimate the continuing pressure, the *internal attack* of that seductive memory, into a compensatory fantasy of inspiration and empowerment by the kite with its exemplary powers of flight, along the lines described by Schapiro, while defensively 'screening out'—repressing—the untranslatable elements that resisted such a defensive revision. Leonardo's fantasy of the kite licensed and energized a scientific discourse and project in which the secret of the kite's aerial acrobatics provided the model for a human flying machine. Leonardo's scientific ambition is itself marked at every point by fantasy: the world will be stupefied, the records filled with its renown and "the great bird . . . will be the eternal glory of the nest where it was born" (ibid., 125). While this last statement can be taken simply to say that the success of the flying machine will reflect credit on its creator, the narcissistic 'high' of its rhetorical crescendo, with its "great bird" and its glorified "nest," speaks the same symbolic language as Leonardo's memorial fantasy with its cradle and the visitation of its own great bird, the originary kite; for the nest, where the adult Leonardo's great bird, his flying machine, and its dream of flying were born, was his kite-visited cradle and the complexities of his infantile situation, however we now reconstruct the latter.

Freud's reconstruction of Leonardo's screen memory and its complexities, despite the error, or *lapsus*, of the vulture and its Egyptological detour, is of considerable interest. It is, as Jean Laplanche observes, one of the rare reappearances of early infantile seduction in Freud's work *after* the abandonment of the seduction theory, although he goes on to add the caveat that it entails merely the factual recognition of maternal seduction rather than a return to the theory of seduction as such.[19] However, *pace* Laplanche, this is not entirely the case, for while the seduction theory is not explicitly invoked as such, Freud's analysis involves a belated implementation of the neglected possibility of the *progressive* screen memory, avoided in all his writings dedicated explicitly to the screen memory phenomenon, which had been explored hitherto only in its retrogressive form. We have here in Leonardo's progressive screen memory the orphan or unrecognized heir of the seduction theory, in which an initial seductive and traumatizing inscription or implantation (to use Laplanche's term) in an originary infantile moment (or 'primal scene', in Freud's particular usage) is reworked in a later moment of translation and binding of the resurgent infantile traces and excitations. Unlike the retrogressive screen memory, Freud's analysis of the memorial fantasy of the 'vulture' does indeed constitute, in Laplanche's words, a "resurfacing of the model of afterwardsness or the two-phase trauma" (Laplanche 1993, 96). In one way at least it represents a development of the seduction theory, as Freud pays some attention to the subjectivity of the seductive other, the nature of the mother's situation and desires (whatever the problems and errors of his reconstruction), in a way that he does not do in the cases of Emma, Miss Lucy R., and the clinical material of the seduction theory.


*Primal Scene as Screen Memory*


Laplanche comments on Leonardo's fantasmatic memory of the bird: "There has been so much interest . . . about which real event it corresponded to, that it has quite simply not been seen for what it is: not a repressed unconscious memory, but a screen memory, to which the model of memorisation as distorting and repressing applies fairly exactly" (1993, 96); and, indeed, it has, as I have tried to demonstrate, the temporal structure of the *progressive* screen memory, the unacknowledged heir of the seduction theory in its later, more developed, but unpublished, version (Draft L and the associated letters to Fliess, discussed in Chapter 4). Laplanche applies to it the model

19. Jean Laplanche, "Sublimation and/or Inspiration," *New Formations* 48 (Winter 2002–3): 44.

of enigmatic signification developed from his revisionary critique of Freud's seduction theory in his General Theory of Primal Seduction. In this model the ordinary gestures of child care and nurturing, which target the child's body in meeting its physical and psychological needs, are carriers of excitations, feelings, and fantasies deriving from the parents' unconscious sexuality. This renders them enigmatic not only to the infantile recipient, who has no means to understand and translate the intensities conveyed, but also to the senders, from whose repressed unconscious they emanate.[20] It is this unconscious, enigmatic dimension of the parental messages targeting the infant's body that provokes the infant's attempts to bind and translate them into its own signifying sequences, 'infantile sexual theories,'[21] fantasies of flying, and so on. The violence of Caterina's caresses, postulated by Freud, constitutes just such enigmatic signifiers whose signification "is partly sexual, perverse, unknown to the mother herself" (Laplanche 1993, 97). In the recipient's attempts to master and assimilate these seductive and traumatizing implantations, "the enigmatic messages of adults undergo a reorganisation, a dislocation. Some aspects of them are translated, while some anamorphotic elements are excluded from translation and become unconscious" (ibid.). The results of this process are, at the conscious level, the fable of the bird, which as a screen memory has the sublimatory and defensive functions described earlier and, at the unconscious level, elements that remain exciting, disturbing, and provoking: "something that turns around a smile, the penetrative kiss . . . a veritable source-object of the drive and of a part of Leonardo's creativity" (ibid., 98).[22]

Maïdani-Gerard, whose book on Leonardo began life as a doctoral thesis supervised by Jean Laplanche at the University of Paris, and who situ-

20. Jean Laplanche, *New Foundations for Psychoanalysis* (Oxford: Basil Blackwell, 1989), esp. chap. 3.
21. Freud, "On the Sexual Theories of Children" (1908c), *SE* 9.
22. Ibid., 98. Laplanche's portmanteau term "source-object" is a transformation of the notions of the 'source of the drive' and the 'object of the drive' in Freud's theory of the sexual drives. For Laplanche it is an object that has become a source: an external signifying element or object that has been translated—"dislocated and reorganised"— through processes of sublimation and repression, into an internal object that acts as the source of the drive, in Leonardo's case to do with the mouth, the enigmatic smile, and the penetrative kiss.

ates his interpretation of Leonardo's childhood memory of the kite in the context of Laplanche's General Theory of Seduction, nevertheless rejects the identification of the scene with the kite as a screen memory. He appeals to the brutality of the kite's action as an act of violent and violating seduction: "a kite came and opened my mouth with its tail, and struck me with such a tail inside of the lips many times" (to cite Almansi's corrected translation, quoted in Eissler 1961 , 13). This brutality, Maïdani-Gerard argues, suggests an interpretation of the scene of the kite "not so much as a 'screen memory'—remodelled and belatedly rendered innocent—as the emergence as if in a raw state of an originary fantasy; here a fantasy of seduction where the male infant becomes the passive object of the aggression of a phallic mother" (Maïdani-Gerard 1994, 11, my translation). Picking up also on Almansi's point that Leonardo's Italian text does not say, as the French and English translations have it, "it seemed to me" but rather "it appeared to me" (*è mi parea ché*), Maïdani-Gerard argues that Leonardo "insists on an event of the order of the figurable, close to a perception, to a dream-vision: a fantasy crudely re-evoked, rather than a screen memory" (ibid., 15, my translation). The scene's qualities of aggressive activity, even violation, and its status as a perceptual and figural reality, a vision or hallucination, as precisely a *scene* (not so much a subjective seeming as an objective appearing), are Maïdani-Gerard's grounds for arguing *against* Laplanche, that rather than a screen memory it is the irruption of an unconscious element, a virtually unprocessed primal or originary representation of seduction in a 'raw' state.

Maïdani-Gerard's argument raises a number of questions. With all formations of the unconscious there is an often undecidable balance or imbalance between conscious elements and the unconscious elements that invest them, as in dreams with their recent 'day's residues' and the archaic infantile scenarios they stand in for, or the repressing and repressed elements that make up the compromise formation of the neurotic symptom. With Leonardo's fantasmatic memory, however, it is clear that the scene is *not* a simple or an unmediated transcription of infantile experience. The very transposition into *a scene with a kite* indicates the symbolic working over of fantasy, and this accords with Freud's comments on the genesis of the wish to fly and his description of the fantasy of flying, with its phallic symbolism of the bird, as a common infantile response to the hints and premonitions of adult sexual activity. Such a translation into the symbolic language of birds indicates the desexualizing work of sublimation; however, this sublimatory symbolization is indeed *compromised* by the qualities that Maïdani-Gerard rightly points to, the intrusive and intimate aggression coming from the kite with its perceptual intensity. This intensity of figuration, however, does not constitute grounds for ruling out the idea of a screen memory, as Freud's analysis (1899a), discussed in Chapter 4, of his own apparent childhood memory of the vivid yellow flowers and the delicious bread, with their heightened, almost hallucinatory, perceptual elements, indicates. The prophetic formula of the infant genius fertilized through the mouth by preternatural agents, established by Meyer Schapiro, is also at work to harness and sublimate the more disturbing sexual elements into a narcissistically confirming and compensatory promise of future greatness. It is this sublimatory legend that manages the seductive violence and intensities that Freud infers and Maïdani-Gerard points to.

## Flying and Painting: Leonardo's Rival Sublimations

To recapitulate, in the previous chapter I argued that in his analysis of Leonardo's fantasmatic childhood 'memory,' Freud has described a complex psychological process that consists of a sequence of moments or levels. Starting from Leonardo's adult scientific preoccupations, especially with the flight of birds (and the associated possibility of building a flying machine), which diverted attention and energy from his pursuit of painting, Freud moves back to the moment of the recollection and recording of the bird memory in Leonardo's scientific notebooks. As the *Standard Edition* translates, "Leonardo inserts a piece of information about his childhood" into his discourse on the flight of 'vultures': "he suddenly interrupts himself to pursue a memory from very early years which had sprung to his mind" (82).[1] What emerges or erupts here in the process of Leonardo's writing

---

1. *Leonardo da Vinci and a Memory of His Childhood*, SE 11 [1910c], 82). Maïdani-Gerard points out that the translation of the verb by 'inserts' in the *Standard Edition* loses

has, Freud goes on to speculate, been formed in an earlier moment of his reading (his encounter with the Church Fathers on the subject of the vulture myth and the Virgin Birth, in which an infantile memory was aroused and turned into the fantasy of the 'vulture'). The internal structure of this formation is that of a scenic palimpsest in which one scene is sedimented beneath another. Behind the imagined scene itself of the bird's visitation of Leonardo in his cradle, with its intimate intrusion into the infant's mouth and aggressive occupation of its inner body space, lies (1) the unlocated and unexplored homosexual fantasy of fellatio, behind which again Freud reconstructs the double scene of maternal seduction, (2) the "innumerable passionate kisses" and "the violence of the caresses" that follow from (3) the suckling at the breast, with its drama of the absent father and the abandoned mother, and we also need to insert into this sequence (4) the infantile fantasy of flying that translates, according to Freud, the infant's encounter with adult sexuality (the primal scene of parental intercourse, in the later psychoanalytic usage restricted to the question of content). This roots the symbolism of the bird in infantile experience, as the first childhood sublimation that is the support for the later adult sublimations of Leonardo's scientific discourse.[2] The driving, determining power of this sequence is the seductive, fixating infantile scene with the violence of its maternal caresses, acting through the successive translations and sublimations of the bird symbolism. In particular, the later scientific discourse of the bird and the fantasy of human flight, authorized by Leonardo's personal myth of initiation by the kite, had the function of translating, that is, both repressing and sublimating, different elements of that originary traumatic experience of maternal seduction, and of managing the continuing excitations that arose from it.

---

Freud's metaphor: *"Leonardo hat . . . eingestreut"*—Leonardo scatters, throws, intersperses—which along with 'interrupts' and 'emerges' (instead of the *SE*'s "springs to mind") implies a previous 'submerging' and suggests a process that is instantaneous rather than considered and premeditated. See Jean-Pierre Maïdani-Gerard, *Léonard de Vinci: Mythologie ou théologie* (Paris: Presses Universitaires de France, 1994), 29–30.

2. "Whenever children feel . . . there is something wonderful of which adults are capable but which *they* are forbidden to know and do, they are filled with a violent wish to be able to do it, and they dream of it in the form of flying, or they prepare this disguise of their wish to be used in their later flying dreams" (1910c, 26). However, this fantasy of the parental primal scene seems at odds with Freud's thesis of the absent father.

*The Bird and the Smile: Leonardo's Rival Sublimations*

Freud gives an account of Leonardo's rival sublimations of his infantile sexual fantasies and scenarios in the competing adult activities of painting and scientific research. Significantly, this locates the symbolic element of the bird exclusively in relation to Leonardo's scientific ambitions. The chain of connections is clear, linking the infantile 'memory' of the kite to the scientific work on the flight of birds (which was the original point of Leonardo's memorandum). Freud inserts into this sequence the fantasy of flying, formed in response to the young child's premonitions of adult sexual activity, as the unconscious support of Leonardo's later adult ambition to build a flying machine. However, neither the primal scene with the kite nor its avian avatars will feature directly in Freud's analysis of Leonardo's two masterpieces, the *Mona Lisa* and the *St. Anne with Two Others*[3] in the Louvre. Indeed, by contrast with Leonardo's extensive studies of the flight of birds (and bats), the figure of the bird, with one major exception, does not seem to feature in Leonardo's pictorial oeuvre at all. If the bird (whether kite, vulture, or whatever else) were predominantly a maternal symbol for Leonardo, as Freud claims, one might have expected to find it as an accessory element in one of his Madonnas or female portraits (a hypothetical *Lady with a Canary* or a *Madonna of the Doves*). Birds appear nowhere in Leonardo's paintings, however, with the one striking exception of *Leda and the Swan* (Figure 1). The possible relation between Leonardo's 'memory' of the kite with the intrusive tail as a scene of seduction and the painting of Zeus's rape of Leda in the form of a swan would indeed have been worth exploring. Freud chose not to do so, for while the scene is clearly one of seduction, if not rape, the swan, with its sinuous neck, questing beak, and embracing wing, is clearly a highly sexualized *male* phallic figure with a distinctly humanoid character, and this would have taken Freud away from his identification of the bird figure as maternal (however phallic). The difference between Leonardo's kite and swan is marked by the fact that the

---

3. This is the SE's translation of the German title of the painting, *'Heilege Anna Selbdrit.'* It is titled in the Louvre catalogue, *The Virgin and Child with St. Anne.* For a discussion of the topos inscribed in the German title, see page 90 in this chapter, and Maïdani-Gerard (1994, 97–101).

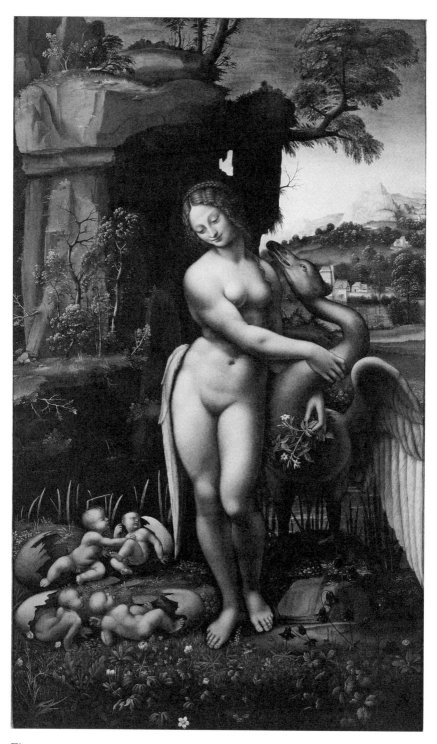

Figure 1
*Leda and the Swan*, Francesco Melzi *after* Leonardo da Vinci Uffizi
Gallery, Florence. PD-Art (Wikimedia Commons)

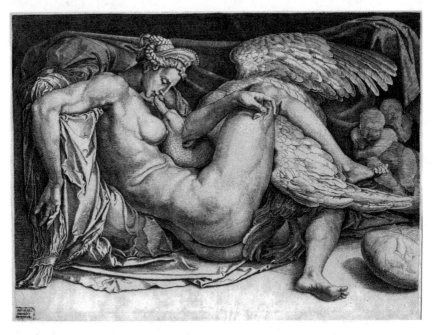

Figure 2
*Leda and the Swan*, Cornelis Bos engraving *after* Michelangelo British
Museum, London © Trustees of the British Museum

swan is not in a *flying* posture but standing upright with the rim of his right
wing embracing Leda and visible along the curve of her thigh (Is this a
short man in a swan suit?), unlike the aerial acrobatics of the kite detailed
in Leonardo's studies.

Michelangelo's treatment of the same subject (Figure 2), lost like Leonardo's and known only through copies, differs strikingly from the latter's,
for Michelangelo's swan 'flies' with spread wings between the prone Leda's
open thighs and with its beak between her lips. The paintings Freud chose
instead to comment on, while discussed in relation to the theme of seduction, have no overt symbolic connection with Leonardo's primal scene with
the kite, like the greater part of his pictorial oeuvre, which remains a virtually bird-free zone.

The importance Freud assigns to Leonardo's screen memory, and the
childhood experiences encoded within it, bears on both Leonardo's rival
sublimations, the artistic and the scientific and the interference of the latter

with the former, "as if the key to all his achievements and misfortunes lay hidden in the childhood phantasy of the vulture" (1910c, 136). However, he proposes a hierarchy of sublimations in which the pictorial comes later at puberty, while the investigative is connected to libido "that evades repression by being sublimated *from the beginning* into curiosity" (ibid., 80, emphasis added). This formulation of an original sublimation is taken from Freud's discussion of three possible outcomes or pathways that radiate out from the repression of the early childhood 'sexual researches' or 'sexual theories': 1. intellectual inhibition, 2. compulsive but inconclusive brooding, 3. transference of the libido from sexual to nonsexual matters, which he calls 'sublimation from the beginning.' Consequently, Leonardo's midlife turning away from his art, when he becomes, in the words of a contemporary report, "obsessed with geometry, being most disgruntled with the brush,"[4] is explained by Freud as a regression from the secondary to the original sublimation:

> The development that had turned him into an artist at puberty was overtaken by the process that led him to be an investigator, and which had its determinants in early infancy. The second sublimation of his erotic instinct gave place to the original sublimation for which the way had been prepared on the occasion of the first repression. (Freud 1910c, 133)

The two paintings Freud describes, however, are *not* derivatives of the screen memory of the kite, and each has a different relation to the scenes of seduction that lie hidden behind it, a relation *not* mediated by the symbolism of the bird, its aggression, its phallic ambition, and Leonardo's consequent investigative drive. The implications of these two different paths from originary seduction to sublimatory end result call into question the hierarchy of sublimations that Freud proposes on purely chronological grounds, as we shall see.

Freud's chapter devoted to the paintings begins by revisiting Leonardo's 'memory' where, to the universal scene of suckling, he adds the particular drama of maternal abandonment and seduction: "My mother pressed innumerable passionate kisses on my mouth" (1910c, 107). This double scene

4. The report of Fra Pietro da Novellara to Isabella d'Este, who was eager for a painting by Leonardo, after his return to Florence from Milan. See Martin Kemp, *Leonardo da Vinci: The Marvellous Works of Nature and Man* (Oxford: Oxford University Press, 2006), 207.

of the aggressively kissed and suckled mouth of the infant Leonardo leads metonymically to the motif of the mysterious Leonardo smile and its centrality to his chosen paintings. Two different symbolic chains or sequences are at stake here. The one sublimates the scene of seduction in the direction of scientific investigation:

> Suckling/penetrative kissing of the mouth (the mother's tongue in the mouth ?)—the bird's tail beating inside the mouth—the tail/penis equation—initiation into birdlike/phallic activity via the mouth—the fantasy of flying—investigation of the kite and its powers of flight (esp. the activity of its tail)—the ambition to fly and the building of a flying machine.

The other sequence sublimates the scene of seduction in the direction of painting:

> Suckling/kissing the mouth—the kiss/smile/gaze of the mother who fondles the infant ("the violence of her caresses")—the smile/gaze of the Mona Lisa—the smiles/gazes of St. Anne and the Virgin Mary (London cartoon, Louvre painting), St. John the Baptist and Bacchus.

The symbol of the bird, which plays such a key role in giving shape and direction to Leonardo's *scientific* interests and ambitions, finds its equivalent or parallel in the alternative sequence of late-period paintings in the motif of the mysterious smile and the accompanying gaze that seems to focus the expression of his *artistic* interests. This motif will be central to Freud's analysis.

Freud's account of the *Mona Lisa* centers on the represented smile of the sitter (he says nothing about any other features of the portrait). It is introduced as an example of the more general phenomenon of the 'Leonardesque' smile to be found across a number of his late paintings: "a remarkable smile, at once fascinating and puzzling, which he conjured up on the lips of his female subjects. It is an unchanging smile, on long curved lips" (1910c, 107). As instanced in the *Mona Lisa*, the motif of the smile is felt to be peculiarly enigmatic, and Freud assembles a small anthology of comments and responses through which to approach the enigma, as if to secure through an apparent consensus some objective grounding of the range of intense subjective effects produced in the (male) viewer by such an elusive image. He traces the enigma to "the idea that two distinct elements are combined in Mona Lisa's smile" (ibid., 108), though these elements are drawn from the commentators' responses rather than from a specification and analysis of the aesthetic features of the painting itself. The combination or alternation of contradictory features includes coldness and seductiveness (Muther), tenderness and coquetry, modesty and sensuousness, reserve and radiance (Müntz quoting de Corlay), kindness and cruelty (Conti), all organized under the topos of the "essence of femininity" (de Corlay) and its traditional theme of femininity as deceit, veil, enigma, "the will to seduce and ensnare," together with more recent Darwinian inflections: "her instincts of conquest, of ferocity, all the heredity of the species" (108–9). Freud's summary of this consensus, however, adds an element of his own: "the contrast between reserve and seduction, and between the most devoted tenderness and a sensuality that is ruthlessly demanding—consuming men as if they were alien beings" (108). Freud here takes to a lurid extreme the figure of the femme fatale as a ruthless consumer of men, sexual difference as predatory otherness and alienness.

Initially he sees the figure of Mona Lisa as presenting a truth, an essence of femininity: "the contrasts which dominate the erotic life of women" (ibid.). However, the main line of Freud's argument will be that the *Mona Lisa* figures not the "the erotic life of women" but, in the words he quotes from Pater's famous celebration of the painting, "what in the ways of a thousand years men had come to desire," that is, not the representation of female desire but of male heterosexual desire, that is, a desiring male fantasy of the woman. In particular, Freud combines Pater's suggestion, that "from childhood, we see this image defining itself on the fabric of his dreams" (ibid., 110), with Konstantinowa's argument that it was Leonardo's encounter with his sitter, Mona Lisa del Gioconda, and her enigmatic smile,[5] that led to its repetition in the figures of St. John the Baptist and especially the Virgin Mary and St. Anne with the Christ Child. This enables Freud to propose the speculative hypothesis of a genetic process that relates the *Mona Lisa* to the other late paintings via the reference back to Leonardo's childhood and in particular to his reconstruction of the

---

5. For a recent scholarly account of the del Gioconda family and the identity of Leonardo's sitter, see Giuseppi Pallanti, *Mona Lisa: The True Identity of Leonardo's Model*, trans. Tim Stroud (Milan: Skira Editore, 2006).

originary maternal seduction on the other side of the screen memory of the kite's visitation.

## Infantile Fantasy and the Creative Process

Two years previously in his essay "Creative Writers and Day-Dreaming" (1908e), Freud had sought to model the role of fantasy in the writing process and its relation to time: "We may say that it hovers, as it were, between three times."[6] In the first moment, "some provoking occasion in the present" arouses "one of the subject's major wishes." This refers back to the second moment of an infantile memory "in which this wish was fulfilled." In the third moment, this process creates "a situation relating to the future which represents a fulfilment of the wish" (ibid., 147). Freud summarizes it as a process in which "the wish makes use of an occasion in the present to construct, on the pattern of the past, a picture of the future" (148). A certain ambiguity, however, haunts Freud's formulations in the essay, as he had begun by proposing as a general principle that "the motive forces of phantasies are *unsatisfied* wishes" (146, emphasis added), before going on to speak of the infantile experience that provides a model or pattern as one in which the wish had been fulfilled. The wish in question throughout all three moments appears to be the same—"one of the subject's major wishes"— which seems to refer to some permanent, quasi-structural element of the writer's subjectivity, dating back to an infantile wish that remains lodged at the very core of the personality. In a final summary Freud speaks of the infantile experience as one "from which there now proceeds a wish which finds expression in the creative work" (149).

The first ambiguity is the role of the infantile: Does it contribute the *unsatisfied* wishes necessary to create the fantasy ("a happy person never fantasies, only an unsatisfied one" (146), or does it contribute the experience of an actual *wish fulfillment* that provides the pattern or model of the future situation of fulfillment that is the fantasy? Freud's hypothetical example of the orphan boy who imagines a future in which he marries the boss's daughter and comes to inherit the business, thus regaining his lost

6. Freud, "Creative Writers and Day-Dreaming," *SE* 9, 147.

childhood happiness of home and parents, in effect locates the unsatisfied wish in the present and the fulfillment in the past as a model for the future. This raises the second ambiguity as to the location of the unsatisfied wish that drives the formation of the fantasy. This is the issue that dogged Freud in his oscillations over the temporal structure of the seduction theory and was replayed in the dialogue between analyst and fictional analysand in his 1899 "Screen Memories" essay. In the model of the dream, it is very clearly the infantile wish that is the 'capitalist' of the dream, which supplies the drive energy that funds its formation and that is transferred to the recent impressions of the day's residues. In the model of the regressive screen memory, however, it is the wishful fantasy of the later moment that borrows the earlier infantile experience to model its disguised fulfillment.

Is it the later wishful fantasy of the present moment that drives and fuels the artwork, only borrowing the infantile wish fulfillment as its pattern or *mise-en-scène*, or is it the primordial infantile wish at the heart of the adult personality? If so, does it contribute its *dissatisfaction* as a motivating force rather than its experience of *fulfillment* as a pattern and model? These ambiguities return also to haunt Freud's account of Leonardo's late paintings and their mysterious and seductive power.

## Leonardo's Primal Objects

> . . . some heads of laughing women . . . and some children's heads . . .
> —GIORGIO VASARI, *Lives of the Artists* (1568)[7]

The same temporal structure of three moments, the present awakening the past as a model of an imagined future, is the conceptual backbone of Freud's genetic hypothesis: "It may well have been that Leonardo was fascinated by Mona Lisa's smile for the reason that it awoke something in him which had long lain dormant in his mind—probably an old memory." The power of this memory was such "for him never to get free of it when it had once been aroused; he was continually forced to give it new expression" (1910c, 110). This tripartite time structure is then tied to a specific theme

7. Quoted in Freud (1910c, *SE* 11, p. 111).

via the coincidence Freud notes between, on the one hand, Vasari's report of Leonardo's earliest artistic creations—"he made some heads of laughing women out of clay . . . and some children's heads which were as beautiful as if they had been modelled by the hand of a master"—and, on the other, "the two kinds of sexual objects that we have inferred from the analysis of his vulture-phantasy" (ibid., 111). The theme is the seductive and erotic power of the mother in relation to the child: "We begin to suspect the possibility that it was his mother who possessed the mysterious smile—the smile that he had lost" (ibid.). This convergence of theme and time structure gives Freud the substance of the genetic connection that he proposes between the *Mona Lisa* and *St. Anne with Two Others.*

> It would best agree with our expectations if it was the intensity of Leonardo's preoccupation with the features of Mona Lisa which stimulated him to create the composition of St. Anne out of his phantasy. For if the Gioconda's smile called up in his mind the memory of his mother, it is easy to understand how it drove him at once to create a glorification of motherhood, and to give back to his mother the smile he had found in the noble lady. We may therefore permit our interest to pass from Mona Lisa's portrait to this other picture. (Freud 1910c, 112)

Freud describes Leonardo's artistic intention in *St. Anne* as "a glorification of motherhood," not surprising for a painting of the Madonna and Child. However, the painting contains *two* mothers, both the Virgin Mary and *her* mother, St. Anne (figure 3), in an iconographical motif known in Italian as the *Anna Metterza* (*Anna Selbdrit* in German, *Anna te Drieën* in Dutch, *Anna Samatreti* in Czech, for which Jean Laplanche suggests the French neologism *Sainte-Anne-en-tierce*).[8] The adjective—a hapax or designation that is used only in this one instance—signifies the third, who makes up a set of three. Lacking an English equivalent, the *Standard Edition* translates the German *'Heilege Anna Selbdrit'* as *'St. Anne with Two Others.'* Both Schapiro and Maïdani-Gerard locate this motif in the history of the development of the cult of St. Anne and its associated theological controversies about the doctrine of the Immaculate Conception of Mary, free from Original Sin, by

8. See Maïdani-Gerard (1994, 97–101) for a lexicographical commentary on these terms.

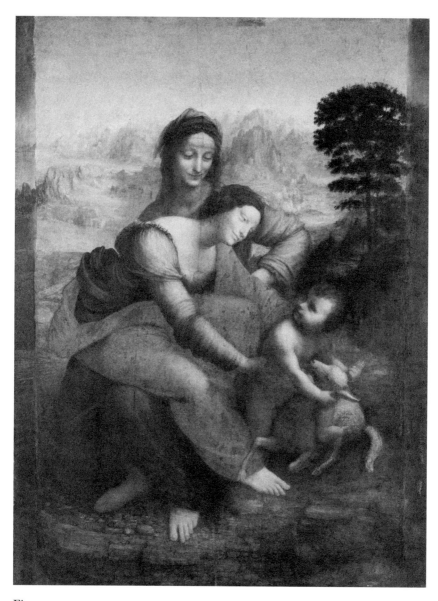

Figure 3
*Leonardo da Vinci*, The Virgin and Child with St. Anne
Louvre, Paris. PD-Art (Wikimedia Commons)

her mother St. Anne.[9] Following Schapiro's lead, Maïdani-Gerard gives an extensive account of its theological contexts and the iconographical variet- ies of the *Anna Metterza* motif in medieval and early Renaissance paintings. Freud seems to have been largely ignorant of the coherence and theological underpinnings of the motif. He takes it as the basis, however, for an analy- sis of the fantasy structure of the painting, and, in particular, with regard to the presence of the two mothers overseeing the small male child, he proposes that "the picture contains the synthesis of the history of his [Leonardo's—JF] childhood" (Freud 1910c, 112).

The synthesis in question is embodied in a particular configuration of the two mothers in relation to the child Jesus who is the object of their double maternal gaze. First, as a mother-grandmother couple, Mary and St. Anne reference Leonardo's own "childhood watched over by mother and grandmother" (ibid., 113), his stepmother, Donna Albiera, and his pa- ternal grandmother, Monna Lucia, both residing in the family household into which he was received. Second, St. Anne, while "portrayed as being a little more mature and serious than the Virgin Mary," is still "a young woman of unfaded beauty" (ibid.). This perception of St. Anne's youthful countenance is supported by Maïdani-Gerard's detailed observations of the women's headgear. Traditionally, St. Anne is portrayed as a matron equipped with a wimple and veil, while the Virgin is bareheaded, a sartorial difference that signifies their different ages and statuses. In the slightly earlier London Cartoon, which reworks the Anna Metterza iconography, both women dress their hair in a similar fashion with a light veil, worn slightly back from the hairline, and they are indistinguishable in two of the four surviving preliminary sketches, while in the other two a markedly aged St. Anne wears a heavy turbanlike headdress. In the Louvre painting we are discussing, the last in the series, St. Anne wears neither wimple nor turban but the same light veil worn previously by both women, while the Virgin appears to be bareheaded. Leonardo attenuates the age-related dif- ferences without abolishing them entirely (see Maïdani-Gerard 1994, 252).

This relative contemporaneity of the two mothers, Freud suggests, par- allels another aspect of Leonardo's childhood circumstances; as well as a

9. This doctrine is often confused by those ignorant of the Catholic tradition of Mariol- ogy with the doctrine of the Virgin Birth of Jesus from Mary.

mother and grandmother, he had two young mothers, Caterina, his birth mother from whom he was taken away, and his young, childless stepmother, Albiera. These two sets of two are synthesized or condensed, Freud suggests, into the composite unity of the Anna Metterza scene. This condensation of three into two is further supported by Maïdani-Gerard's observation that in two preparatory sketches *three* female heads can be seen, unclearly related to a fused maternal group (those of the Venice Anna Metterza preliminary sketch, and less clearly a much earlier sketch of a "Madonna with the Cat" [Maïdani-Gerard 1994, 190, 202, 205]). Freud thus distributes the three maternal figures of Leonardo's childhood across the two figures of Leonardo's painting. St. Anne, the grandmother, the figure more distant from the young boy, references both the actual grandmother from the first set and the birth mother from the second set, leaving the figure of the Virgin Mary reaching out to catch hold of him as the reference to Albiera, the young stepmother.

In a pair of footnotes added in 1919 and 1923, Freud addresses the question of the fused maternal group. In 1919 he observes of the figures of St. Anne and Mary in the Louvre oil painting: "They are fused with each other like badly condensed dream-figures, so that in some places it is hard to say where Anne ends and where Mary begins" (1910c, 114). What from one perspective might be considered an aesthetic defect from a psychoanalytic perspective "is vindicated . . . by reference to its secret meaning . . . the two mothers of his childhood were melted into a single form" (ibid.). By 1923, however, Freud's attention had been drawn to the great London Cartoon (figure 6), which reworks the Anna Metterza motif into a very different composition from that of the Louvre painting: "Here the forms of the two mothers are fused even more closely and their separate outlines are even harder to make out, so that critics . . . have been forced to say that it seems 'as if two heads were growing from a single body'" (ibid., 115). This engagement with the earlier composition forces Freud to rethink the question of the fused maternal group in the later oil painting and he now proposes that

> Leonardo must have felt the need to *undo* the dream-like fusion of the two women—a fusion corresponding to his childhood memory—and to separate the two heads in space. . . . From the group formed by the mothers he detached Mary's head and the upper part of her body and bent them downwards. To

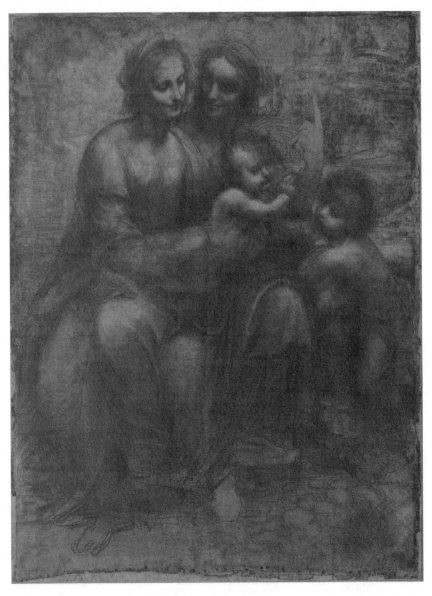

Figure 4
Leonardo da Vinci, *The Virgin and Child with St. Anne* and *St. John the Baptist*
National Gallery, London. PD-Art (Wikimedia Commons)

provide a reason for this displacement the child Christ had to come down from her lap onto the ground. There was no room for the little St. John, who was replaced by the lamb. (Freud 1910c, 114–15, emphasis added)

The later painting, in comparison to the earlier cartoon, is now the site of a process of *undoing* the "dream-like fusion" of the maternal group, and Freud locates this in the rearrangement of the figures of Mary and the child to differentiate her from St. Anne, on whose lap she somewhat awkwardly half sits in the earlier composition. This implies a progression from cartoon to painting in which the fused maternal grouping represents an earlier and more archaic psychic complex of memorial elements, representations, and associations subjected to a process of working over and differentiation, resulting in a less compacted and monumental but more dynamic later composition. This is the core of Freud's insight into Leonardo's painting, an insight that is properly psychoanalytic, drawing both on the model of the dream-work, with its primary processes of condensation and displacement in the formation of the manifest dream-scene (or pictured scene) and its figures, as well as on the paradigm of maternal seduction. The latter theme is not just applied from the outside but reworked and rethought in terms of its consequences, through Freud's engagement with both Leonardo's life and work.

## The Return of Seduction: Oedipus in Reverse

This reworking from cartoon to oil painting can be seen in the narrative of maternal seduction that Freud weaves around his commentary on the paintings. I have in a previous section commented on the premature sexualization of the young Leonardo by his mother's excessive targeting of the mouth with "the violence of her caresses," which Freud infers from the 'vulture' fantasy. This constitutes a traumatic excess that provides the insurgent inner pressure for the defensive and sublimatory formation of the screen memory of the kite. Here I will merely refer to the ambiguity that haunts Freud's account and the way it produces an overturning of the standard male oedipal paradigm. The Leonardo narrative of maternal abandonment, which involves the son taking the place of the missing husband for the unsatisfied mother and the mother taking the place of the missing father for the son, with the consequent forfeiture "of a part of his masculinity" (Freud 1910c, 117), has a puzzling conclusion. Freud segues without remark or explanation into a *generalization* of this excessive mother–infant relation, such that it exemplifies not just the abnormal peculiarity of Leonardo's situation but the mother–infant relation as such. According to Freud, the mother–infant relation of its very nature is exclusive, excessive, and perverse. If it is "in the nature of a completely satisfying love-relation" and "represents one of the attainable forms of human happiness," this is because for the infant it "not only fulfils every mental wish but also every physical need," while for the mother it offers the possibility "of satisfying, without reproach, wishful impulses which have long been repressed and which must be called perverse" (ibid.). While the contributions of Melanie Klein on the psychotic and psychoticizing dimensions of early infantile experience might suggest that Freud's description is a highly selective and idealizing account of a mother–son romance, what is notable is the way Freud builds an inescapably seductive and perverse dimension into the maternal relation in general.

Leonardo's particular narrative of father–son substitution is then matched by a *bouleversement* of the normal oedipal relations between father and son. This is a direct result of the scenario of maternal seduction. Instead of an explanatory narrative that begins with the parricidal impulses of the jealous oedipal son, as in the standard Freudian paradigm, we are told:

> In the happiest young marriage the father is aware that the baby, especially if he is a baby-son, has become his rival, and this is the starting point of an antagonism towards the favourite which is deeply rooted in the unconscious. (Freud 1910c, 117)

As Laplanche comments, here is an "anti-Oedipus," but one that is located at the very roots of the Oedipus.[10] The seductions of the mother and the antagonism of the father are accorded here a primary status, a situation in which the maternal favorite takes the place of the husband. It is as if the peculiarities of Leonardo's primal situation as reconstructed by Freud are not so much a perverse *alternative* to the norm of "the happiest young marriage" as they are its very dynamic of seduction and substitution writ large.

---

10. Jean Laplanche, *Problématiques III: La sublimation* (Paris: Presses Universitaires de France, 1980), 91.

The effect of Freud's return to and working through the problematic of seduction in the material of Leonardo's life and art is to decenter the oedipal subject and to recenter the Oedipus complex on the seductive and/or rivalrous transmissions of the parents. Through his engagement with Leonardo, Freud momentarily reverses the dominant 'Ptolemaic' model of the Oedipus, centered on the spontaneous incestuous and jealous impulses of the infant subject. He recaptures something of what I have argued in Chapter 5 is the Sophoclean drama of Oedipus with its 'Copernican' perspective, an Oedipus who is positioned by and responding blindly to the parental fate, or *tuche*, visited upon him.

### Oedipal Transgressions

> All women become like their mothers, that is their tragedy.
> No man does, that is his.
> —Oscar Wilde[11]

It is in the immediate wake of such an overturning of the oedipal paradigm that usually works to produce culturally normative outcomes that Freud pens a quite extraordinary celebration of male femininity as embodied in the two late paintings of *Bacchus* and *St. John the Baptist* (Figure 5).

> These pictures breathe a mystical air into whose secret one dares not penetrate. . . . They are beautiful youths of feminine delicacy and with effeminate forms; they do not cast their eyes down, but gaze in mysterious triumph, as if they knew of a great achievement of happiness, about which silence must be kept. The familiar smile of fascination leads one to guess that it is a secret of love. (Freud 1910c, 117)

Freud's lyrical prose poem hails these male figures as representatives of an erotic enigma, whose smiles certainly repeat and so relate them back to the figures of the Virgin and St. Anne, as do their upward pointing gestures. The latter have distinct theological meanings in traditional Catholic iconography—St. Anne referencing the absent Divine Father of the Christ

---

11. Oscar Wilde, *The Importance of Being Earnest* (Act I), in *The Importance of being Earnest and Other Plays*, (Harmondsworth: Penguin Books, 1954): 270.

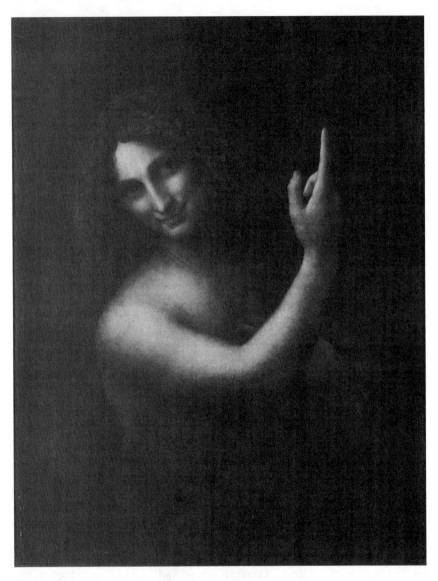

Figure 5
Leonardo da Vinci, *St. John the Baptist*
Louvre, Paris. PD-Art (Wikimedia Commons)

Child, and St. John indicating the Messiah who is to come and whose herald, preparing the way, he is. However, these late paintings seem to sit loose
with respect to the theological traditions from which they emerge, as the
repainting as Bacchus of what had formerly been another St. John, a half-
naked male figure sitting in his curious cross-legged posture, indicates.
The knowing half smiles, the softly fleshed youthfulness, and the ambiguous erotic glow that surrounds Leonardo's Baptist figures contrast strikingly with the traditional representation of St. John as a lean, muscular,
and eremitical embodiment of austerity and penitence. Freud locates their
youthful smiles in relation to "an inhibition which forbade him [Leon-
ardo—JF) ever again to desire such caresses from the lips of women"
(Freud 1910c, 117), and from which he infers the consequent "unhappiness
of his erotic life" (ibid., 118) now overcome in his art. "The great achievement of happiness, about which silence must be kept," indicates a deviant
sublimation that converts the unavailable maternal object into a cross-
gendered identification. This androgyny that clearly fascinates, one might
say even seduces, Freud in these paintings, and in the figure of Leonardo
more generally, is interpreted by him as "representing the wishes of the boy,
infatuated with his mother, as fulfilled in this blissful union of the male and
female natures" (ibid.).

## Fusion and Defusion: The Dynamics of Sublimation

If the implications of maternal seduction for Freud's metapsychology are
surprising, its implications for a psychoanalytic understanding of Leonardo's late paintings are less clear. Freud had suggested that it was St. Anne,
the maternal grandmother, who figured both Leonardo's grandmother (who
was in fact his *paternal* grandmother) and also Caterina, the abandoned and
seductive birth mother, a disturbing figure around whom a number of intense and negative feelings accumulate in Freud's account: "The artist
seemed to have used the blissful smile of St. Anne to disavow and to cloak
the envy which the unfortunate woman felt when she was forced to give up
her son to her better-born rival, as she had once given up his father as well"
(ibid., 113–14). The trouble with this is not just that the novelization of
Freud's reconstruction has no evidence whatsoever from which to infer

Caterina's feelings but, more importantly, that it has no plausible connection to either the figure of St. Anne, as represented, or with the atmosphere of serenity that characterizes the painting.

Freud himself comments that Leonardo had given the key motif of the smile to both Mary and Anne: "both are endowed with the blissful smile of the joy of motherhood" (ibid., 113). The pictorial configuration, in which Anne sits behind Mary, is interpreted by Freud, plausibly enough, as the birth mother's displacement by the stepmother. This, however, ignores the drama being enacted between Mary and the child Jesus. Freud does not comment on either of these figures, but it is clear that the difference between the cartoon and the painting involves a radically different dramatic situation in each. In the earlier cartoon, St. Anne looks toward Mary, who holds the child on her lap as he looks down toward the figure of his slightly older cousin, St. John, and blesses him. As Laplanche comments, there is a play of both fusion and defusion between Mary and her son, as well as between the two mothers:

> "The son who is soldered to the maternal couple in the drawing which is
> earlier, and who by contrast in the painting escapes, to the point where his
> mother is obliged to recapture him . . . seizes a kind of autonomy . . . but turns
> back, fascinated, towards her in the same way that, Freud supposes, Leonardo
> was fascinated by the maternal gaze and by that of Mona Lisa." (Laplanche
> 1980, 88–89, my translation)

The drama of escape and fascinated turning back that Laplanche perceptively describes develops Freud's insight into the fusion and defusion of the compositions' figures (and which is elaborated more extensively in Maïdani-Gerard's study of the whole Anna Metterza sequence of five sketches, the London Cartoon and the Louvre oil painting). This would suggest, however, that it is precisely the Virgin Mary and *not* St. Anne who represents the primal maternal figure, in Freud's account the abandoned and seductive birth mother, Caterina, in relation to whom the child's bid for autonomy and continuing fascination is played out.

A certain ambiguity also haunts the question of the smile, for while Freud asserts along with Konstantinowa that "the smile that plays on the lips of the two women is unmistakably the same as that in the picture of Mona Lisa," he also observes that "it has lost its uncanny and mysterious character; what it expresses is inward feeling and quiet blissfulness" (Freud 1910c, 112). On the one hand, it is the same smile; on the other hand, it is not. One might rather argue that while it bears a strong family resemblance to the *Mona Lisa*, it has been transformed. The difference is captured in Freud's opposition between the uncanny element of "sinister menace" in the Mona Lisa's smile and the "quiet blissfulness" of the smiles of St. Anne and the Virgin. Freud had suggested that Leonardo had "used the blissful smile of St. Anne to disavow and to cloak the envy that the unfortunate woman felt when she was forced to give up her son to her better-born rival, as she had once given up his father as well" (113–14). However, the smile of "quiet blissfulness" is shared by *both* women as Freud had earlier observed, so it would be necessary to propose that the whole composition of the painting, the Anna Metterza situation of the small son with two smiling mothers, functions to ward off or to disavow that disturbance represented by the imago of the abandoned and seductive mother. In fact, Freud's whole narrative of maternal seduction, with its inhibiting, fixating, and emasculating effects, derives from the uncanny, *unheimlich* doubleness of the Mona Lisa's smile. It is hard for it to find a purchase on the *heimlich* serenity of the St. Anne painting. Although Freud does not correlate his two observations, it would be possible to suggest a connection between the painting's *defusing* of the highly condensed maternal group of the cartoon (not to mention the even more radically confused maternal grouping in the preliminary sketches), which differentiates the Virgin from St. Anne and the child from both of his mothers, and the *heimlich* reduction of the uncanny doubleness of the Mona Lisa's smile, with its sinister menace.

This defusion, differentiation, and reduction of the ambiguities of the fused maternal and child figures result in the serenity and blissfulness of Leonardo's final realization of the Anna Metterza topos. It is accomplished in a triangular situation of differentiated 'thirds,' in which the child descending from his mother's lap escapes his position as maternal phallus or part-object. The artistic process of composition and recomposition of the fatherless, mother–son threesome in fact *puts into reverse* the screen memory of the kite's traumatic visitation (one might note, however, that in the Cartoon St. Anne's right hand—or an enlarged but unfinished right arm and hand that emerge from the fused maternal group—gestures upward to God the Father, a gesture that has disappeared from the oil painting but has reappeared in the painting of St. John the Baptist). The final recomposed Anna Metterza grouping outflanks or goes behind the defensive symbolization of the kite to access and rework the emotionally fraught ambiguities of the fused maternal imagoes and the infant's possession by and absorption in them.

As a sublimatory symbolization, that is quite independent of his screen memory of the flying predator with its invasive tail, Leonardo's final form of the *Anna Metterza* iconography reopens and readdresses the enigma of the maternal smile and gaze. It does so in a situation that stages both distance and continuing attachment on the part of the child, along with serenity and containment on the part of the maternal figures. This sense of containment can be located in the outstretched gesture of Mary, which is not just an attempt to repossess the errant child but which intervenes in the child's rather violent stranglehold on the unfortunate lamb that has been substituted for the figure of the little St. John of the Cartoon. The lamb carries a traditional theological signification: it is the Paschal *Agnus Dei* or Lamb of God, which looks forward to Christ's sacrificial role as conceived by traditional Christian theology. Nevertheless, the lamb's traditional emblematic function is somewhat displaced by Leonardo's naturalistic drama of childish aggression and 'naughtiness' vis-à-vis the lamb as family pet. This eruption of violence and aggression in the figure of the Christ Child in the lower right-hand corner of the painting is quite extraordinary, a breach of all the representational conventions and decorum of the Madonna and Child topos, where the Child is always framed, positioned and contained by the maternal figure. One might wonder whether to recognize here the return and discharge of the aggression—"e molte volte *mi percuotesse* con tal coda dentro alle labbra"[12]—directed toward the cradled Leonardo by the intrusive *nibio*. It testifies to the continuing need for maternal holding and containment of those unruly impulses, a containment that is implemented through the seductive power of the smiling gaze of the mother that draws the child's return gaze back to her even as he eludes her grasp.

12. See Almansi's translation "and struck me with such a tail inside of the lips many times" (Eissler[o] 1961, 13) and the discussion in the previous chapter of the invasive violence of this act at the centre of Leonardo's primal scene.

# Part IV  Prototypes and the Primal

## The Transference and Its Prototypes

> "For when all is said and done, it is impossible to destroy anyone *in absentia* or *in effigie*."[1]

Freud's cryptic final proposition, quoted above, closes the first of his three major short papers on transference published between 1912 and 1915. Despite arguing in the 1912 paper that the transference is implicated in the resistance to the analytic treatment, Freud nevertheless presents the transference as rendering "the inestimable service of making the patient's hidden and forgotten erotic impulses immediate and manifest" (Freud 1912b, 108). What was first experienced by Freud as an obstacle, often leading to the analysand's premature exit from the treatment if neglected or misinterpreted (the case of Dora is only the most famous of such flights), is now to be considered as the very mainspring of its success: "Every conflict has to be fought out on the field of the transference. . . . It is on that field that the victory is to be won" (ibid., 104, 108). The object of the analysis is not something at a distance, *in absentia*, a remote infantile reality, but something

---

1. Sigmund Freud, "The Dynamics of Transference" (1912b), *SE* 12, 108.

that is in the present, alive again in the analytic situation and in direct relation to the analyst; nor can it be resolved *in effigie*, for the German phrase is a legal idiom referring to the practice of punishing absconding criminals in simulacrum, burning or beheading a straw-filled dummy of the guilty person. Sentencing someone to death *in absentia* or executing them *in effigie* is merely a gestural act, lacking in material reality and in, at least immediate, effectiveness. If what the transference bears on is neither in the past and so absent, nor present merely *in effigie*, the question is raised as to what kind of present or virtual reality the transference can claim, especially when it is understood as a repetition *of something else*.

In the first paper of 1912, "The Dynamics of Transference," the transference is mapped initially through a pair of terms—stereotype plates, prototypes—whose operation is described thus:

> It must be understood that each individual . . . has acquired a specific method of his own in his conduct of his erotic life—that is, in the preconditions to falling in love which he lays down, in the instincts he satisfies and the aims he sets himself in the course of it. (Freud 1912b, 99)

The notion goes back at least to the 1910 paper "A Special Type of Choice of Object Made by Men" (1910h). Here Freud is concerned with what he calls "necessary conditions for loving" (ibid., 165) that are expressed in a strikingly abnormal object-choice: the requirement that an injured third party be involved, who "can claim right of possession" of the woman "as her husband, fiancé or friend" (166), or that the woman be promiscuous or a *cocotte*, liable to take, or at least flirt with, other lovers, often accompanied by the urge to rescue the woman from some real or imagined disgrace. Although a demand on himself for fidelity is made, the male lover's passionate attachment is repeated with different women, again and again, so that "*a long series of them is formed*" (168). Like normal object-choice, however, Freud argues, these abnormal "conditions for loving and behaviour in love do in fact arise from the psychical constellation connected with the mother" (169). The childhood experience of the mother as involved in a prior relation to the father or in other relations to siblings, or in a realm of sexual relations unavailable to the child, forms a template for later adult object-choice. Whereas displacement of the libido from the mother has normally been in large part achieved, this type reveals "an infantile fixation" to "the

maternal prototype of the object-choice" (168–69). "The maternal characteristics remain stamped on the love-objects that are chosen later," which
are "easily recognizable mother-surrogates" (169). This idea of an infantile
prototype that is compulsively reproduced in later adult object-choices, often in a repetitive series, a prototype that involves not just an isolated figure
but one caught up in a web of preexisting relations, becomes central to
Freud's account of the transference.

The notion of the prototype in the papers on transference is supplemented by the metaphor of the "stereotype plate," taken from engraving
and printing, where later objects and the impulses directed at them are
described as reproductions or new "editions" of the infantile pattern. In
"The Dynamics of Transference," this "stereotype plate . . . is constantly
repeated—constantly reprinted afresh—in the course of the person's life so
far as circumstances . . . permit" (1912b, 99). The same metaphor occurs
in Freud's first full statement of the indispensable nature of transference in
the therapeutic process, made in his self-critical reflections on his failure in
the case of Dora to recognize and deal with the transference:

> What are transferences? They are new editions or facsimiles of the impulses
> and phantasies which are aroused and made conscious during the progress of
> the analysis; but they have this peculiarity, which is characteristic of their
> species, that they replace some earlier person by the person of the physician . . .
> a whole series of psychological experiences are revived, not as belonging to the
> past, but as applying to the person of the physician in the present moment.[2]

Closely associated with the stereotype plate is the idea of the constant repetition of this infantile prototype in the experiences of adult object-choice,
of which the analytic transference of the prototype onto the analyst and
the analytic situation is but a specialized subset. Two further qualifications
are added, although not developed: that a given individual might have more
than one such stereotype plate, and that, in a somewhat minimal conces-
sion, these prototypes are "not entirely insusceptible to change in the face
of recent experiences" (1912b, 100). In his earlier statement in the Dora
case, Freud had been more sanguine about this susceptibility of the prototype to change and had used his printing metaphor to suggest a potentially

2. Sigmund Freud, "Fragment of Analysis of a Case of Hysteria" (1905e), *SE* 7, 116.

important distinction. While some transferences are exact repetitions that merely substitute the person of the analyst and are "merely new impressions or reprints," others have been "subjected to a moderating influence—to *sublimation*, as I call it," by consciously taking advantage of "some real peculiarity in the physician's person or circumstances and attaching themselves to that." They are not "new impressions, but revised editions" (1905e, 116).

Freud's starting point in his 1912 essay is that if someone's need for love is unsatisfied, "he is bound to approach every new person whom he meets with anticipatory libidinal ideas" (1912b, 100). Hence it is inevitable that the analyst will be the object of these anticipatory libidinal fantasies that will seek to "introduce him into one of the psychical 'series' which the patient has already formed" (ibid.) on the basis of his prototypes and stereotype plates. Freud suggests that it is the prototype of the father-imago that is most commonly projected onto the (male) analyst, but the transference is not confined to that alone, as it may act via other prototypes such as the mother-imago or brother-imago. These anticipatory ideas will include "impulses which . . . have passed through the full process of psychical development," are consequently "directed towards reality," and are "at the disposal of the conscious personality" (ibid.). However, they will also include "libidinal impulses" that have been "kept away from the conscious personality and from reality," and these have "either been prevented from further expansion except in phantasy or remained wholly in the unconscious" (ibid.). It is to these latter *unconscious* dimensions of the patient's infantile prototypes that Freud points in order to explain that peculiarity of the analytic transference, its excessiveness, "both in amount and nature," with regard to any rational or sensible response to the person of the analyst. In any neurosis the balance between conscious and unconscious deployments of the libido has shifted in favor of the latter, which "has entered on a regressive course and has revived the subject's infantile imagos" (ibid., 102). It is the task of the analytic treatment to "track down the libido . . . withdrawn into its hiding-place," which will provoke the emergence of resistances against the analytic work in order to preserve the state of intensified unconscious libido, now invested in and bound to the infantile prototypes (ibid.).

Freud's final emphasis in the essay is on the 'presentness' of these unconscious impulses and their resistance to being remembered and assigned a place in the patient's life history:

The unconscious impulses do not want to be remembered in the way the treatment desires them to be, but endeavour to reproduce themselves in accordance with the timelessness of the unconscious and its capacity for hallucination. Just as happens in dreams the patient regards the products of the awakening of his unconscious impulses as contemporaneous and real; he seeks to put his passions into action without taking into account the real situation. (Freud 1912b, 108)

We can see here Freud once again encountering the strange virtual reality he had struggled to make sense of in his early work on hysteria with his model of traumatic seduction, discussed at length in the first four chapters of this book. Something reproduces itself that the patient claims to have no conscious memory of. It does so with such compelling, even compulsive, power that the impulses, and the scenario that encodes them, that con-script the patient into an acting out are relived as a present reality. The analogy with the dream, and the way it also is lived by the dreamer as a present reality, is very striking, all the more so as Freud had used the term 'transference' to describe precisely the relation between the infantile sources, the 'capitalist' of the dream that funds its formation, in Freud's metaphor, and the previous day's residues. In the dream, the unconscious infantile dream-wish exercises its power on an existing preconscious idea, through the primary processes of condensation and displacement. It does this, Freud argues,

> by establishing a connection with an idea that already belongs to the precon-scious, by transferring its intensity onto it and getting itself 'covered' by it. Here we have the fact of 'transference,' which provides an explanation of so many striking phenomena of the mental life of neurotics.[3]

The dream is not the unconscious itself or 'in person' but a derivative or formation of the unconscious. It is formed through transference of uncon-scious wishes onto the day's residues, those charged, leftover fragments of the dreamer's most recent experience, that are the provoking occasion of the dream and that help determine its manifest dream-scene. As a result, the dream is lived by the dreamer as a present reality in the timeless and hallu-cinatory mode of the unconscious.

3. Sigmund Freud, *The Interpretation of Dreams* (1900a), *SE* 5, 562–63.

Similarly, this hallucinatory putting of the passions into action might remind us of Charcot's *attitudes passionelles*, or 'scenes of passionate movement,' as Freud described the third phase of Charcot's schematization of *la grande hystérie*, the hysterical attack. However, if the dream, the hysterical attack, and its clinical double, the remembering of trauma under hypnosis, can all be grouped with the nonhypnotic clinical transference as forms of repetitive reenactment outside of the cognizance and control of ordinary consciousness, the differences between them are also crucial. Hence it is precisely with a revisiting of his work with Breuer and of the cathartic model of treatment they shared in the early to mid-1890s that Freud begins the richest and most important of the three essays. His aim is to contrast his developed understanding of the clinical transference with the old practice of catharsis and abreaction under hypnosis.

## Repetition and the Transference-Neurosis

Freud begins by setting out in a simplified schema three stages through which the clinical treatment had developed. First, he cites what he calls "Breuer's catharsis," which consisted in "bringing into focus the moment at which the symptom was formed," and especially "the mental processes involved in that situation." The verb used here, as often in the texts of 1895–96, is not 'remember' but 'reproduce' (*reproduzieren*), with its suggestion of an affective reenactment of memories, "in order to direct their discharge along the path of conscious activity."[4] Freud summarizes the clinical aim as "remembering and abreaction, with the help of the hypnotic state." Here the technical term 'abreaction,' as elaborated in the texts of 1893,[5] suggests, beyond the activity of cognitive recollection and recognition, an economic dimension, a cathartic purging of an excessive quota of affect that is tied to a set of traumatic memory traces and associated ideas, whose retention has kept those ideas both active and unconscious.

4. Sigmund Freud, "Remembering, Repeating and Working-Through" (1914g), *SE* 12, 147.
5. Sigmund Freud, "On the Psychical Mechanism of Hysterical Phenomena: A Lecture" (1893h), *SE* 3; Josef Breuer and Sigmund Freud, "On the Psychical Mechanism of Hysterical Phenomena: Preliminary Communication" (1893a), *SE* 2.

In the second stage hypnosis is given up as the means of access to the situations behind the symptom and "the task became one of discovering from the patient's free associations what he failed to remember" (Freud 1914g , 147). Where previously the patient's resistance had been overcome by hypnosis, now "the resistance was to be circumvented by the work of interpretation and by making its results known to the patient" (ibid.). Where previously the patient's role had been to remember and abreact, purging the "strangulated affect" (1893a, 17) of the scenes recalled under hypnosis, now "abreaction recedes into the background and seemed to be replaced by the expenditure of work which the patient had to make to overcome his criticism of his free associations" (Freud 1914g, 147). This seems to shift the emphasis away from an affective revival and reliving of past experience, a catharsis, to an "expenditure of work" by the patient on his own resistance to the process of free association, perhaps more a cognitive than an affective activity.

In the third stage of development the immediate focus is no longer directly concerned with a particular problem or situation, a particular symptom and the moment of that symptom's appearance, but with "whatever is present for the time being on the surface of the patient's mind" (ibid.). The analyst's interpretation addresses not the traces of a past situation but the patient's resistances as manifested in his speech and free associations in the present. In a rather ideal schema, Freud announces a new division of labor in which the analyst uncovers the patient's resistances and "the patient often relates the forgotten situations and connections without any difficulty" (ibid.). The ultimate aim remains the same as in the earlier forms of the treatment: "to fill in gaps in memory," not now with the aid of hypnosis but through the overcoming of "resistances due to repression" (ibid., 148).

As if in response to the simplicities of this ideal general schema, Freud inserts a brief excursus that entails in effect a rewriting of the common-sense understandings of forgetting and remembering: a survey of phenomena described by psychoanalysis in which nothing is ever really forgotten, but nothing is ever really remembered as such; nothing is ever quite lost, but nothing is ever quite recovered. Where forgetting is commonly understood as the wearing away of the mental records or traces of an experience or event, Freud insists that "forgetting impressions, scenes or experiences nearly always reduces itself to shutting them off," that is, they remain present in the mind but inaccessible to conscious recall. The patient characteristically comes to acknowledge their presence with this or a similar statement: " 'As a matter of fact I've always known it; only I've never thought of it' " (ibid.). The patient's eagerness to recover such 'forgotten' things is often rewarded, Freud adds, especially in the case of conversion hysterias, where bodily symptoms and malfunctions come to stand in for experiences that have been repressed. By contrast with this forgetting as symptomatic substitution in hysteria, in obsessional neurosis, the other major category of neurosis, "forgetting is mostly restricted to dissolving thought-connections, failing to draw the right conclusions and isolating memories" (ibid.).

With the phenomenon of screen memories, the scope of forgetting is restricted even further, as the familiar forgetting of childhood experiences is entirely counterbalanced by them: "Not only *some* but *all* of what is essential from childhood has been retained in these memories. . . . They represent the forgotten years of childhood as adequately as the manifest content of a dream represents the dream-thoughts" (ibid.), that is, distorted by the primary processes of condensation and displacement.

In the case of "purely internal acts," as distinct from impressions and experiences of external events and situations, often "something is 'remembered' which could never have been 'forgotten' because it was never at any time noticed—was never conscious" (ibid., 149). Of these internal psychical processes Freud asserts: "The conviction which the patient obtains in the course of his analysis is quite independent of this kind of memory" (ibid.). Where with these internal acts an apparent memory is really a first coming into consciousness, in contrast Freud picks out a special class of important external experiences of which *no* memory ever appears: "These are experiences which occurred in very early childhood and were not understood at the time but which were *subsequently* (*nachträglich* – JF) understood and interpreted" (ibid.). Again Freud asserts that, like the previous group, the patient's conviction as to the existence of these experiences is not dependent on a memory of them—they are understood and interpreted in the analysis, but as a reconstruction, not in the form of a memory.

To sum up Freud's survey: with neurosis, the power of 'forgetting' is reduced by the displaced and disguised return of the forgotten material in conversion symptoms or isolated, obsessional ideas and rituals. In the case of internal mental acts and processes, it is often not a question of 'remembering' but of a first belated coming to consciousness, whereas with certain early infantile experiences, which were not understood at the time but remain active in dreams and symptoms, no memory is possible. More generally, in the case of what Freud usually calls 'childhood amnesia,' the essential elements of early experience are retained in the disguised form of screen memories. All of this troubles Freud's ideal of a clean, almost surgical removal of resistances by the analyst's interpretation, followed by the transparent recall "without any difficulty" of causal experiences and situations by the patient (as appeared to be the case in the early trauma theory of hysterical symptom formation). The experiences in question, although they might not have been understood or even consciously noticed at the time, have certainly not been abolished; on the other hand, they are mostly known through their derivatives: symptoms, screen memories, dreams.

As Freud ruefully notes, in the hypnotic treatment "the process of remembering took a very simple form. The patient put himself back into an earlier situation, which he seemed never to confuse with the present one" (ibid., 148). With a technique focused on the transference, however, it is precisely in and through its confusion with the present situation of the treatment that access to the earlier situation is gained:

> The patient does not *remember* anything of what he has forgotten and repressed, but *acts* it out. He reproduces it not as a memory but as an action; he *repeats* it, without, of course, knowing that he is repeating it. (Freud 1914g, 150)

Freud instances this repetition with the examples of a patient who does not remember being defiant or hostile to the authority of his parents but who behaves defiantly toward his analyst; or who does not recall being ashamed and secretive about his sexual feelings and activities but is intensely ashamed and secretive about his entering into analytic treatment. Like the screen memory and the range of neurotic symptoms, the transference onto the analyst and the analytic situation is both an unavoidable alternative to remembering and a point of access to what is not being remembered: "As long as the patient is in the treatment he cannot escape from this compulsion to repeat, and in the end we understand that this is his way of remembering" (ibid.). As the editor of the *Standard Edition* notes, this is the first appearance of Freud's formulation of "the compulsion to repeat." We will consider it in Chapter 11 at greater length in its relation to the death drive, but it is significant that it is Freud's reflection on the transference that is the occasion of its first formulation.

Freud's clinical aim is still to "fill in the gaps of memory," to turn the compulsion to repeat into "a motive for remembering" by a handling of the transference that gives the compulsion "the right to assert itself in a definite field." The transference becomes "a playground in which it is allowed to expand . . . to display to us everything in the way of pathogenic instincts that is hidden in the patient's mind" (ibid., 154), of which the analyst becomes the new object.

> We regularly succeed in giving all the symptoms of the illness a new transference meaning and replacing his ordinary neurosis by a 'transference-neurosis'[6] of which he can be cured by the therapeutic work. The transference thus creates an intermediate region between illness and real life through which the transition from one to the other is made. The new condition has taken over the features of the illness; but it represents an artificial illness which is at every point accessible to our intervention. It is a real piece of experience. (Freud 1914g, 154)

This is an extraordinary conception of a hybrid formation that is artificially induced so that the patient's unconscious "pathogenic instincts" can be put into play and made manifest vis-à-vis the analyst, but within the artifice of the analytic situation and its conventions (free association, speech rather than action, regular attendance at agreed times only, the couch, the fees, etc.). At the same time, however, it is "a piece of real experience," but one whose function is to actualize anew something else that had already existed before the treatment. The original conflict emerges from the unconscious and its deposits from the past, into the space of the transference, as a now-present object of what Freud elsewhere calls the 'free-floating attention' of the analyst, and on the part of the patient of "a certain tolerance for the state of being ill." The rationale for this is pragmatic: "One cannot overcome an

6. The term 'transference-neurosis' has a double reference in Freudian theory: to those neuroses—hysteria, anxiety hysteria, obsessional neurosis—that produce transferences from one set of objects onto another (thus excluding what Freud calls the 'narcissistic neuroses' or psychoses), and to the later thesis that in the treatment the transference takes the form of a special 'transference-neurosis,' centering on the analytic situation and the analyst. It is only a transference-neurosis of the first kind that can produce a transference-neurosis of the second kind.

enemy who is absent or not within range" (ibid, 152). Neither *in absentia* nor *in effigie*, the presentness of the repetition in relation to the analyst allows a new kind of therapeutic intervention. Freud's clinical claim is that the absent infantile conflict can be targeted and resolved, as it were by proxy, through the artificial transference-neurosis that replaces it in the present moment of the analysis—a proxy that is not, however, *in effigie* but a derivative that is also a *representative* and not just a likeness or mimetic *representation*.

In this 1914 essay little attention is given to describing exactly what is being repeated, beyond the statement that the patient "repeats everything that has made its way from the sources of the repressed into his manifest personality—his inhibitions, and unserviceable attitudes and his pathologi-cal character-traits" (ibid., 151). The emphasis here is on the ego, its habit-ual attitudes and symptoms, as derivatives of the repressed, "everything that has already made its way from the sources of the repressed into his manifest personality," which sounds like a description of the resistance and its forces. This is rather different from the emphasis in the previously dis-cussed essay of 1912, which was on unconscious infantile prototypes, rela-tions to family and especially parental figures, and their repetition in the transference. Indeed, the passage quoted earlier, and the claim it makes in relation to the transference-neurosis, presupposes just such a notion of a self-replicating unconscious prototype or template. Here instead, however, Freud cites briefly the inhibited, unserviceable, and pathological features of the resisting ego as the material of repetition, without connecting the two. This leaves it to later analysts to distinguish between different types of the transference. Notably, Jean Laplanche has distinguished between the 'filled-in transference' (*transfert en plein*), with its repetition of the ego's standard self-representations, defensive maneuvers, and self-justificatory narratives, which must be worked through and dismantled to release the 'followed-out transference'(*transfert en creux*). It is in the latter that the original relation to the enigmatic desire of the parental figures is re-peated, of which the filled-in transference is a defensive and only partial translation.[7]

---

7. Jean Laplanche, *New Foundations for Psychoanalysis* (1987) (Oxford: Basil Blackwell, 1989), 159–62; also see "Transference: Its Provocation by the Analyst" (1992), in *Essays on Otherness*, ed. John Fletcher (London: Routledge, 1999).

*True Love*

Freud's emphasis, in the three texts I am concerned with, falls then on the transference as a derivative or formation of the unconscious, specifically in the form of a transference-neurosis centering on the analyst. In elaborating this thesis he displays considerable ambiguity as to the reality status of the transference. He attempts to grasp this through three sets of oppositions: between the real and the unreal, between the conscious and the unconscious, and between the present and the past (or absent). They do not map neatly onto each other, however, and any attempt to distinguish the real from the unreal in terms of the other two oppositions only serves to demonstrate the instability of all three; for if the real might appear at first to be what is conscious and what is present, what is unconscious cannot be said to be either unreal or absent. What is at stake here is what one might call the ontology of repetition, or at least of the kind of repetition entailed in the compulsion to repeat—a repetition in which what is repeated is present in (not absent from) its repetition; a repetition which is not to be considered merely a simulacrum or mimesis of what it repeats. Given the timelessness of the unconscious (as the detemporalized product of a time-bound repression), the compulsion it generates reproduces not just an effigy or a reference to something *in absentia* but a derivative, which functions as an agent or a representative rather than just as a representation. The relation of repetition is not just a metaphorical one, of likeness or similitude, but a metonymic one, that of contiguity or continuity, of a part to a whole for which it stands in. The repetition compulsion is such that the analyst's intervention in the adult repetition, in effect, constitutes a therapeutic action on the infantile prototype that is being repeated.

The tension between what is present and so real and what belongs to the past is at work throughout these essays. In "Remembering, Repeating and Working-Through," there is a constant affirmation that the transference repetition "implies conjuring up a piece of real life" (1914g, 152) as opposed to reenactment under hypnosis; that, although an "artificial illness," the transference-neurosis is also "a piece of real experience" (ibid., 154). However, the insistence that "we must treat his [the patient's] illness, not as an event of the past, but as a present-day force" is soon contradicted by the statement that "while the patient experiences [the illness] as something real and contemporary, we have to do our therapeutic work on it . . . tracing it back to the past" (151–52). If the reality of the transference is in the present, its truth lies in the past. However, the more Freud stresses the unrevised clinical aim to recover past memories, the more the affective reality of the present relation to the analyst is in danger of being drained of 'realness,' of coming to be seen as merely a necessary subjective illusion.

In his 1915 essay "Observations on Transference-Love," the importunate demand for love by the (female) patient caught up in the throes of the transference pushes this aporia, of the reality or otherwise of the transference, to the limit. At first the eruption of the patient's transference-demand for love from the analyst is described as if it were the displacement of the theater of the analysis by a superior reality, "as though it had been interrupted by some elemental phenomenon."[8] The patient gives up her treatment, declares she is well, and demands to have her love returned:

> There is a complete change of scene; it is as though some piece of make-believe had been stopped by the sudden irruption of reality—as when, for instance, a cry of fire is raised during a theatrical performance. (Freud 1915a, 162)

The analysis is a theatrical performance in which the demand for love turns make-believe suddenly real and stops the performance. However, the real illusion here would be "that the treatment is at an end." The analyst avoids this by neither acquiescing in the demand for love nor repelling it but by allowing it to persist in the face of his own withholding of a response. "He must keep firm hold of the transference-love, but treat it as something unreal, as a situation that must be gone through in the treatment and traced back to its unconscious origins" (ibid., 166). Rather than a superior elemental reality—the cry of fire—the transference is now what is unreal, while reality is, in contrast, the "unconscious origins," "the infantile roots of her love." However, it is not at all clear why the intermediate realm brought into being by the analyst's refusal to return the demand for love, the analysis as theater or performance, the realm of repetitions, should have its reality denied—"all her preconditions for loving, all the phantasies springing from her sexual desires, all the detailed characteristics of her state

8. Sigmund Freud, "Observations on Transference-Love" (1915a), *SE* 12, 160.

of being in love" (ibid.). It is, after all, the actualization in the transference of these modes of object-choice and object-relation rather than their acting out outside the analysis, which opens the way and gives access to the infantile prototype that generates the repetition.

Freud's recommendation to treat the erotic transference "as something unreal" is elaborated as he mounts a series of arguments with an imaginary patient against the genuineness of the transference-demand that her love be returned. First, such a demand means the end of the analysis, as what she wants is incompatible with its continuance. Consequently, "she is bringing out a resistance in the guise of being in love with him" (ibid., 167), for she will either withdraw from the analysis in order to have the proposed love affair with her analyst, or she will do so out of revenge and resentment as a woman scorned when he refuses her love. Freud's second argument against the genuineness of the transference-love involves a return to the question of the prototypes: "It exhibits not a single new feature arising from the present situation but is entirely composed of repetitions and copies of earlier reactions, including infantile ones" (ibid.). Here the notion of repetition is being invoked, not as previously, to establish the present reality of the transference, but to call its genuineness into question—it is unreal, only a copy, of something earlier, somewhere else.

It is at this point that Freud performs a spectacular 180-degree about-turn. "Can we truly say," he asks, "that the state of being in love which becomes manifest in the analytic treatment is not a real one?" (ibid., 168). He then reviews the two arguments he has just advanced: the argument that cites the resistance and the argument that cites the prototype. Of the first, he states: "The resistance did not, after all, *create* this love; it finds it ready to hand, makes use of it and aggravates its manifestations. Nor is the genuineness of the phenomenon disproved by the resistance" (168). However, it is over the question of the relation of the transference-love to the infantile prototype, the weaker of the two arguments he now claims, that he executes his most striking reversal:

> It is true that the love consists of new editions of old traits and that it repeats infantile reactions. But this is the essential characteristic of every state of being in love. There is no such state that does not reproduce infantile prototypes. It is precisely from this infantile determination that it receives its compulsive character, verging as it does on the pathological. (Freud 1915a, 168)

The fact that transference-love repeats an infantile prototype, if anything, confirms its genuineness, as that is "the essential characteristic of every state of being in love." It is precisely this infantile dimension of 'falling in love' that accounts for its compulsiveness and puts it on the verge of pathology. Transference-love has "perhaps a degree less freedom" than "normal" love, is more clearly dependent on the infantile prototype, and is "less adaptable and capable of modification" (ibid, 168). However, these deviations from normality are "not what is essential." The essential is then precisely the infantile prototype and the compulsive love to which it gives rise.

In summary, Freud affirms that transference-love "has the character of a 'genuine' love." Paradoxically, it is this that makes it seem "so lacking in normality," precisely because "being in love in ordinary life . . . is also more similar to abnormal than to normal mental phenomena" (ibid.). Freud allows to transference-love, however, "a special position" due to three characteristic features: first, "it is provoked by the analytic situation"; second, "it is greatly intensified by the resistance, which dominates the situation"; and, third, "it is lacking to a high degree in a regard for reality, is less sensible, less concerned about consequences and more blind in its valuation of the loved person," the latter a classical characteristic of all romantic love. In a final deconstructive twist, Freud disaligns the genuine and the normal by reminding us "that these departures from the norm constitute precisely what is essential about being in love" (ibid., 169). Consequently, it is the very exorbitance of the demand for love that testifies to its genuineness, not as a function of its response to its present object but of its revival and repetition of its source in a past infantile love. The analyst has "evoked this love by instituting the analytic treatment" (ibid.), and "the work then aims at uncovering the patient's infantile object-choice and the phantasies woven around it" (ibid., 167). The analytic situation acts to capture these fantasies in their very action as stereotype plates and prototypes, as they replicate themselves in the present moment of the transference.

# The Wolf Man I: Constructing the Primal Scene

*Prelude: Of Primal Scenes and Primal Fantasies*

The concept of the transference with which we have been concerned in the previous chapter is part of Freud's attempt to understand forms of repetition that express the action in the present of scenes not available to consciousness and memory. It has strong, if partial, analogies—family resemblances—with the screen memory, the dream, and the neurotic symptom: if the analyst and the analytic situation are like the day's residues of the dream that attract the investments of the infantile dream-wish, so transference-love could equally be called 'screen love' or even 'dream love.' Freud began his work on trauma with the model of a 'scene' as the representation of a specific traumatic event to be relived under hypnosis and not to be confused with the present. This model became progressively more complicated, as I have shown in previous chapters, both with respect to the material to be repeated, the appearance or form of the repetition, and the temporal structure of the process of repetition. In particular, what is being repeated comes to be described as a fixed scenario, a stylized scene or memory fragment that condenses the formative identifications and object-choices of infantile life, hence the 'stereotype plates' and 'prototypes' of the essays on transference. The transference neurosis is first cousin to Leonardo's screen memory of the intrusive bird, and both have affinities with the Wolf Man's dream of wolves. Behind each of them lies something else: Freud infers, respectively, the action of an infantile prototype in the transference, of a repeated scene of maternal seduction behind Leonardo's screen memory, and the 'activation' of what in the Wolf Man's case he calls a 'primal scene,' which might or might not be a fantasy (Freud oscillates between the alternatives of memory and fantasy), underlying his dream of wolves. Like his analysis of Leonardo's screen memory, Freud's case history of the Wolf Man is a tour de force demonstration of the centrality of a given scene—a marvelous 'memory' scene in Leonardo's case, a dream scene in the Wolf Man's—to a range of psychical productions, from symptoms to artworks. He also seeks to demonstrate the determining power, in the formation of a whole subjective history with its structuring identifications and its habitual emotional and sexual object choices, of whatever lies behind and has produced these personal myths of the bird or the wolves.

## Primal Scene as Prototype

As the notion of the prototype in the transference papers morphs into the notion of a primal fantasy in the 1915 paper on the paranoid woman,[1] which is taken up again in the Wolf Man case study (written approximately at the same time), some preliminary clarification of terminology is necessary. The forerunner to the term *Urphantasie* (primal fantasy) is the term *Urszene* (primal scene), which emerges as a component of the conceptual arsenal of the seduction theory, in May 1897, in Draft L of the theoretical manuscripts that form part of the correspondence with Wilhelm Fliess. It appears in both Draft L and the accompanying letter, unfortunately somewhat obscured by

---

1. Sigmund Freud, "A Case of Paranoia Running Counter to the Psychoanalytic Theory of the Disease" (1915f), *SE* 14.

being translated differently each time by Masson. In the letter Freud proposes that in hysteria what are repressed "are not in reality memories . . . but impulses that derive from primal scenes [*Urszenen*]."[2] In the opening sentence of Draft L itself, the term occurs again: "The aim seems to be to reach the earliest [sexual] scenes," which translates differently the same German term as in the letter—*Urszenen*; but by translating the prefix 'Ur'/'primal' by the word 'earliest,' Masson reduces it to a question of chronology. The formulation in the letter is glossed in the immediately following sentence by the phrase "*impulses* (derived from memories)." Clearly Freud is using it to indicate the memory of an actual moment or event. This is distinguished from but related to the idea of fantasy, as in the following sentence in the accompanying Draft L Freud writes of his aim in treatment: "In a few cases this [access to *Urszenen*—JF] is achieved directly, but in others only by a detour via fantasies . . . psychic facades produced in order to bar access to these memories" (Masson 1985a, 240). For the most part, known only through the derivative fantasies that defend against them, these scenes are obviously disturbing, both in themselves and in the 'impulses' to which they give rise, which are consequently repressed. The term 'primal scene'/*Urszene* first appears then as part of the theory of traumatic seduction, in particular in its late unpublished form, where, as I have demonstrated in Chapter 4, memory and fantasy appear in intimate connection with each other rather than as polarized alternatives to be chosen between.

The prefix *Ur* relates the primal scene to two other terms, *Urphantasie*/primal fantasy and *Urverdrangung*/primal repression, where the prefix indicates a primacy, as both ground and model, over what comes later (conscious daydreams and fantasies, secondary repression, and perhaps one can add auxiliary scenes and screen memories). *Urszene* does not, however, become a standard term in Freud's theoretical lexicon until the Wolf Man case history. In its first usage in May 1897, a primal scene does not have a particular content, beyond being a sexual scene that is outside the comprehension of the child and one that carries an excitation that is excessive, that cannot be mastered or contained; a sexual trauma, therefore, a component of the temporal structure of afterwardsness (*Nachträglichkeit*), as outlined in

2. *The Complete Letters of Sigmund Freud to Wilhelm Fliess 1887–1904*, trans. and ed. J. M. Masson (Cambridge, Mass.: Harvard University Press, 1985), 239.

Chapter 3, but not tied to the same fixed persons or scenario. Seventeen years later, Freud picks up the term again to designate the scene that he reconstructs as the disturbing event behind the Wolf Man's dream. He continues to use it in the plural as in the original usage, where it might refer to a range of different actions and actors, only one of which is the particular content Freud there reconstructs, that of a scene of parental intercourse, witnessed or overheard by the child. Freud had often attributed importance to such a parental scene, discussing it on a number of occasions in the seventeen-year period between Draft L and the Wolf Man case, but he had never referred to it as a primal scene—let alone as *the* primal scene—as he does throughout the case study.

It is important, however, to distinguish Freud's own usage of this term from what has become the now-standard psychoanalytic usage, at least in English, where it is used simply to reference the content of the scene: the spectacle of parental intercourse with its own peculiar soundtrack. This reduction to content loses the distinctive conceptual status signaled by the prefix *Ur*, that of a *Vorbild*, precisely a prototype or protoscene that has its primal status in relation to scenes that are to come later, and only through which scenes it can be known. This reduction to content is clear in the *Standard Edition*, where 'primal scene' is often indexed as "see parental intercourse," and refers to passages where the actual formulation 'primal scene' does not occur as such. In the French literature, there is a twin usage, *scène primitive* and *scène originaire*, which may be used as synonyms. However, there is a tendency to use the first for the specific parental scene and the latter for the more general conception of an infantile traumatic scene that lays the basis for what is to come, governed by the logic of *après coup*. An originary scene is one that is at the origin and has the power to originate, of which the parental scene would be a specific instance. It is significant that in Freud's later discussions of the scene of parental intercourse, whether as memory or fantasy, outside of the time structure of trauma as analyzed in the Wolf Man case, he does *not* refer to it as 'the primal scene.' The term implies a specific temporal structure independent of a specific content, as the very form of the word in German indicates. Freud paraphrases primal scenes as "the earliest experiences of childhood that are brought to light in analysis," that is, they are experiences that function as a *Vorbild*, as a prototype, and he adds: "In the present case the content of the primal scene is a picture of sexual intercourse between the boy's parents in a posture espe-cially favourable for certain observations."[3] The temporal structure that constitutes a scene as 'primal' may well be exemplified in the parental scene, but it is not identical with it, nor is it confined to it.

### Primal Fantasy as Prototype: The Paranoid Woman

The term 'primal fantasy' (*Urphantasie*) first appears in a paper of 1915, "A Case of Paranoia Running Counter to the Psychoanalytic Theory of the Disease," just after the publication of the transference papers discussed in the previous chapter, and the writing up of the Wolf Man case in 1914 (not to be published until 1918). In the 1915 paper the parental scene figures as a prototype for the production of paranoid symptoms, as one of a triptych of primal fantasies, but it is not yet designated as *the* primal scene.

The case is a brief one concerning a woman of thirty, who lived alone with her mother after her father's death and was her sole support. It con-sisted of two sessions. In the first session the patient reports that during an intimate encounter with her lover in his rooms she was frightened by the sound of a knock or click, which he explained as probably coming from a small clock on his writing desk, by a heavily curtained window. On leaving his apartment she met two men on the stairs, "who whispered something to each other when they saw her" (1915f, 264), one of whom was carrying what looked like a small box. On her way home she rapidly put together an expla-nation: the box might have been a camera, the man a photographer who had been hidden behind the curtain, the click the sound of the shutter as he took a photograph of her in a compromising position. Thereafter she pur-sued her lover with reproaches and demands for explanation, none of which satisfied her, and which led to her engaging a lawyer who brought her to see Freud. Freud's interest in this case of paranoia "running counter to the psychoanalytic theory of the disease," as the title indicates, was due to the fact that the young woman's accusations of persecution were being directed toward a male persecutor, whereas the psychoanalytic hypothesis was that paranoia was based on repressed homosexuality, such that the former same

---

3. Sigmund Freud, "From the History of an Infantile Neurosis" (1918b [1914]), *SE* 17, 55.

sex love-objects reappeared as persecutors within the paranoid fantasy. Freud asked her to see him for a second session, where she revealed that in fact she had visited the young man on two occasions but that on the first visit there had been no problems. On the day after this first visit, however, something had in fact happened. At her workplace where the young man also worked, she had a superior, an older woman with whom she had an affectionate relation and whose favorite she was, and whom she described as having "white hair like my mother" (ibid., 266). The young man appeared in the office, the day after her first visit to his rooms, to discuss some business with her white-haired superior. As she watched them talking quietly together (like the two whispering men on the stairs after her second visit), she became convinced that he was telling her superior of their encounter the day before. It also occurred to her that the unlikely matched couple had been having a love affair that she had hitherto, unaccountably, overlooked. The result was that, in Freud's words, "the white-haired motherly old lady now knew everything" (ibid.) and disapproved.

Freud traces the development of the paranoid fantasy through two stages. In the first stage the superior is clearly a mother-substitute, and the young woman's lover, against all probability, is promoted to her father's position as the older woman's partner in their suddenly postulated love affair. Freud argues that "her love for her mother had become the spokesman for all those tendencies which, playing the part of a 'conscience,' seek to arrest a girl's first step along the new road to normal sexual satisfaction—in many respects a dangerous one" (ibid., 267). Though the term has yet to be invented, the concept of the maternal superego is clearly operative here, untheorized but in implicit or practical form. Freud also insists that "the lover had not become the persecutor directly but via the mother and in virtue of his relation to her" (268). In this stage the superior as mother-substitute and the young man as her partner form the parental couple, whispering together, sharing a sexual secret, which shifts as she watches them, from being the secret of the young woman's meeting with her lover the day before to being the secret of the older woman's prior sexual relation with him. The younger woman has been evicted from the relationship with the man and is now on the outside looking in at the parental couple. In the second stage of the paranoid delusion, on her second visit, she had rejoined her lover on the couch in the young man's rooms but is now being watched by another gaze. As Freud plots the transformation of the delusional structure: "The patient's lover was still her father, but she had taken her mother's place. The part of the listener had then to be allotted to a third person" (ibid., 269). As Freud states, "she herself *became* her mother," and he sketches the unconscious train of thought implied by such a rivalous oedipal identification: "If my mother does it, I may do it too; I've just as good a right as she has" (ibid., 269–70).

The noise or click that interrupted the second love scene is not just an accidental circumstance that gave rise to the fantasy of being watched and photographed, "but something inevitable . . . something which was bound to assert itself compulsively in the patient, just as when she supposed that there was a *liaison* between her lover and the elderly superior, her mother-substitute" (ibid., 269). The compulsion arises from an underlying fantasy as prototype, which gives its structure to both stages of the paranoid delusion. So Freud formulates the concept 'primal fantasy':

> Among the store of unconscious phantasies of all neurotics, and probably of all human beings, there is one which is seldom absent and which can be disclosed by analysis: this is the phantasy of watching sexual intercourse between the parents. I call such phantasies—of the observation of sexual intercourse between the parents, of seduction, of castration, and others—primal phantasies. (1915f, 269)

The conceptual profile of the primal fantasies is only lightly sketched in here in a preliminary way, as a core set of fantasy scenes found with a certain predictability among "all neurotics, and probably all human beings." The notion of a prototype or stereotype plate for individual fantasy production is given briefly a social or collective dimension. This will receive a further theoretical elaboration in Lecture 23 of the *Introductory Lectures on Psycho-Analysis* (1916–17) and the later 1918 additions to the Wolf Man case.

What is important here, however, is Freud's structural analysis that enables one to understand the delusions as scenes constituted by a set of positions in a structure. In the first delusion the young woman is in the position of the childish watcher, looking on enviously at the parental couple with their shared sexual secret, whereas in the second delusion there has been a permutation of positions in the structure such that the patient has moved from the third outsider position to take the mother's place, evicting her from the parental couple, as she had herself been evicted in the first phase of her paranoid fantasy. The price to be paid for this, as Freud notes, is that "the part of listener had then to be allotted to a third person" (ibid., 269). The two men on the stairs repeat the motif from her first delusion of the whispering couple with a secret that concerns her, and though she accuses her lover of setting up the photographer, he only holds his persecutory position by virtue of his relation to the offstage figure of the motherly superior. Consequently, behind the photographer it is the mother who now occupies the third position, and her gaze has the power to break up the young woman's relation with the man. This had been prefigured in the first delusional scene as from her place in the parental couple, "the superior knew about the girl's love affairs, disapproved of them, and showed her disapproval by mysterious hints" (ibid., 266–67). In both scenes, therefore, "the mother thus became the hostile and malevolent watcher and persecutor" (268), whether in her relation to the man (scene I) or evicted from it (scene II).

In Freud's scenographic analysis, the triangular parental scene functions as a template or prototype for the young woman's production of successive paranoid fantasies and delusions. It is a three-term structure in which she moves from one subject position to another, as the first delusory scene is reformulated as the second. While it represents a certain gain for the paranoid subject, as Freud suggests, in that she asserts her right to sexual enjoyment— "I've just as good a right as she has"—in the face of the elderly superior's imagined disapproval (and, indeed, the superior appears to drop out of the manifest fantasy structure altogether, in its second stage), nevertheless, it is something of a Pyrrhic victory. The price paid for the eviction of the mother's surrogate is high. The whispering 'photographers' clearly reference the whispering 'parental' couple, and the continuing gaze "of the hostile and malevolent watcher and persecutor," now delegated to the imagined camera, has the power to compromise her lover and break up the lovers' relationship.

It is, however, only with the Wolf Man case that the parental scene is promoted by Freud to being designated as *the* primal scene, and here its status as the record of a real event is both affirmed and at issue throughout, precisely because it cannot be remembered as such by the Wolf Man.

*The Wolf Man's Primal Scene: Memory versus Transference*

The case of the Wolf Man is central to the development of Freud's thought because it radiates out into key theoretical topics and concerns and seems to give the impulse to a number of new developments. Strachey, in his editorial introduction to the case in the *Standard Edition*, lists the areas for which it is crucial—the early oral organization of the libido and its importance for a psychoanalytic understanding of incorporation, identification, and the formation of the ego-ideal; and even more striking the exploration of the subject's anal sexuality and its relation to the topic of bisexuality, and so the more elaborated version of both positive and inverted Oedipus complexes. This presentation of the earlier pregenital phases of infantile sexuality constitutes its primary importance for Freud, as the case appears to provide clinical evidence and support for the theory of infantile sexuality, in his polemic with both Adler and Jung after their recent breaks with Freud, and their repudiations of the centrality of either sexuality (Adler) or the infantile dimension (Jung).

For the purposes of this book, however, the importance of the case arises from the return of the old, officially repudiated trauma theory and Freud's explicit theoretical recognition of it (unlike its only implicit and largely subtextual presence in the Leonardo study, as demonstrated in Chapters 6 and 7, in the unacknowledged form of the progressive screen memory and the thematic of seduction). In particular, the case presents the most elaborate scenography of trauma, the most painstaking reconstruction of the scenario of a traumatic event in the whole Freudian corpus, and the most problematic.

There are a number of striking features about Freud's reconstruction of what he designates as 'the primal scene' at the center of the case. First and most striking is the starting point for his reconstruction, for the scene manifested itself in the *first* instance, not in a neurotic symptom, nor a screen memory, but in a dream. It was a manifest dream scene—to which the analysand kept returning again and again—that gradually emerged as, in Freud's view, the key to both his patient's adult neurosis and the childhood neurosis to which it pointed. As a childhood anxiety dream, it occurred immediately before the appearance of the wolf phobia, which it seems to have precipitated. Through his analysis of the dream, Freud sought to reconstruct the causes of the phobia and the obsessional neurosis that soon after took its place. Certain features of this manifest dream scene, Freud argued, themselves did not just point to latent dream-thoughts composed of infantile wishes stirred up by the day's residues of recent events, as in the standard model of the dreaming process formulated in *The Interpretation of Dreams* (1900a), but they also referenced an actual traumatic event, for the memory of which the dream acted as a substitute. The temporal sequence that then emerges as significant for Freud's analysis stretches from the infancy to the adult present of his patient: primal scene→anxiety dream→childhood neurosis (animal phobia, obsessional neurosis)→adult neurosis.

Freud's ambition was to reconstruct the Wolf Man's childhood neurosis that at a later point was to act as the prototype of the adult neurosis that had brought him into analysis. In particular, he sought to locate its causes through his analysis of the transformative childhood wolf dream that precipitated the formation of the child's neurosis. Nevertheless, this temporal sequence has a second striking and indeed puzzling feature: the absence of a key moment in the treatment that Freud's work on transference and the analytic process, contemporary with the case, would have led us to expect— the transference neurosis. The Wolf Man case is notable for its minimal reference to the transference (at most, a few remarks), and in its place, instead, we find the consequent centrality of a project of memorial reconstruction, based on the analysis of the patient's wolf dream. This has been the basis for criticism by later generations of psychoanalysts for whom analysis of the transference has become a central part of psychoanalytic technique, and for whom the construction of past events and the recovery of past memories have become problematic where not impossible, at best secondary by-products of analysis rather than first-order aims.[4] The absence of a sustained presentation of the Wolf Man's transference, however, is not the result of a failure to recognize it, as in the case of Dora. One can only infer a deliberate attempt by Freud to exclude anything other than a focus on the formation of the infantile neurosis, which is the main object

4. See the flippant dismissal of Freud's major case study in half a page by a contemporary American historian of psychoanalysis: George Makari, *Revolution in Mind: The Creation of Psychoanalysis* (New York: HarperCollins, 2008), 302–3.

and end point of the study. This privileges the dream, its interpretation, and the consequent reconstruction of the primal scene, which in Freud's account had acted via the dream as the generative matrix for the consequent phobia and infantile obsessional neurosis. With the exclusion of any sustained account of the later adult neurosis, many of the aftereffects of the infantile neurosis as prototype—including its acting out in the transference—were also excluded.

*A Dream of Wolves*

The text of the Wolf Man's dream runs as follows:

> I dreamt that it was night and that I was lying in my bed. (My bed stood with its foot towards the window; in front of the window there was a row of old walnut trees. I know it was winter when I had the dream, and night-time.) Suddenly the window opened of its own accord, and I was terrified to see that some white wolves were sitting on the big walnut tree in front of the window. There were six or seven of them. The wolves were quite white, and looked more like foxes or sheep-dogs, for they had big tails like foxes and they had their ears pricked like dogs when they pay attention to something. In great terror, evidently of being eaten up by the wolves, I screamed and woke up. My nurse hurried to my bed, to see what had happened to me. It took quite a long while before I was convinced that it had only been a dream; I had such a clear and life-like picture of the window opening and the wolves sitting on the tree. At last I grew quieter, felt as though I had escaped from some danger, and went to sleep again. The only piece of action in the dream was the opening of the window; for the wolves sat quite still and without making any movement on the branches of the tree, to the right and left of the trunk, and looked at me. It seemed as though they had riveted their whole attention upon me.[5]

Freud's first approach to the wolf dream was in a specialized article, "The Occurrence in Dreams of Material from Fairy Tales" (1913d), and he begins his analysis in the case study simply by quoting from his earlier article. The result is to connect the dream's manifest wolf scene with traditional folktales in which wolves play a central role. The patient refers in particular

5. Freud (1918b), *SE* 17, 29.

to the tales of "Little Red Riding-Hood," "The Wolf and the Seven Little Goats," and an anonymous tale told by his grandfather that might be called "The Wolf and the Tailor." The wolf tales function as an extended equivalent to what Freudian dream theory calls 'the day's residues,' that is, contemporary material from the dreamer's life whose impact awakens earlier infantile experiences and wishes that, in Freud's well-known metaphor, act as the capitalist of the dream, providing the psychic energy that funds the formation of the dream. The dreamer's association that Freud lists first is his fear of the picture of a wolf from a book of fairy tales. His elder sister used to tease him by holding up the picture before him, to terrify him and make him scream: "In this picture the wolf was standing upright, striding out with one foot, with its claws stretched out and its ears pricked" (1918b, 30). This particular image of the wolf will be crucial in Freud's construction of the primal scene behind the dream, as it is only in this upright, striding posture that the wolf terrified the little boy (wolves on all fours carried no such emotional charge). Freud infers: "The effect produced by these stories was shown in the little dreamer by a regular animal phobia" (ibid., 32), adding the significant observation that the anxiety animal was not a familiar object, such as a dog or horse, but one known only from stories and picture books.[6] This attributes the formation of the wolf phobia directly to the influence of the wolf stories, and certainly the picture on which it centered was an illustration from the story "The Wolf and the Seven Little Goats." The Wolf Man himself simply correlated the dream with the period of his fear of the wolf picture, establishing no clear chronology, unsure whether the crucial grandfather's story "The Wolf and the Tailor" was told him before or after the dream. Freud's one interpretative comment in this self-quotation from his earlier article interprets the wolf as "a first father-surrogate," and reads both the little boy's dream and the wolf tales as sharing the same unconscious content of "the infantile fear of the father." This infantile fear clearly acts as a prototype (though Freud does

6. In a letter to Freud in 1926, the Wolf Man, Serge Pankejev, writes: "The Wolf-dream always appeared to me to be central among childhood dreams, if for no other reason, the Wolf dominated my childhood fantasy. However, when I later on saw a real wolf in the menagerie, I was quite disappointed, and I did not recognize in it the Wolf of my childhood." See S. Pankejev, "Letters Pertaining to Freud's 'History of an Infantile Neurosis'" (1926), *Psychoanalytic Quarterly* 26 (1957): 449.

not use the word) for both the later adult neurosis and the transference: "His fear of his father was the strongest motive for his falling ill, and his ambivalent attitude towards every father-surrogate was the dominant feature of his life as well as of his behaviour during the treatment" (ibid.). The dream's central symbol—the wolf—and its unconscious signification—the fear of the father—are already present in the fairy-tale material prior to the dream. Consequently, these traditional wolf stories provide both the dream's manifest scene and its *dramatis personae*, together with a significant amount of its latent content.

Although the patient related the dream at the beginning of the analysis and recurred to it often throughout, it was only in its last months, when Freud had set a final date for the end of the analysis, that he was able to construct an interpretation of the dream with the help of various spontaneous initiatives taken by the Wolf Man. The dreamer had always stressed three strong impressions left by the dream, which he communicated in three supplementary comments on it. The first was the intense sense of reality with which the dream had left him: "It took quite a long while before I was convinced that it had only been a dream; I had had such a clear and life-like picture of the window opening and the wolves sitting on the tree." The second impression was the stillness and immobility of the wolves: "The wolves sat quite still and without making any movement on the branches of the tree." The third impression was the gaze of the wolves fixed upon the dreamer: "It seemed as though they had riveted their whole attention upon me" (ibid., 29). To these one should perhaps add the comment on the wolves that forms part of the dream text itself: "The wolves were quite white, and looked more like foxes or sheep-dogs, for they had big tails like foxes and they had their ears pricked like dogs when they pay attention to something" (ibid.). This makes it plain that the 'wolves' were what Freud's dream theory calls composites, the end result of the condensing of a number of figures under a single rubric: they were white, which reminded him of sheep, but they looked more like sheepdogs or foxes, with the pricked ears of the former and the bushy tails of the latter, while they were experienced in the dream under the concept 'wolf,' with its reference to the wolf stories and the terrifying wolf picture.

Freud's leading inference from the first of these impressions is to frame his entire interpretation of both the dream and the case study as a whole:

The lasting sense of reality . . . assures us that some part of the latent material of the dream is claiming in the dreamer's memory to possess the quality of reality, that is, that the dream relates to an occurrence that really took place and is not imagined. (Freud 1918b, 33)

The reality in question was not something with which the dreamer was already familiar, Freud argues, but was something unknown and "very strongly emphasized as being in marked contrast to the unreality of the fairy tales." This "unknown scene," Freud insists, was not recent but "must have belonged to an even earlier period" (ibid., 33). The dreamer's other two impressions of the manifest dream scene, the wolves' fixed attention and their immobility, Freud also infers, reproduce "the unknown material of the scene in some distorted form, perhaps even distorted into its opposite" (ibid., 34).[7] The latter suggestion is to play a major part as an interpretative strategy in Freud's reconstruction of this unknown and soon to be designated 'primal' scene.

Freud's first provisional sketch of the outlines of the unknown scene contains the following elements:

A real occurrence—dating from a very early period—looking—immobility— sexual problems—castration—his father—something terrible. (Freud 1918b, 34)

What is obvious here is that two related thematic elements dealing with sexuality have appeared that have not been apparent at the manifest level of the dream. The basis for Freud's importation of these elements is given by two sets of associations that are recorded in the first presentation of the dream in the earlier article, one set bearing on the wolves–sheep connection and the second set on the grandfather's tale of the tailor and the wolves. The first set of associations, dealing with the unusual whiteness of the normally grey wolves, called to mind for the dreamer the large flocks of sheep in the neighborhood of the family estate that he sometimes visited with his father. Two specific associations occurred to him: "His father occasionally took

7. In the next chapter of the case study, Freud refers us in a footnote to his earlier formulation of the memory-dream relation for another patient: "A few days earlier I had explained to the patient that the earliest experiences of childhood were '*not obtainable any longer* as such' but were replaced in analysis by 'transferences' and dreams." *The Interpretation of Dreams* (1900a), *SE* 4, 184.

him to visit these flocks, and every time this happened he felt very proud and blissful" (ibid., 30). The second was an epidemic among the sheep: "His father sent for a follower of Pasteur's who inoculated the animals, but after the inoculation even more of them died than before" (30). Freud does not explore either of these potentially interesting trains of thought, at least as written up in the case study: one, a little drama of emotions connected with his father ("he felt very proud and blissful"), and the other, a little story of the doctor's cure that had only made things worse, which echoes the Wolf Man's experience so far with doctors for his own illness, and so is potentially a piece of negative transference to Freud. Freud ignores these associations, however, and leads the wolves–sheep connection in a different direction: "Behind the mention of the sheep-breeding, evidence was to be expected of his sexual researches, his interest in which he was able to gratify during his visits with his father" (ibid., 34). The clinical notes from which Freud wrote up his case study might indeed have contained extra material that supports this introduction of the theme of 'sexual researches,' but the associations recorded in the case study fall somewhat short of it. The dreamer's references are to the large numbers of sheep, the epidemic and the deaths of the sheep, but not directly to 'sheep-breeding,' which as a theme might well have signified the child's 'sexual researches,' his curiosity as to sexual difference and reproduction. Consequently, the signifying link of sheep-breeding with sexual researches seems a construction based more on what Freud admits he *expected* to find than on the dreamer's actual associations as given in the case material as we have it.

It is the theme of castration, however, that is to play the major role in Freud's construction of the primal scene behind the dream, and to provide the occasion for the return of the 'old trauma theory' from the 1890s. According to Freud, "the most obtrusive thing in the dream, the wolves in the tree," references the grandfather's story, of which he asserts: "What was fascinating about this story and capable of provoking the dream can scarcely have been anything but its connection with the theme of castration" (ibid.). Now the grandfather's tale involved two meetings between a tailor and a wolf. In the first, the wolf leaped through the tailor's open window while he was working, then in an interesting hesitation that Freud does not comment on, the tailor either hit him with his yard or "caught him by his tail and pulled it off, so that the wolf ran away in terror" (ibid., 31). In the second scene, the tailor walking in the forest encountered a pack of wolves and climbed into a tree to escape them. The maimed wolf then proposed that the other wolves should climb one upon another so the last one could reach the tailor, and that he would be the base of the pyramid. The tailor recognized the tailless wolf and cried out, "Catch the grey one by his tail," with the conclusion, as Freud retells it, "The tailless wolf, terrified by the recollection, ran away, and all the others tumbled down" (ibid.). Freud's unpacking of the implications of this wolf story will eventually play a leading role in his construction of the primal scene. His preliminary interpretation in the earlier article had proposed that the tale "contains an unmistakable allusion to the castration complex. The *old* wolf was docked of his tail by the tailor. The fox-tails of the wolves in the dream were probably compensations for this taillessness" (ibid.). The connection to castration might be supported by the fact that the German for 'tailor'—*Schneider*—derives from the verb 'to cut'—*schneiden*—so that the tailor who docked the old grey wolf of his tail was a 'cutter.' However, what Freud is interpreting at this point is not so much the dream as the wolf story and its latent dimension (castration anxiety) and the dream's derivation of a key detail from it. With characteristic dream logic the many bushy tails (foxtails rather than wolftails) disavow and compensate for the wolf's traumatically docked tail in the story.

It is not until an initiative from the Wolf Man himself takes up the dream again that further progress with its interpretation takes place. The original dream text had run: "Suddenly the window had opened of its own accord, and I was terrified to see" (ibid., 29). The dreamer now thinks that the window is not just the window through which the wolf leaps in his grandfather's story of the tailor and the wolf, but that it requires translation: "It must mean: 'My eyes suddenly opened.' I was asleep, therefore, and suddenly woke up, and as I woke I saw something: the tree with the wolves" (34). Freud aligns this comment of the dreamer on the relations of looking in the dream with the looked-at object, the tree full of wolves, and so with the wolf-tree connection from the story of the tailor. He draws a crucial implication for the organizing principle of the dream: both the function of looking and the wolf-tree connection had undergone a reversal. Where in the original scene he had woken up and looked intently at something, in the dream he woke up and found the wolves looking in at him. The look had been transposed onto the wolves, and he had become the object of their gaze. So also, where in the grandfather's story the castrating tailor had been in the tree, while the wolves had been underneath unable to climb up into it, now in the dream the wolves were in the branches of the tree (What had happened to the tailor?). Extrapolating this organizing principle of reversal from these two instances to the other key impression that the dream had left behind in the dreamer, Freud asks:

> What, then, if the other factors emphasized by the dreamer were also
> distorted by means of a transposition or reversal? In that case instead of
> immobility . . . the meaning would have to be: the most violent motion.
> That is to say, he suddenly woke up, and saw in front of him a scene of
> violent movement at which he looked with strained attention. In one case the
> distortion would consist in an interchange of subject and object, of activity
> and passivity: being looked at instead of looking. In the other case it would
> consist in a transformation into the opposite: rest instead of motion. (Freud
> 1918b, 35)

Where previously "the only piece of action in the dream was the opening of the window" (ibid., 29), which represented the dreamer's waking up in the dream to gaze at a scene of stillness and staring, now behind the dream scene the unconscious memory of a shadowy scene of "violent motion" is inferred, one that has been subjected to transformation and reversal by the processes of the dream-work. Three scenes of waking are superimposed here like a palimpsest. The real waking *from* the dream, screaming in fear of being eaten by the wolves, which followed the waking *in* the dream to the scene of the immobile and staring wolves in the tree ("The only piece of action in the dream was the opening of the window"), and finally the obscurest scene of all, the earliest awakening long *before* the dream to a scene of "the most violent motion" (ibid., 35).

A further late contribution from the Wolf Man helps establish with more specificity the immediate context of the dream: "The tree was a Christmas tree," from which Freud infers, "He now knew that he had dreamt the dream shortly before Christmas and in expectation of it." As Christmas Day was also his birthday, "he had gone to sleep, then, in tense expectation of the day which ought to bring him a double quantity of presents" (ibid.). In the wake of the Wolf Man's association that the wolf tree was a Christmas tree, the wolf dream was revealed as a *Christmas dream* that had gone badly wrong. As Freud comments: "So it was already Christmas in his dream; the content of the dream showed him his Christmas box, the presents which were to be his were hanging on the tree. But instead of presents they had turned into—wolves, and the dream ended by his being overcome by fear of being eaten by the wolf (probably his father)" (ibid.). Although the link to the theme of Christmas is introduced by the dreamer himself, it is not clear what role, if any, he then played in the drawing of the subsequent inferences from that link. The transformation of presents on the Christmas tree into wolves on the walnut tree is both striking and plausible as a visual representation of the negation of his Christmas wishes, or their reversal into something threatening, with the subsequent production of anxiety, although it seems to be largely Freud's work of inference.

Freud's interpretative dominance is all the more obvious in the immediately succeeding steps in the process of interpretation. He identifies the Christmas wishes/presents (to be received from his parents) as sexual wishes, specifically "the wish for the sexual satisfaction that he was at that time longing to obtain from his father" (ibid.). The context that supports this inference Freud had given in considerable detail in the previous section of the case study on the seduction of the Wolf Man by his elder sister in his fourth year. Freud's analysis of that episode had resulted in the conclusion that the seduction by his sister, of which he had a clear memory, had given him the passive aim of being touched on the genitals. When in a seductive display he had masturbated in front of his beloved Nanya, he received from her both a rejection and a warning, amounting to a threat that "children who did that . . . got a 'wound' in the place" (ibid., 24). This rejection produced a regression from genital activity to sadomasochistic behavior and fantasy in the register of anality (tormenting behavior that drove his Nanya to tears, cruelty to small animals and insects, fantasies of boys, including the "heir to the throne," being punished, beaten especially on the penis). Freud traces a development from his sister's seduction via his Nanya's rejection to a turn to his father. The little boy's change of character took place earlier that year in his parents' absence, from a relative docility to irascibility and proneness to tantrums, in the wake of both his seduction by his sister and the disturbed and aggressive behavior of their English governess. On his father's return, they were now directed at the latter:

When his father came home in the late summer or autumn the patient's fits of rage and scenes of fury were put to a new use. . . . By bringing his naughtiness forward he was trying to force punishments and beatings out of his father, and in that way to obtain from him the masochistic sexual satisfactions that he desired. (Freud 1918b, 27–28)

It was the strength of this wish, Freud argues, that "made it possible to revive a long-forgotten trace in his memory of a scene which was able to show him what sexual satisfaction from his father was like" (ibid., 36). A revulsion from its consequences, however, turned the Christmas presents on the tree into anxiety-wolves and resulted in repression of the wish and a flight from his father. Freud poses the question: "What picture can the nightly workings of his sexual desire have conjured up that could frighten him away so violently from the fulfilment for which he longed?" (ibid.). He claims that "it is the material of the analysis that shows there is one condition which this picture must satisfy," that is, that it must "create a conviction of the reality of the existence of castration." Consequently, it is "fear of castration" that provides "the motive power for the transformation of the affect" (ibid.), of desire into fear and anxiety, specifically, in the dream, the fear of being eaten by the wolves.

Up to this point, however, castration has not been a *manifest* element in the material of the analysis. In the grandfather's story of the tailor, Freud detects its presence through interpretation as an unconscious signification of the tailor's act of pulling off the tail from the wolf. This was not, however, an interpretation made consciously by the small recipient of the story. Similarly, when Freud lists a set of memories that he claims present the child with "the problem of castration" (ibid., 25), it is not at all obvious that the memories cited carried that meaning for him, as distinct from the adults involved: the governess's fantasy about chopped-up snakes, the father's killing a snake, another story about a wolf losing its tail, and "the names by which horses are distinguished, according to whether their sexual organs are intact or not" (ibid.), are all instances of practices, messages, fantasies of the adult culture that surround him rather than examples of his assumption of that meaning. Indeed, the one instance where the question of sexual difference is explicitly posed, an observation of two girls urinating, he interprets quite differently: "He rejected the idea that he saw before him a confirmation of the 'wound' with which his Nanya had threatened

him, and he explained to himself that this was the girls' 'front bottom'"
(ibid.). Somewhat tendentiously, Freud interprets the boy's description of
the vagina as a "front bottom," not as a description by analogy from a part
of the body with which he himself is familiar but as the *denial* of the
'wound' resulting from masturbation, as threatened by his Nanya, as if the
boy's description of the girls' genitals were a disavowal of castration. At
least, it is not clear that the denial of the 'wound' is actually reported as a
thought by the Wolf Man himself rather than imputed to him by Freud,
hence Freud's final comment: "Thus he was occupied with thoughts about
castration, but as yet he had no belief in it" (ibid.). However, the only instance Freud cites where the theme of castration is at all explicit is the question of the nomenclature of horses,[8] where the distinction is between
geldings and stallions, and not between the sexes. It is not at all clear, from
the material Freud provides, that the child's one encounter with castration
as a specific cultural practice had in fact been generalized into a constant
preoccupation with it as an explanatory motif.

### Freud's Leap: Constructing the Primal Scene

> I have now reached the point at which I must abandon the support I have
> hitherto had from the course of the analysis. I am afraid it will also be the
> point at which the reader's belief will abandon me. (Freud 1918b, 36)

Freud's statement indicates his awareness that the construction he is about
to embark on goes beyond anything that can be plausibly inferred from the

---

8. Although one should add that in a later addition made by the Wolf Man in 1926, in a
letter to Freud after his analysis, he refers to a childhood memory "from my earliest
days" of "a conversation with a coachman about the operation that is performed on
stallions," making it not just a matter of nomenclature but of a surgical operation (see
Pankejev, "Letters Pertaining to Freud's 'History of an Infantile Neurosis,'" 451). It is
important to note at this point, however, that the practice of animal castration involves
the loss of the testicles, whereas the castration complex and its associated fantasies, as
described by psychoanalysis, center on the cutting off of the penis as an organ of excitation and pleasure. Freud himself acknowledged the absence of interest in the former
and the exclusive focus on the latter in the fantasies that emerge in analysis (see "The
Infantile Genital Organization"[1923e], n. 142). For a recent discussion of this, see
Catherine Bates, "Castrating the Castration Complex," *Textual Practice* 12, no. 1
(1998): 101–19.

dream and the material of the analysis alone. His opening proposition frames the construction that follows: "What sprang into activity that night out of the chaos of the dreamer's unconscious memory-traces was the picture of copulation between his parents, copulation in circumstances which . . . were especially favourable for observation" (ibid., 36). The details of this outline are then colored in: the dreamer's age at the time of his observation of the scene as one and a half years, established indirectly from attacks of malaria that he suffered at that age, according to family tradition, and at the same hour every day. These Freud connects to the symptom, recurrent from his tenth year up to the time of the analysis, of moods of depression that intensified toward five o'clock in the afternoon. Malaria implies a summer occurrence, so, having been born on Christmas Day, he must have been $n + \frac{1}{2}$ years. Six months is ruled out as too early, and $3 + \frac{1}{2}$ is too close to the time of the dream at 4 years. With the recovery of the Grusha memory at $2 + \frac{1}{2}$ years later on in the analysis, the timing of the parental scene at $1 + \frac{1}{2}$ years is considered the most likely alternative. The child's cot is in the parental bedroom due to his illness (the unlikelihood of which for wealthy Russian gentry, with an army of servants and the child's Nanya, has been pointed out). Thus the scene is set by Freud the scenographer:

> He had been sleeping in his cot, then, in his parents' bedroom and woke up, perhaps because of his rising fever, in the afternoon, possibly at 5 o'clock, the hour which was later marked out by depression. It harmonizes with our assumption that it was a hot summer's day, if we had supposed his parents had retired, half-undressed [Freud's note: "in white underclothes: the *white wolves*"], for an afternoon *siesta*. When he woke up, he witnessed a coitus *a tergo*, [from behind], three times repeated [Freud's note: "a spontaneous association, exempt from further criticism"]; he was able to see his mother's genitals as well as his father's organ; and he understood the process as well as its significance. (Freud 1918b, 37)

Perhaps somewhat defensively Freud insists that the *content* of the scene he has constructed should not be the occasion for any doubts as to its credibility, as it is a plausible domestic scene; indeed, "such an event would, I think, be something entirely commonplace and *banal*" (ibid., 38). The only doubts Freud will countenance bear on the crucial question of time-structure, of afterwardsness (*Nachträglichkeit*) as the temporality of trauma, which now reappears so strikingly in Freud's account from the hitherto abandoned theory of seduction of the 1890s, and which Freud addresses more fully in his subsequent chapter. For the moment I want to trace Freud's exposition of the relations between the content of the reconstructed primal scene and its aftereffects in both the dream and the Wolf Man's subsequent life and symptoms.

The crucial element in Freud's scenographic mapping of the primal scene is the postures of the participants. These postures are crucial for its essential meaning that is reprised in the dream scene, crucial for understanding the transformation of the former into the latter, and crucial for the symptoms that were to dominate the Wolf Man's adult life. These are "the postures which he saw his parents adopt—the man upright, and the woman bent down like an animal" (ibid., 39). Within a few pages Freud is to shift his Latin formula for the mode of parental intercourse from "*a tergo* [from behind]" (37) to "*more ferarum* [in the manner of animals]" (41). While the latter designation entails logically that to mount from behind as much as to be mounted from behind is to act in the manner of animals, it is, nevertheless, notable that Freud's formulation shifts the burden of animality entirely onto the woman. An implicit and unreflective opposition is also tacitly at work here, between the male posture that is described as 'upright' (rather than bent over his partner), so retaining the dignity of that animal who goes upright on two feet, and the female posture that is on all fours, the very image of animality.

The Wolf Man himself connects the male posture in Freud's reconstructed scene with the image that embodied his fear of the wolf, inflicted on him so often at the hands of his sister: "He thought that the posture of the wolf in this picture might have reminded him of that of his father during the reconstructed primal scene" (39). This seems, however, less a spontaneous memory than a compliant speculation—"might have reminded him"—helping Freud out with a connection that confirms his construction. More to the point, although the image in the picture book, that of "The Wolf and the Seven Little Goats," assiduously tracked down by the Wolf Man in the secondhand bookshops of Vienna during his analysis, presents an 'upright' posture, it is not, on the face of it, that of a male engaged in intercourse, from behind or indeed from any other direction. In Freud's own description, "the wolf was shown standing upright, with one foot forward, with its claws stretched out and its ears pricked" (39). The outstretched foot suggests not so much a standing as a striding wolf, which is supported by a later dream when he was seven or eight years old, about a new tutor he was to meet the next day: "He dreamt of this tutor in the shape of a lion that came towards his bed roaring loudly and in the posture of the wolf in the picture" (39). Whether wolf or lion, the boy's anxiety animal adopts not so much a rutting or even a standing posture as an aggressive striding posture, like the mythic prototype from whom Wilhem Jensen's Gradiva, so beloved of Freud, takes her name: "Mars Gradivus, the wargod going out to battle."[9] A *Lupus* (or later a *Leo*) *Gradivus*, then, rather than a *Lupus a tergo*, and definitely not *more ferarum*, but in a distinctively human, two-footed posture, albeit belligerently if not predatorily male (one might think of Leonardo's upright swan in his distinctly unavian posture vis-à-vis Leda in his painting of that mythic scene; see Chapter 7).

However, whatever its relation to Freud's construction, the threatening wolf figure certainly seems to have cast a long shadow over the Wolf Man's life and to have generated a range of later symptoms. The *nachträglich* aftereffects of the wolves with their human and animal postures are the chief exceptions to Freud's exclusion of the Wolf Man's later adult pathology and its analysis. Freud mentions his "paralyzing fear" (ibid., 40) of a Latin master at his secondary school, fortuitously named 'Wolf,' and a mistake in translation over which he was severely reprimanded. Freud reports but does not analyze the mistake, which was that of translating the Latin *filius* (son) with the French *fils* rather than the Russian *CbIH* (syn). Freud concludes: "The wolf, in fact, was still his father" (ibid.). However, it is less a *mistake* in translation—*fils* is an accurate translation of *filius*—than the symptomatic attempt to keep the role of 'son' in a foreign language (French), a refusal to allow it home into his mother tongue (Russian). Indeed, the meaning of the symptom might be interpreted as the attempt *to deny* his role as son of the Wolf-father. A more linguistically nuanced analysis at this point might have explored the significance of the missing signifiers 'iu' in

9. Wilhelm Jensen, *Gradiva: A Pompeiian Fantasy* (1904), trans. Helen M. Downey (Los Angeles: Sun and Moon Press, 1993), 5. 'Gradivus' (masculine), one who strides or marches forth, is from the Latin verb *gradior*, "I step or march."

the slippage from Latin to French, and their possible relation to the Russian 'syn,' but this line of thought requires the associations of the Wolf Man for any access to the unconscious processes of his boyhood self.

Furthermore, one of Freud's rare citations in the case study of a transference symptom occurs in relation to the story "The Wolf and the Seven Little Goats," the source of the picture of the striding wolf at the heart of his phobia. In Freud's consulting room, the patient lay on a sofa with his back to Freud and opposite a large grandfather clock, a situation, one might have thought, designed to provoke paternal transference, if not to induce the persecutory anxiety it seems to have done. Freud noted the patient's recurrent reaction: "I was struck by the fact that from time to time he turned his face towards me, looked at me in a very friendly way as though to propitiate me, and then turned his look away from me to the clock." Freud's commonsense inference was that "he was in this way showing his eagerness for the end of the hour" (ibid.). It is only toward the end of the analysis that the Wolf Man himself reminded Freud of "this piece of dumb show" and interpreted it in terms of the "seven little goats," six of whom were eaten by the wolf, while the seventh saved himself by hiding in the grandfather clock. Freud then translates this transference behavior as saying: "Be kind to me! Must I be frightened of you? Are you going to eat me up? Shall I hide myself in the clock-case like the youngest little goat?" (ibid.). It is a striking glimpse of the way the Wolf Man, years later in his analysis, still lived out his fears and anxieties through the wolf stories of his childhood. He seems, unsurprisingly, to have had a special difficulty with tailors:

> Among the most tormenting, though at the same time the most grotesque, symptoms of his later illness was his relation to every tailor from whom he ordered a suit of clothes: his deference and timidity in the presence of this high functionary, his attempts to get into his good books by giving him extravagant tips, and his despair over the results of the work however it might have turned out. (Freud 1918b, 87)

As Freud reports, *Schneider*, or "cutter," and its association with the tailor/cutter who docked the old grey wolf of his tail, is clearly at work here.

These instances certainly testify to the aftereffects of the wolf symbol in the Wolf Man's life, to his fear of the wolf and his later avatars such as the lion, and to the connection of this phobia with the father and his surro-gates. Nevertheless, their relation to Freud's construction of the primal scene remains somewhat underdetermined. The slight link that Freud re-lies on is the fact that "his fear of the wolf was conditional upon the creature being in an *upright* posture" (ibid., 40, emphasis added), as wolves on all fours, or tucked up in bed in Grandma's nightcap, as in "Little Red Riding Hood," called up no such fear. 'Uprightness' becomes the verbal point of contact, then, between the wolf phobia and (despite the picture apparently representing a striding, not a rutting, posture) the parental scene of *a tergo* intercourse. However, one might wonder whether the ghost of a sexual meaning does not haunt the word 'upright,' signifying 'erect' in both senses, although Freud does not appear to register this. Freud's German term is *'aufrecht'*, which is used of both the upright striding wolf who terrified him and his father's posture in the reconstructed primal scene.[10] It is also a term used for erection in the sexual sense. Such a double meaning would entail that the 'upright' wolf would be an erect wolf in both senses, and that the terrifying posture was, after all, a male sexual posture. The other features of the wolf's stance, the foot thrust forward, the claws outstretched, the ears pricked (reproduced in the 'pricked ears' of the dream-wolves), all in-stances of bodily arousal, might also hint by displaced analogy at a state of erection and engorgement.

In contrast, the woman's posture is limited exclusively to the sexual sphere, and Freud relates it plausibly to "his liability to compulsive attacks of falling physically in love, which came on and disappeared again in the most puzzling succession" (ibid., 41). This compulsive love was subject to a specific condition of which he was not consciously aware, and in recogniz-ing it Freud returns to the notion of the 'prototype' (though without the term itself), and its determining effect on later sexual object-choice:

> It was necessary that the woman should have assumed the posture which we have ascribed to his mother in the primal scene. From his puberty he had felt large and conspicuous buttocks as the most powerful attraction in a woman; to copulate except from behind gave him scarcely any enjoyment. (Freud 1918b, 41)

10. *Aus der Geschichte einer infantilen Neurose* (1918[1914]), *Gesammelte Werke: Werke aus den Jahren 1917–1920*, Band 12 (Frankfurt am Main: Fischer Taschenbuch Verlag, 1999), 39, 66, 68.

This is the same terrain as the 1910 paper "A Special Type of Choice of Object Made by Men" (1910h), discussed in the previous chapter on transference, where the term 'prototype,' along with the term 'Oedipus complex' appears for the first time, signaling the emergence of a structural understanding of the Oedipus (as distinct from being merely a set of incestuous or parricidal feelings and themes). In the 1910 paper the oedipal configuration acts as the common prototype for the later formation of a series of apparently perverse and unrelated adult object-choices. In the Wolf Man case study, however, it is a single traumatic event, encoded in a primal scene and its postures that Freud excavates as the active prototype in the formation of the Wolf Man's adult object-choice.

These postures, which resonate throughout the Wolf Man's later life and loves, are also the link between the primal scene and the dream scene. It is noticeable that Freud works from what he says he *expects* to have been the child's desire and hence the content of the dream: "this picture of sexual satisfaction afforded through his father's agency, just as he had seen it in the primal scene," which was "a model of the satisfaction that he himself was longing to obtain from his father" (ibid., 41). We have again the notion of a prototype or model (*Vorbild*), the mother's supposed sexual satisfaction from the father, which acts as the model for his own imagined satisfaction. Instead of an infantile memory of maternal *jouissance*, however, the material of the grandfather's story appears in the dream: "the tree, the wolves, and the taillessness (in the overcompensated form of the bushy fox tails of the putative wolves)" (ibid., 41–42). The "associative bridge" is "provided once again by the postures and only by them. In the grandfather's story the tailless wolf asked the others *to climb upon him*. It was this detail that called up the recollection of the picture of the primal scene, and it was in this way that it became possible for the material of the primal scene to be represented by that of the wolf story" (ibid., 42). So it is the sequence: primal scene—grandfather's story of the tailor (the tailor in the tree, the tailless wolf being climbed upon)— "Seven Little Goats" (six of the seven little goats eaten by the wolf, the picture of the upright and striding wolf), Freud argues, that indicates the sequence of the latent dream-thoughts: "longing for sexual satisfaction from the father—realization that castration is a necessary condition of it—fear of his father," and, he adds, "It is only at this point, I think, that we can regard the anxiety-dream of this four-year-old boy as being exhaustively explained" (ibid.).

Castration, then, is the turning point of the sequence of dream-thoughts as Freud reconstructs them, the point at which the wishes that drive the dream are repudiated, wishes for the presents from his parents on the Christmas tree and the homosexual wishes they stand in for, directed at his father. These wishes are reversed and negated in the dream image of the immobilized and staring (potentially devouring) wolves, which have also taken the place of the castrating tailor in the tree (Have they eaten him and taken his place?), and which now appear on the walnut tree outside the child's bedroom window. The upright-erect wolf and the climbed-on-tailless wolf on all fours, the postures taken from the two different wolf stories, are the switch points that enable the young dreamer's sexual yearnings to be given a lupine symbolization, to be at once fulfilled and repudiated in the same terrifying, reversed scene. While repression–repudiation does take place, its failure is also indicated by the outbreak of anxiety that wakes the dreamer, despite the unthreatening behavior of the becalmed, whitened, bushy-tailed, un-wolf-like 'wolves.' Fear of being devoured by the wolf (like six of the seven little goats), nevertheless, is the dream's outcome, a transformation of his sexual wish for the father, Freud argues. Henceforth, fear of the Wolf-father, as we have seen, will cast a shadow over his life. The driving force of the repression that coproduces the dream, Freud infers, "can only have been his narcissistic genital libido, which, in the form of concern for his male organ, was fighting against a satisfaction whose attainment seemed to involve the renunciation of that organ" (ibid., 46).

In Freud's account, repression is a defense against wishes that entail castration and is powered by genital narcissism, the basis for the little boy's imperiled masculinity. His wishes and their repudiation in the dream are very plausibly located by Freud at the intersection of the wolf material with a sequence of actually remembered experiences—seduction by his sister, attempted seduction of and threat from his Nanya, tantrums and provocations directed toward his father. The wolf material puts into circulation figures of phallic aggression and phallic deprivation, which in the wake of the dream come to function as prototypes, achieving a repetitive fixation in the dreamer's subsequent life history. However, Freud also seeks to reconstruct, on the other side of this carefully assembled network of connections, a specifically *parental* primal scene, whose traces emerge not in the form of a memory (like the remembered scenes with the maid, Grusha, his sister, his Nanya, and his father) but in the form of the dream of wolves. The reality of this parental scene becomes intimately connected, in the Wolf Man case study, to the thematic of castration, which is the vehicle of a set of arguments about sexual difference, and which is also accorded the status of a real event. Indeed, the questionable, individual reality of the Wolf Man's never remembered primal scene leans heavily not on the anatomical reality of sexual difference but on a symbolic interpretation of it, together with a supplementary appeal to prehistory as the solution to its own uncertainty.

## The Wolf Man II: Interpreting the Primal Scene

"The old trauma theory of the neuroses, which was after all built up
upon impressions gained from psycho-analytic practice, had suddenly
come to the front once more."[1]

Freud's return to his "old trauma theory"—or at least to elements of it—is
evident throughout his attempt to reconstruct the primal scene behind the
Wolf Man's dream, a scene postulated in the face of the failure of any
memory of it to emerge. It therefore joins the host of excessive and unassimilated scenes, acted out through their translations and derivatives,
momentarily captured in a scenography they exceed, but denied and not
remembered, with which this book has been concerned. The nonappearance of any memory of the primal scene as reconstructed by Freud has been
taken by many (not least the Wolf Man himself) as a sign of both interpretative error and clinical failure. By contrast, a 'deconstructionist' commen-
tator like Ned Lukacher reproaches Freud from the opposite position: "We
might wish he could have openly acknowledged that with the notion of the

---

1. Sigmund Freud, "From the History of an Infantile Neurosis" (1918b [1914]), *SE* 17, 95.

primal scene he had formally and finally moved beyond recollection."[2] What both positions fail to understand is that the inability to recall the earliest scenes, combined with their prolific repetition in various forms, defines the clinical problem Freud encountered and struggled with theoretically from the early 1890s onward. His first use of the term '*Urszenen*' (primal scenes, and in the plural) in Draft L (May 2, 1897) stresses the unlikelihood of direct access: "In a few cases this is achieved directly [i.e., through memory], but in others only by a detour via fantasies. For fantasies are psychic facades produced to bar access to these memories" (Masson, 1985a, 240). In his 1899 "Screen Memories" essay, Freud concludes, "It may indeed be questioned whether we have any memories at all *from* our childhood: memories *relating to* our childhood may be all that we possess" (1899a, 322). I have previously quoted Freud's similar statement that "the earliest experiences of childhood were '*not obtainable any longer* as such' but were replaced by 'transferences' and dreams" (Freud 1900a, 184). Similar arguments are made by Freud in his papers on transference that certain earliest experiences repeat themselves and can only be accessed in analysis in the form of derivatives, dreams, and transferences, which are representatives but not transparent representations, of those experiences. Analogous to Freud's claim that transferential acting out is both substitute and equivalent to memory—"in the end we understand that this is his way of remembering" (1914g, 150)—is Freud's statement in the case study that "dreaming is another kind of remembering" (1918b, 51). Lukacher criticizes this statement, and Freud's equation of memory and repeated dreams as sources of subjective conviction in the analysand, as a "misrepresentation of clinical experience" (Lukacher 1986, 140). However, Lukacher's accusation against Freud, based on a reductive reading of the Wolf Man case predominantly in terms of Freud's battle with Jung (a battle that certainly takes place) isolates the case study from its theoretical hinterland in the history of the formative configurations and refigurations of the Freudian conceptual field, and especially from his earliest models of traumatic seduction onward. As a result, Lukacher fails to see Freud's argument in the Wolf Man case as another theoretical manifestation of his continuing attempt to

2. Ned Lukacher, *Primal Scenes: Literature, Philosophy, Psychoanalysis* (Ithaca, N.Y.: Cornell University Press, 1986), 139.

grapple both clinically and theoretically with the generative *Vorbild*, or prototype, that can only be reconstructed "gradually and laboriously from an aggregate of indications" (Freud 1918b, 51), from its epistemologically treacherous derivatives, repetitions, facades, and screen memories (even if Freud leaves the door slightly ajar to the possibility of occasional recollection but with diminishing expectations; see the late "Constructions in Analysis" [1937d]).

It is therefore significant that Freud's explicit acknowledgment of the return of his trauma theory, in the epigraph to this chapter, should take place not in relation to his construction of the primal scene itself but prompted by the scene with the nursery maid, Grusha, which to Freud's great satisfaction does emerge as a spontaneous memory in the process of the analysis and toward its end. It is as if Freud's explicit acknowledgment of the trauma theory at this point in his argument relates only to its earliest forms, such as the cases presented in *Studies on Hysteria* of 1895, where the traumatic scenes emerge finally as memories confirmed by the analysand, and their verbalization readily brings about the liquidation of symptoms. However, Freud's model of trauma and its action, as I have argued in Chapters 2–4, evolved away from the relatively straightforward causal relation of the 1893 "Preliminary Communication" through the impasses of the published seduction theory papers of 1896 to the late unpublished developments in the letters and drafts sent to Wilhelm Fliess. These later developments are marked by Freud's constant wrestling with the anomaly of his patients' reproduction in hysterical attacks and symptoms, hallucinations and transferential repetitions, emotionally charged scenarios—scenes—of which they deny having any memory. Freud initially responded to this anomaly with a determination to establish the reality of the earliest scenes of abuse, combined with increasing doubts as to their status as either memory or fantasy. This led, as we have seen, to a theoretical oscillation, evident throughout his letters to Fliess in the late 1890s, between the earliest infantile scenes or later postpuberty scenes as the key determinants in the production of neurotic symptoms. Consequently, the return of the trauma theory implies not just the gratifying emergence, from behind the child's phobic reaction to the striped butterfly, of the scene with the maid, Grusha, but also a return of the same problems and tensions of the 1890s played out again in the material of the wolf dream and the parental scene it supposedly refigures.

Freud's defense of his construction of the primal scene turns on a distinction between the content of the scene and the question of its time structure, its deferred action from the infant's encounter with the parental scene at eighteen months to its traumatic reprise on the eve of his fourth birthday in the anxiety dream from which he awakens screaming, and which provokes his wolf phobia and consequent infantile neurosis. In a rhetorically prophylactic gesture, Freud attempts to deflect any doubt away from the content of his construction, especially the details of its *a tergo* postures—"something entirely commonplace and *banal*" (1918b, 38)—directing it instead toward its proposed temporal structure.

> Doubts as to its probability will turn upon three other points: whether a child at the tender age of one and a half could be in a position to take in the perceptions of such a complicated process and to preserve them so accurately in his unconscious; secondly, whether it is possible at the age of four for a deferred revision of the impressions so received to penetrate the understanding; and finally whether any procedure could succeed in bringing into consciousness coherently and convincingly the details of a scene of this kind which had been experienced and understood in such circumstances. (Freud 1918b, 38)

It is in this "deferred revision" that we can recognize the motif of *Nachträglichkeit*, which, as noted by Laplanche, the foremost contemporary theorist of this motif, appears fifteen times in adjectival–adverbial form in the case study (*nachträglich*) and twice as an abstract substantive (*Nachträglichkeit*).[3] The motif of a combined deferral and retroaction characterized Freud's trauma theory in its most developed form, emerging first in the particular cases in *Studies on Hysteria*, then elaborated theoretically under the rubric of 'pathological defence' and the 'hysterical *proton pseudos*,' in the case of Emma in the unpublished "Project for a Scientific Psychology," (1950a [1895]), then both invoked and put at risk in the run of seduction theory papers published in 1896.

At the end of *Studies on Hysteria* Freud admitted that, while the cathartic method that Breuer and he pioneered could explain and treat successfully the "psychical mechanism" of hysterical symptom formation, "it cannot

3. Jean Laplanche, *Problématiques VI: L'après-coup* (Paris: Presses Universitaires de France, 2006), 124.

affect the underlying causes of hysteria: thus it cannot prevent fresh symptoms taking the place of the ones that had been got rid of."[4] With the seduction theory, however, Freud believed that he had found in early infantile sexual abuse the specific causes of hysteria as an underlying condition, and more generally what he called triumphantly the *'caput Nili* of psychopathology,' or source of the Nile for all psychoneuroses, as distinct from the 'actual neuroses' with their physiological causes. As I have argued in Chapter 4, the seduction theory papers are marked by conflicting tendencies produced by Freud's adherence to an etiological model inherited from Charcot. This privileges a category of specific causes, specific to each pathological condition, and so found in no other, and which cannot be absent in any instance of the condition. This privileging of a single, uniform earliest causal event—which Freud always thinks of as a "scene"—reduces all later events and their scenes to being merely concurrent or precipitating causes, that can only act quantitatively to intensify the primary and specific cause, thus depriving the later events of their codetermining and form-giving powers. This undermines and puts at risk the more complex understanding of traumatic temporality (and its theoretical corollary, the thesis of overdetermination) that Freud developed, haltingly and unevenly, under the rubric of afterwardsness *(Nachträglichkeit)*, with its double dimension of deferral and retroaction between the successive scenes that orchestrate the emergence and continuing afterlife of the trauma.

The conflict between the etiological privileging of the reconstructed primal scene at one and a half years and an adequate account of the complexities of its *nachträglich* operation in the dream at four years marks the Wolf Man case throughout, as with the seduction theory papers of 1896. The word that Freud uses on a number of occasions is precisely "activation," a term that he is concerned, in section IV of his case study, with distinguishing from memory: "The activation of this scene (I purposely avoid the word 'recollection') had the same effect as though it were a recent experience" (1918b, 44); *"Aktivierung"* versus *"Erinnerung."*[5] Even more striking, later on in section IX we find:

4. Sigmund Freud, *Studies on Hysteria* (1895d), *SE* 2, 261.

5. *Aus der Geschichte einer infantilen Neurose* (1918[1914]), *Gesammelte Werke: Werke aus den Jahren 1917–1920*, Band 12 (Frankfurt am Main: Fischer Taschenbuch Verlag, 1999), 71.

It was at that point [the boy's fourth birthday] that the dream brought into deferred operation his observation of intercourse at the age of one and a half. It is not possible for us completely to grasp or adequately to describe what now ensued. The activation of the picture, which, thanks to the advance in his intellectual development, he was now able to understand, operated not only like a fresh event, but like a new trauma, like an interference from outside analogous to the seduction. (Freud 1918b, 109)

There is a tension in the terms Freud uses to characterize the processes at work in the second moment of his three-term temporal schema, and he admits to his difficulty with it.[6] If the description of this moment in section IV talks of a "deferred revision" of the primal scene's "impressions" (1918b, 38), the term "activation," especially when opposed to "recollection," suggests a process that is an unconscious, even involuntary, repetition. The terms "activation" and "revision," however, are also paired with "understanding." In the earlier passage quoted the "revision" (38), which might be thought to be a critical or at least an interpretative process, is said "to penetrate the understanding" ("*zum Verständnis vordringende*," *GW* 12, 65) rather than to be the product or work of understanding. What, then, carries out this penetrating revision if it is not the understanding? Something else that comes from the outside? In the later passage quoted (109) the "activation," the repetition of the primal scene outside the process of conscious memory, is in contrast the *object* of understanding. However, the understanding of an activation of an "observation" and its "picture" is not quite the same thing as a "deferred revision," especially one that "penetrates the

6. Indeed, at a number of points where he attempts to describe the complexities of the second moment of his schema, Freud makes not just different but sometimes conflicting statements. Following his model of the dream as wish fulfillment, he states: "The strength of this wish [to receive sexual satisfaction from his father] made it possible to revive a long-forgotten trace in his memory of a scene which was able to show him what sexual satisfaction from his father was like" (ibid., 35–36). A few pages later, this is contradicted by the claim: "In his grandfather's story the tailless wolf asked the others *to climb upon him*. It was this detail that called up the recollection of the picture of the primal scene" (42), whereas the model of the dream would require that the wish called up the memory trace of the primal scene, in which the mother's posture rhymed with and so in turn called up the tailless wolf's offer to be climbed on. The term "recollection" ('*Erinnerung*' again [*GW* 12, 69]) here also contradicts Freud's distinction between "activation" and "recollection" two pages later.

understanding." The revision, however deferred, implies a resymboliza-
tion, a resignification—parents into wolves (both upright/erect and on all
fours)—while in the later passage an activation of a picture that is, "thanks
to the advance in his intellectual development" (ibid., 109), now understood,
implies a meaning that is latent or inherent, just awaiting its belated acknowledgment. Like the scenic reproductions Freud encountered in the
1890s in the form of hysterical attacks, hypnotic reenactments, transference
repetitions, this activation is also experienced as a "recent experience," a
"fresh event," but even more he now suggests "a new trauma." One might
recall the cases of Katharina and Miss Lucy R., discussed in Chapters 2 and
3, where a scene both reactivates earlier, highly charged, and unprocessed
material while being toxic in its own right. In other words, it is not just a
repetition of the immediate experience of being overwhelmed by the excessive excitations of the parental scene,[7] which retains its freshness and power
due to its split-off or repressed status but something new, a trauma associated
with a new "understanding." It is, Freud adds, something that comes to the
child subject from the outside, but it does so forcefully, if not violently, "like
an interference," which is analogous to his seduction by his sister. In this
sense it might indeed be conceived as being able to "penetrate the understanding" rather than just being the child's own work of understanding.[8]

*Castration as the Real Event*

If understanding is the subsuming of experiential data under a concept,
Freud insists repeatedly throughout the study that the 'interfering' and

---

7. "It is, I may say, a matter of daily experience that sexual intercourse between adults
strikes any children who may observe it as something uncanny and that it arouses anxiety
in them. I have explained this anxiety by arguing that what we are dealing with is a sexual
excitation with which their understanding is unable to cope and which they also, no
doubt, repudiate because their parents are involved in it, and which is therefore transformed into anxiety." See Sigmund Freud, *The Interpretation of Dreams* (1900a), *SE* 5, 585.
8. Laplanche, in his lectures on *Nachträglichkeit*/Afterwardsness, stresses both the revival of the two-scene schema from the 1890s and also the fact of the second moment
being an interior event, a dream that is described as both a trauma and like a seduction
that comes from the outside. He does not, however, interrogate in detail the psychological processes ascribed by Freud to that moment. See Laplanche 2006, 134–39.

traumatizing concept in the Wolf Man's case is castration. Freud makes a very strong assertion as to what the content of this new understanding consisted in: "What was essentially new for him in his observation of his parents' intercourse was the conviction of the reality of castration—a possibility with which his thoughts had already been occupied" (1918b, 45). Castration is an example of the primitive *lex talionis* (or law of retaliation), as Freud elsewhere explains it,[9] which punishes the sinful member for its participation in the incestuous wish to disrupt the parental scene in order to possess the mother. Castration is a punitive and precisely targeted return-to-sender of the incestuous genital wish (compare the cutting off of the thief's hand, ordained by Sharia law). This punishment fantasy bearing on the child would certainly represent a *revision* and not just an activation of the primal scene. The wolf stories, 'day's residues' out of which the manifest scene of the dream is formed, especially the grandfather's story of the Tailor and the Wolf, are established by Freud as the carrier of the idea of castration, of the violent cutting off of a bodily part. This would, indeed, make the moment of the dream an instance of 'deferred revision,' a traumatic interference from the outside, in the form of the wolf stories, in the little boy's erotic investment (however that is to be described) in the parental scene.

Freud extends the motif of castration, however, from a question of punishment played out between the Wolf-father and son to being a representation of sexual difference. The woman does not just have a different genital from the man, but she *lacks* the penis (the result of the phallic stage assumption that all humans of either sex have or should have a penis), and this lack is the result of an act of violence—castration. In what is to become the standard account of the castration complex, the idea of castration is then belatedly realized by the boy as a real possible punishment through the coincidence of his phallic stage expectation with his perception of the alternative genital formation of the female, and the latter's consequent designation as a phallic lack or deprivation. This phallic-stage infantile fantasy

---

9. "The self-blinding of the mythical criminal Oedipus, was simply a mitigated form of the punishment of castration—the only punishment that was adequate for him by the *lex talionis*" ("The Uncanny" (1919h), *SE* 17, 231); "To make the punishment fit the crime," in the words of Gilbert and Sullivan's Mikado.

of sexual difference governed by a binary logic (having or not having the penis) would also count as a 'deferred revision' of the parental scene, one specific to the four-year-old Sergei's stage of sexual development and not just as an 'activation' of the memory traces of that scene. He would have constructed, through the received cultural code of the wolf stories, an anxiety-laden "understanding" (Freud's repeated term)—one might prefer "representation" or "symbolization"—of parental sexuality and his own endangered relation to it, which constituted a *Vorbild*, sufficiently traumatizing and pathogenic to give rise to the infantile and adult neuroses he later brought to Freud's couch.

What is surprising, however, is that Freud endorses and naturalizes the Wolf child's phallic-stage fantasy as an "understanding," in the normative sense, of the biological significance of sexual difference: "The activation of the primal scene in the dream brought him back to the genital organisation. He discovered the vagina and the biological significance of masculine and feminine" (ibid., 47).[10] In Freud's account, however, the vagina is the last thing the four-year-old boy could be said to have discovered. The "biological significance" of sexual difference has been completely rewritten in terms of the punitive drama of castration, such that the latter is said to inhere in the very nature of biological reality:

> We have been driven to assume that during the process of the dream he
> understood that women are castrated, that instead of a male organ they have a
> wound that serves for sexual intercourse and that castration is the necessary
> condition of femininity; we have been driven to assume that the threat of this
> loss induced him to repress his feminine attitude to men, and that he awoke
> from his homosexual enthusiasm with anxiety. (1918b, 78)

Freud goes on to speak of "this comprehension of sexual intercourse, this recognition of the vagina" (ibid., 78). However, it is obvious that the drama

10. The various forms of this claim throughout the case study—"the dream which gave him a deferred comprehension of the scene he had experienced when he was one and a half, and an explanation of the part played by women in the sexual act"—a comprehension, recognition, and understanding that he did not have before the dream—would seem to contradict one of the essential theses of Freudian dream theory: "The dreamwork is not simply more careless, more irrational, more forgetful and more incomplete than waking thought. . . . It does not think, calculate or judge in any way at all; it restricts itself to giving things a new form" (1900a, *SE* 5, 507).

of castration is not a biological description and does not function within the register of biological discourse at all. Neither a "comprehension" nor a "recognition," it is a fantasy deriving from the wolf stories as carriers of the idea of mutilation, loss, and punishment from the erect and devouring Wolf-father and reinforced by his Nanya's threat of a genital 'wound' for his masturbation. It is striking that of the infantile sexual theories recorded by Freud, the scene of parental intercourse viewed by the child as an act of violence, the idea of anal birth of the *lumf*-baby ("Little Hans", 1909b), are always clearly described by Freud as misleading, as a *misrecognition* determined by the child's own anal-stage sadistic impulses, while in contrast the fantasy of castration, especially in its application to sexual difference, is hailed as a recognition of biological reality (in *Inhibitions, Symptoms and Anxiety* of 1926, the castration threat is considered a "real danger").[11] When the parental scene was translated or 'revised' by the dream-work in the terms introduced by his grandfather and his Nanya—the severed tail and the threatened wound—it indeed "operated not only like a fresh event, but like a new trauma, like an interference from the outside analogous to the seduction" (ibid., 109).

These slippages in Freud's description of the work of the second moment of his three-moment schema, in particular the tension between "activation," "understanding," and "revision," signal the tendency, evident throughout the 1896 seduction theory papers, to reduce the retrospective action of

11. This touches on the much larger question of the undoubted phallocentrism of Freudian thought. In his development of the important idea of 'childhood sexual theories' and his later formulation of the 'phallic stage' with its assumption that both men and women have a penis, the polarity is between phallic and castrated, not penis and vagina. Fetishism is then explained as the phallic stage *denial* that the woman is castrated, by affirming that the woman, some women, are phallic and do have a penis (those equipped with the fetish). Freud's own thought is then caught up in this fetishist logic, by turns asserting that women are either castrated (the vagina is a wound) or phallic (the clitoris is a stunted penis), though unlike his co-thinker Little Hans, Freud does not expect that the latter will grow any bigger. For the intermittent presence of an alternative to the dominant thesis of phallic primacy in Freud's work, see Jacques André, "Feminine Sexuality: A Return to Sources," *New Formations* 48 (Winter 2002–3): 77–112. For a recent discussion of psychoanalytic phallocentrism and an exit from it, see John Fletcher, "Gender, Sexuality and the Theory of Seduction," in *Women: A Cultural Review* 11, nos. 1 and 2 (2000): 95–108, revised and reprinted in L. Braddock and M. Lacewing, *The Academic Face of Psychoanalysis* (London: Routledge, 2007).

later moments—revision—to the merely delayed action of the parental scene itself—understanding (that is, misunderstanding). The complexities of this second moment of Freud's temporal schema, the wolf dream, are thereby reduced to a delayed 'understanding' of a primal scene that carries its own meaning—castration—always already inscribed within it, and needing only to be 'recognized' and 'understood' and defended against. Thus the double temporal dimension of afterwardsness is thereby reduced to the single dimension of deferral or postponement, by the privileging of the all-determining moment of the parental scene and its *pregiven* meaning. This tendency actually enters into the very construction of the content of the parental scene as one of intercourse from behind, which in Freud's account makes it a spectacle in which nothing is lost or in shadow—everything is to be seen:

> When he woke up, he witnessed a *coitus a tergo*, [from behind], three times repeated; he was able to see his mother's genitals as well as his father's organ; and he understood the process as well as its significance. (1918b, 37)

This passage comes from Freud's long and detailed scenographic reconstruction of the parental scene, and it is symptomatic of his tendency to include everything—the anatomical facts, their supposed 'significance' and, here for a moment, even the wolf child's own 'understanding' of them as well—in the one foundational moment. He does then immediately go on to correct himself in a footnote: "I mean that he understood it at the time of the dream when he was four years old, not at the time of the observation" (ibid., 37). This slip, however, betrays the tendency to construct a 'primal' moment whose meaning is always already inscribed in the facts, thus a 'significance' without a signifying agent. As Jean Laplanche points out (Laplanche 2006, 144, 165–71), Freud does not conceive of the scene as itself transmitting a message, a meaning from the parents to the infant, demanding translation—"You will be castrated, if . . ."—but a scene where the meaning is another fact, alongside what he sees—"the woman is castrated; she lacks a penis and has a wound instead." The 'fact' of the woman's castration precedes, and indeed founds, any implication or threat the scene might have for the child: "Because she is castrated, so will you be if you persist in wanting to take her place with the father."

Hence Freud's insistence on the importance of that first moment of seeing and the full availability of what is to be seen: "a picture of copulation between his parents, copulation in circumstances which were not entirely usual and were especially favourable for observation" (ibid., 36). It is surprising, as Patrick Mahony has observed, that the plausibility of this 'realist' construction has so rarely been challenged. As Mahony points out, the first was Serge Viderman, who noted, "The position *a tergo* is the least favourable to observe the female genitals, unless the child enjoyed the optimal position, neither behind nor before the couple, but at their very junction"; and he adds, tellingly that not only is it "the least favourable to observe the genital organs" but also "the most favourable to maintain the confusion with the anal region."[12] The confusion may not have been entirely the Wolf Man's, as Freud is to go on in section V to claim of the picture of parental intercourse operative in the Christmas dream, that "the first view of it to come up was the old one, according to which the part of the female body which received the male organ was the anus"; furthermore, he adds, "And, indeed, what else could he have supposed when at the age of one and a half he was a spectator of the scene?" (Freud 1918b, 79). Gone is the widescreen vision of the parental genitalia (Cinerama in the bedroom)! Freud's extraordinary rewriting of his previous, somewhat implausible construction of the parental scene as a spectacle of total visibility here seems to concede Viderman's criticism in advance that, on the contrary, it could only have been a spectacle of anal-genital confusion: "And, indeed, what else *could* he have supposed?"(emphasis added).

Freud's unacknowledged revision of his primal scene construction is motivated by the context in which it appears, that is, his consideration of the relation between the dream's implementation of the boy's castration complex and the predominance of an anal-sadistic sexuality in the period before the dream. This rewriting does not just bear on the content of the primal scene as the site of supposed perceptual clarity (actual confusion), and so an all-determining source of delayed effects. The self-evident equation, maternal vagina = castration, can no longer hold as the parental scene of traumatic 'understanding.' Instead, the motif of castration emerges only

---

12. Serge Viderman, *Le Céleste et le Sublunaire* (Paris: Presses Universitaires de France, 1977), 306, 314, quoted in *Cries of the Wolf Man* (New York: International University Press, 1984), by Patrick Mahoney, who goes on to observe that "the perceptual acrobatics . . . assigned to the Wolf baby's angle of vision would exceed the ingenious staging of any pornographic film producer" (52).

through a network of later scenes, whose key elements and dramatis personae are the upright/aroused *lupus gradivus*, the tailless, climbed-upon wolf, the seventh little survivor goat watching from the insides of the grandfather clock, the wound threatened by Nanya for his masturbation, the angry figure of the maid, Grusha, on all fours washing the floor, and rebuking the urinating Sergei. The postulation of a 'real' primal scene of adult–child encounter on the other side of this network of mixed mythic and actual figures could only ever have been, at its best, speculative. Whatever form it took, whatever other figures it included, and while the father is indeed a leading candidate for inclusion, central place must surely be given to the sister: the sister who played with her three-year-old brother's penis, who terrorized him with the Wolf picture, who was his rival for the father's love, good opinion, and family fortune, who rejected his first adolescent sexual overtures but was suspected by him of not refusing their father's, with whom he claimed a "very deep, intimate and personal relationship" as "my only comrade,"[13] and whose suicide provoked such an elaborately displaced mourning, played out at the grave of the poet Lermontov. One of the unheard 'cries of the Wolf Man' was: "this sister complex is really the thing that ruined my entire life."[14]

## Freud's Oscillations

I admit that this is the most delicate question in the whole domain of psycho-analysis . . . no doubt has troubled me more; no other uncertainty has been more decisive in holding me back from publishing my conclusions. I was the first . . . to recognize both the part played by phantasies in symptom-formation and also the 'retrospective phantasying' of late impressions into childhood and their sexualization after the event. If, in spite of this, I have held to the more difficult and more improbable view, it has been as a result of

13. Sergei Pankejev, *The Memoirs of the Wolf Man*, trans. Muriel Gardiner. In *The Wolf-Man and Sigmund Freud*, ed. Muriel Gardiner (Harmondsworth: Penguin Books, 1973), 40.
14. Karin Obholzer, *The Wolf-Man: Sixty Years Later*, trans. Michael Shaw (London: Routledge and Kegan Paul, 1982), 37.

arguments such as are forced upon the investigator by the case described in these pages or by any other infantile neurosis. (1918b, 103)

This "troubled" footnote at the end of section VIII of the Wolf Man case study sums up succinctly the clinical and theoretical dilemma that this book has traced Freud struggling with from the early 1890s. He goes on to mention *The Interpretation of Dreams* and the Rat Man case as sites for his formulation of 'retrospective phantasying' (*Zurückphantasieren*, the very term Jung was later to use in his polemic against Freud's theory of infantile sexuality and its etiological centrality)[15]. As we have seen in the previous chapters, he might as aptly have mentioned *Studies on Hysteria*, his letters and drafts to Fliess (had he had them to hand), especially his first use of the term *Urszenen* in Draft L, the "Screen Memories" essay of 1899, and his analyses of the childhood memories of Leonardo and Goethe, not to mention the ambiguous virtual reality of transference love and the transference neurosis.

Freud's 'trouble' manifests itself again in the two additions he makes in 1918, the year of final publication, to his original text of 1914, written after the termination of the Wolf Man's treatment. The first occurs in section V, as if an afterthought to his argument with Jung's claim that what look like infantile memories are simply retrogressive fantasies through which the neurotic takes refuge in childhood and shies away from the tasks of adjustment and adaptation in adult life. For Jung it is a matter of "the peculiar use that he [the neurotic] makes of his infantile past. It looks as if he exaggerated its importance and attributed to it a wholly artificial value."[16] As a result, Jung claimed, "the *regression of libido abolishes to a very large extent the aetiological significance of childhood experience* . . . neither the infantile sexual trauma nor the incest complex present in everyone causes hysteria. Neurosis occurs only when the incest complex is activated by regression."[17] In response, Freud chose to focus primarily on the reconstruction of a childhood

15. Sigmund Freud, *Gesammelte Werke*, 12, 137, n1.
16. C. G. Jung, "Psychoanalysis and Neurosis" (1913), in *Freud and Psychoanalysis: The Collected Works of C. G. Jung*, vol. 4, ed. Herbert Read, Michael Fordham, and Gerhard Adler (London: Routledge and Kegan Paul, 1961), 246–47.
17. C. G. Jung, "The Theory of Psychoanalysis: 7. The Aetiology of Neurosis," (1915) in *Collected Works*, vol. 4, 168.

neurosis and its precipitation by a traumatic dream that itself reprised even earlier infantile experience, but in doing so he worked backward from a clinical starting point in a contemporary adult neurosis. This unusual strategy was obviously determined by his attempt to disprove Jung's claims about the etiological irrelevance of childhood traumas and complexes. However, regression and retrospective fantasy, as Freud insisted in the epigraph to this section, and Jung duly acknowledged, was an essential component of Freud's account of hysteria in particular and neurosis in general. Jung's argument had merely reactivated the long history of Freud's own theoretical travails, to which all the texts listed in the previous paragraph bear witness. In the "Screen Memories" essay, as I have argued, Freud stages an imaginary dialogue between himself as analyst and his alter ego as analysand, each of them at different moments of the dialogue voicing a proto-Jungian retrospective position, which in practice became Freud's dominant version of the screen memory. A moment of theoretical amnesia in which Freud's earlier insight into the internal relations between fantasy and traumatic memory, the double temporal dimension of afterwardsness, was lost—until its unacknowledged reemergence in the form of the *progressive* screen memory in the Leonardo study.

So Freud chose experimentally to construct *his own* retrospective rearrangement of the clinical evidence from the Wolf Man case, but within the time frame of his infantile phobia and obsessional neurosis, both of which were based on family testimony, as if to demonstrate the operation of the retrogressive tendency but within the field of infantile experience and thus to disable Jung's mutually exclusive opposition of the two. Reenter the sheepdogs. The parental scene now becomes the canine scene: "It is true that we cannot dispense with the assumption that the child observed a copulation, the sight of which gave him a conviction that castration might be more than an empty threat"—so the combination of threat and perception remains—"But what the child observed was not the copulation between his parents but copulation between animals, which he displaced onto his parents, as if he inferred that his parents did things in the same way" (1918b, 57). The primal scene now becomes a composite scene of parents and dogs, the product of a dreamlike condensation, "searching out in his memory a real scene in which his parents had been together" and driven by "the inquisitive child's subsequent wish, based on his experiences with the

dogs, to see his parents at their love-making" (ibid., 58). The advantage for
Freud is that his elaborate scenographic reconstruction is preserved: "It
really was on a summer's afternoon while the child was suffering from
malaria, the parents were both present, dressed in white . . . but—it was innocent" (ibid.). The dream-trauma's formative sequence now goes:

sheep-dogs > parents > wolves

One might observe that in this rewriting the wolves are somewhat back-
grounded, no longer mentioned as such, being replaced at the beginning by
a brief and unspecific mention of a castration threat, while Freud seems to
assume that a brief glance at the female genitals in either dogs or humans is
enough to either suggest or confirm the idea of castration. It also is not
clear why anal-genital confusion at three years, instanced by his reference
to the urinating girls' 'front bottoms,' should be any less at one and a half.
The claim of a "deferred understanding of the impressions he may have
received a few weeks or months earlier" (ibid.), rather than a traumatized
misunderstanding, is no closer to being established. Nevertheless, the postulation of an imagined but repressed scene with full traumatic powers is
significant:

> The scene which was thus imagined [the composite canine–parental scene—JF]
> now produced all the effects that we have catalogued, just as though it had
> been entirely real and not fused together out of two components, one earlier
> and indifferent, the other later and profoundly impressive. (1918b, 58)

However merely speculative the basis of this sheepdog-into-parent meta-
morphosis might seem, or unconvincing Freud's claims for it as a scene of
"deferred understanding," nevertheless, a line of thought is taken up again,
from his earliest attempts, in Drafts L, M, and N from the correspondence
with Fliess, to think the trauma–fantasy relation in a way that gave originary power to unconscious fantasy. This will lead us to the great essay on
'beating fantasies' written a year later, to which we will turn in the final
sections of this chapter. However, the outcome of Freud's thought experi-
ment in constructing an alternative back-projected account of a composite
primal scene is puzzlingly indeterminate. His first retrospective addition
concludes: "I intend on this occasion to close the discussion of the reality of
the primal scene with a *non liquet*," which the *Standard Edition* informs us

means: " 'It is not clear'—a verdict where the evidence in a trial is inconclusive" (ibid., 60), which is followed by the promise, to a reader who is assumed rhetorically to be unconvinced by the main argument for the actuality of the parental scene, that "a factor will emerge which will shake the certainty which we seem at present to enjoy" (ibid.).

The unspecified "factor" turns out in section VIII to be the spontaneous emergence of two of the Wolf Man's childhood memories; first, a moment of panic when chasing a butterfly with yellow stripes, from behind which there gradually comes to light the second memory of a scene between him and the nursery maid, Grusha. With the latter on all fours scrubbing the floor and scolding the two-and-a-half-year-old boy, her figure relates back to his mother (significantly, in the first version of the memory he thought she had the same name as his mother, which he later corrected) and to her posture *more ferarum* in the reconstructed parental scene. She also relates forward to a series of later young women with whom he fell violently in love, having discovered them working in the same posture. From the last in this series, Matrona, he caught the gonorrhea that had precipitated his mental breakdown and the psychic prostration that led eventually to his going into analysis with Freud. As we have seen, this posture had become the prototype and necessary condition for his falling in love. From other associations (Grusha's birch broom, the firewood with which Johan Huss was burned at the stake, thus becoming "the hero of people who at one time suffered from enuresis" [ibid., 92]) Freud makes—some might think leaps to—the inference that the boy, sexually excited by the memory of his mother's similar posture in the parental scene, urinates and is threatened with castration by Grusha. The gonorrhea in his eighteenth year thus comes to represent the threat to his genitals made by the ancient castration threat from Grusha and his Nanya and implemented by the wolf dream. This unsolicited memory of a real scene of excitation and danger, at the age of about two and a half, appears to ground and complete a sequence that connects the Wolf Man's adult sexual crisis to the sexual fixations of his object choice, via the wolf dream and the reconstructed parental scene to which it lends some of its remembered actuality.

At this very point Freud inserts his second addition of 1918. However, instead of fulfilling his earlier promise of challenging the skeptic's certainty based on the retrogressive perspective about the reality of the primal scene, and providing the confirmation we might have expected, Freud proceeds instead to challenge the reality of the very scene he himself has just laid out in detail. He entertains another retrogressive alternative, this time to the infantile sexual reality of the Grusha scene. Was the child's urinating proof of sexual excitation, evidence then of an earlier impression that itself might have been the actual experience of either the parental scene or perhaps the observation of animals? "Or are we to conclude that the situation as regards Grusha was entirely innocent, that the child's emptying of his bladder was purely accidental, and that it was not until later that the whole scene became sexualized in his memory?" (ibid., 96). Astonishingly, Freud delivers what he himself acknowledges to be an "unsatisfactory conclusion": "On these issues I can venture upon no decision" (ibid., 97, 96).

Freud's oscillations, which we have already seen played out in the texts and letters of the 1890s, here reach back four years, from the moment of delayed publication of the Wolf Man case to the apparently finished and concluded text of 1914, to destabilize the apparent certainty of its dominant argument. Laplanche, in his recent commentary on the Wolf Man case, in relation to the problematic of afterwardsness, notes the repeated pattern of expectation and disillusion with regard to a naively conceived material reality of a primal scene that would progressively determine what comes afterward. This can be found in both the supposed turning point of 1897 and again in the period 1914–18:

> It is striking to observe that the same crisis, over the same themes, is reproduced a second time. The same determined search aiming to reconstitute the scenes in their least details. The same conviction that there, as with the old theory of trauma, lies the secret of neurosis. Then the same doubts and the same disillusion. In 1897, Freud no longer believed in his 'Neurotica,' while in 1917 he doubts, in exactly the same way, the primal scene that he had taken such trouble to reconstitute. (Laplanche 2006, 159, my translation)

In the crisis of 1897, Freud had noted to Fliess, albeit reluctantly:

> It seems once again arguable that only later experiences give the impetus to fantasies, which [then] hark back to childhood, and with this the factor of an hereditary disposition regains a sphere of influence from which I had made it my task to dislodge it. (September 21, 1897; Masson 1985a, 265)

Here the hereditary disposition had been Charcot's inherited hysterical constitution. In the various texts from 1916 to 1918, however, Freud postulates an 'archaic heritage' of 'primal fantasies' (*Urphantasien*), which he had first named in the 1915 paper on the case of paranoia that we have looked at in the previous chapter. It is by recourse to the primal fantasies that Freud now seeks to stabilize his oscillations between the polarized retrogressive and progressive dimensions, and to provide a grounding in a real event that had itself regressed from infantile prehistory to the prehistory of the species.

## From Afterwardsness to Phylogeny

In both these additions of 1918, in the intermediate Lecture 23 of *The Introductory Lectures on Psycho-Analysis* (1916–17) and, finally, in the closing pages of section IX, Freud proposes that the parental scene has a particular status. In section V, he states: "Scenes of observing intercourse between parents at a very early age (whether they be real memories or phantasies)" are frequent among both neurotic and non-neurotic subjects: "Possibly they are part of the regular store in the—conscious or unconscious— treasury of their memories" (1918b, 59). However, he then adds that when it takes the form of "*coitus a tergo*, which alone offers the spectator the possibility of inspecting the genitals," then what we are dealing with is "only a phantasy, which is invariably aroused, perhaps by an observation of animals" (ibid.). Undecidability inhabits the very phrasing of Freud's propositions: "real memories or phantasies" become "memories," then the supposed full visibility of *a tergo* intercourse, which once had vouched for the possibility of a really observed event, is now the guarantee of its being a "phantasy." It is by invoking phylogenesis—the evolutionary development of the species—and by seeing these scenes as a phylogenetic endowment that Freud seeks, in Lecture 23 and in later sections of the case study, to lay to rest this invasive undecidability. Certain scenes—parental intercourse, the threat of castration, seduction—appear so frequently and are of such a general incidence that they are given a structural status: while they often occur as real events in the life of the subject, when they do not, however, "they are put together from hints and supplemented by phantasy" (1916–17, 370). Freud calls this essential repertoire of scenes *primal fantasies*, but he might equally have called them *primal memories*, for the ground of their necessity is, what Laplanche and Pontalis in their classic essay on the primal fantasies have called, "the bedrock of the event."[18] What are "told to us today as phantasy . . . were once real occurrences in the primaeval times of the human family, and that children in their phantasies are simply filling in the gaps in individual truth with prehistoric truth" (Freud 1916–17, 371). The hitherto opposed terms are just identified by speculative *fiat*. Fantasies just *are* memories, and not even progressive or retrogressive screen memories. What may be fantasies with respect to the individual's own life history are inherited memory-traces of real events from the barbaric times of the *Urvater* (the primal father) and the primal horde, as elaborated in the notorious fourth chapter of *Totem and Taboo* (1912–13). In Freud's search for the bedrock of the originating event, a reconstructed personal history gives way to an imaginary anthropology.

In his final restatement in section IX of the primal fantasies as "phylogenetically inherited schemata," Freud draws an analogy with Kant's transcendental categories of space, time, and causality, that organize the influx of sense-data: "Like the categories of philosophy [they] are concerned with the business of 'placing' the impressions derived from actual experience. I am inclined to take the view that they are precipitates from the history of human civilization" (1918b, 119). However, their structurally overriding or overdetermining power is more forcefully stated here, as it is not just a matter of filling in gaps (the nonappearance of these scenes as real events), with the hereditary schema supplementing the lived experience in fantasy. With the Wolf Man case we can witness "the independent existence of the schema . . . triumphing over the experience of the individual," for the boy's father becomes in fantasy the castrating figure and threat to his sexuality, despite the boy's *inverted* Oedipus complex and a literal castration threat from his Nanya and the nursery maid, Grusha.

Freud further relates the primal fantasies—now extended to include the Oedipus complex—to the question not just of an inherited but of an *"instinctive* endowment" (ibid., 120, emphasis added), which he locates in the child's reactions to both the parental scene at eighteen months and the

---

18. Jean Laplanche, and J-B. Pontalis, "Fantasy and the Origins of Sexuality," (1964), translated in *International Journal of Psychoanalysis* 49 (1968): 17.

reactivated scene at four years: "Some sort of hardly definable knowledge, something, as it were, preparatory to an understanding, was at work in the child at the time," which he compares to "the far-reaching *instinctive* knowledge of animals" (ibid.). The *Standard Edition* footnotes the word "instinctive" to inform us that the repeated German word in this passage is not Freud's usual term '*triebhaft*' (translated as "instinctual") but '*instinktive.*'[19] So also, when in his metapsychological paper "The Unconscious" (1915e) Freud considers whether "inherited mental functions exist in the human being," he sees them as "something analogous to instinct [*Instinckt*] in animals" (1915e, 195). It is not the sexual drives (*Triebe*) that are analogous to instinct in animals but rather the inherited primal fantasies, and these "inherited mental formations" form "the nucleus of the unconscious" (1918b, 121).

In Freud's speculative construction, inherited phylogenetic schemas, said to be collective memory-traces of real archaic events, function in an instinct-like way (i.e., preprogrammed, predetermined, not like the *Trieb*, contingent and variable) to produce subjective fantasies that are lived as real events. This is a version of recapitulation theory current in nineteenth-century zoology and biology, as formulated in Haeckel's biogenetic 'law': "Ontogeny recapitulates Phylogeny," the development of the individual recapitulates the development of the species, a proposition Freud explicitly cites in his 1915 introduction to the third edition of the *Three Essays* (1905). In Freud's deployment of this thesis, it is combined with a stubborn attachment to a discredited (by 1918) Lamarckianism in which acquired characteristics are directly transmitted genetically to succeeding generations. In a species of 'psycho-Lamarckianism' Freud extends this recapitulation from inherited dispositions characteristic of all living organisms—"the capacity and tendency, that is, to enter particular lines of development and to react in a particular manner to excitations, impressions and stimuli"[20]—to actual experiences, memories, and associated states of feelings. Indeed, he gives as the basis of this extension children's "reactions to early traumas,"

19. What is at stake here is the untheorized but implicit distinction between the human sexual *Trieb* (drive) and *Instinkt* in Freud's usage. For two clear discussions of these terms, see Jean Laplanche, "Drive and Instinct: Distinctions, Oppositions, Supports and Intertwinings," and "Sexuality and Attachment in Metapsychology," both in *Freud and the Sexual*, ed. John Fletcher (New York: International Psychoanalytic Books, 2011).
20. Sigmund Freud, *Moses and Monotheism* (1939a), *SE* 23, 98.

and especially their reactions to their parents in the Oedipus and castration complexes, "which seem unjustified in the individual case and only becomes intelligible phylogenetically": "Its evidential value seems to me strong enough for me to venture on a further step and to posit the assertion that the archaic heritage of human beings comprises not only dispositions but also subject-matter—memory-traces of the experience of earlier generations" (ibid., 99). It is this phylogenetic grounding in an archaic heritage of memories and scenes that enables Freud to state in a footnote in the concluding pages of his case study, "It is also a matter of indifference in this connection whether we choose to regard it [the parental scene] as a primal *scene* or a primal *phantasy*" (1918b, 120).

With this recourse to phylogenesis as an emergency exit from the undecidability of the progressive and the retrogressive, Freud reduces afterwardsness, with its previous interplay and translation of scenes, to a bald schema of phylogenetic repetition, and this in the very case study where the vocabulary of *Nachträglichkeit* and its variants is reiterated more than in any of his other texts. The *internal* relations of traumatic memory and fantasy have been lost, and the latter has become conceived as an unproblematic reproduction of an archaic scene, but one so formulaic as scarcely to qualify as a particular event or lived experience. Once Freud had talked of fantasies and, behind them, of "the auto-erotic activities and the caresses or punishments that stimulated them";[21] of the mother whose feelings were "derived from her own sexual life" and whose "marks of affection were rousing her child's sexual instinct and preparing for its later intensity," thus "fulfilling her task in teaching the child to love" (1905d, 23). The adult other of seduction, with his caresses and punishments, possessed of an unconscious with all its particularities, has now been replaced by the schematic blankness of the *Urvater* and his cartoonlike activities.

## Coda: Beating Fantasies as Originary Fantasies

Within months of the publication of the Wolf Man case study in 1918, with its two late additions, Freud was, in January 1919, working on a paper on

---

21. Sigmund Freud, "Notes upon a Case of Obsessional Neurosis" (1909d), *SE* 10, 206–7.

childhood sexual fantasies to be published later that year.[22] His analysis of a common beating fantasy both in childhood and into adulthood, conceived as a study specifically of masochism, develops into an extraordinary if temporary overturning of a number of dominant Freudian theses, whose radical alternatives seem to pass unnoticed. It has consequently attracted considerable commentary, two of the most productive being by Jean Laplanche and his cothinker, Jacques André. Freud's analysis is elaborated confidently, without a trace of the repeated hesitations between memory and fantasy that marked the Wolf Man study. André most strikingly demonstrates in Freud's account of feminine beating fantasies an implicit alternative account of female (early vaginal) sexuality to Freud's dominant phallocentric model, and indeed he draws from Freud's essay a provocative account of the 'feminine' sources of all sexuality in both male and female.[23] However, I wish to examine Freud's essay in the wake of Laplanche's reading of it as an alternative theorization to the model of phylogenesis and the primal fantasies, with which the Wolf Man case concluded.[24]

Freud's essay begins with the beating fantasy in its final conscious form as reluctantly presented in analysis, summed up in the formulation given in the essay's title: 'a child is being beaten.' In adolescence and adulthood this bare and impersonal formula can be elaborated into quite complex narratives, as demonstrated in Anna Freud's extraordinary structural analysis of the fantasy's further development by a teenage girl.[25] The final form in girls, from whom most of Freud's material is taken, involves a number of children, usually boys, being beaten by an adult authority figure. The fantasy is persistent and sexually charged, being usually accompanied by masturbation. The fantasizing child does not appear as such in the fantasy, and in reply to questioning states, "I am probably looking on" (1919e, 186).

22. Sigmund Freud, "'A Child Is being Beaten': A Contribution to the Study of the Origin of Sexual Perversions" (1919e), *SE* 17.

23. Jacques André, "Feminine Sexuality: A Return to Sources," *New Formations* 48 (Winter 2002–3): 77–112.

24. Jean Laplanche (1991), "Interpretation between Determinism and Hermeneutics: A Restatement of the Problem" in *Essays on Otherness*, ed. John Fletcher (London: Routledge, 1999), 138–165.

25. Anna Freud, "Beating Fantasies and Daydreams" (1922), *The Writings of Anna Freud*, vol. 1 (New York: International Universities Press, 1974).

Freud traces this back to a first phase that can be formulated as "my father is beating a child (usually brother or sister)." Both of these are consciously remembered and entertained. However, he explains the derivation of the final phase of the fantasy from the first phase via a second *unconscious* phase, formulated as, "I am being beaten by my father." The first phase Freud describes as proto-fantasy barely to be distinguished from memory and the reactions to actual events: "It is perhaps rather a question of recollections of events which have been witnessed, or desires which have arisen on various occasions" (ibid., 185). Of the second phase he observes that while the person beating remains the father, the child being beaten has changed into the child producing the fantasy, which is accompanied by intense pleasure of a masochistic character. Most strikingly, he says of the second phase:

> This second phase is the most important and the most momentous of all. But we may say of it in a certain sense that it has never had a real existence. It is never remembered, it has never succeeded in becoming conscious. It is a construction of analysis, but no less a necessity on that account. (1919e, 185)

Laplanche's argument is that the second phase exemplifies the specificity of *unconscious* fantasy, in that it is different from the memory from which it has arisen, as well as from the conscious fantasy that derives in turn from it. The virtually permanent repression of the second phase is not a form of memorization of an actual scene or scenes, but is the production of a new and different 'psychical reality,' which is not a copy of the events preceding it. Laplanche notes that Freud terms the second unconscious scene an 'original fantasy' (*ursprüngliche Phantasie*), partly because it is here that fantasy proper begins. Also such a formulation, as he puts it, "competes with and even invalidates the conception of 'primal fantasies' [*Urphantasien*] of phylogenetic origin, formulated two or three years earlier." Despite Freud's allusion to man's 'archaic heritage' elsewhere in his paper, his analysis of the beating fantasy indicates, in Laplanche's words, that "unconscious fantasy can be *'original' without ceasing to be the product of an individual process*" (Laplanche 1991, 156).

It is also important to note that the status of the 'real event' of the first phase is very different from that object of intense archaeological detective work, the Wolf Man's primal scene, which we have just considered at length in this and the previous chapter. Rather than a single traumatic event to be meticulously reconstructed, Freud refers to 'various occasions' and the desires to which they gave rise. As Laplanche observes, "Different circumstances, we shall say, have been able to convey one and the same message, and it has been possible for this to be repeated in different ways" (ibid., 156). Furthermore, the familial drama between father and siblings is not simply a material sequence of events, for these events are *presented* to the child. Laplanche dryly observes: "If a little brother or sister is beaten in the presence of the child in question, it is not like beating an egg white in the kitchen" (ibid.). This is clear from the addition Freud makes to the beating formula that locates it in the drama of sibling jealousy: "My father is beating the child *whom I hate*" (1919e, 185). In this emotionally loaded context, the father's act is not innocent; it sends a message, part of which has been translated by the child. This can be seen from the further transformations of the beating formula that Freud suggests. For what makes the scene so gratifying for the watching child, and so a likely candidate for further elaboration in fantasy, is the translation of it that Freud's further addition makes: "The idea of the father beating this hateful child is therefore an agreeable one . . . it means: 'My father does not love this other child. *He loves only me*' "(ibid., 187).

Indeed, Freud sets up the transformation of the material from the first phase into the unconscious fantasy of the second phase, in terms of an imagined dialogue between different translations of the father's implicit message:

> The fantasy of the period of incestuous love had said: 'He (my father) loves only me, and not the other child, for he is beating it.' The sense of guilt can discover no punishment more severe than the reversal of this triumph: 'No, he does not love you, for he is beating you.'
> (Freud 1919e, 189)

If this punitive translation is driven by guilt, Freud also sees it symptom-like as a compromise-formation that is driven as well by the incestuous wish being punished by beating and defended against by repression. Repression brings with it a regression from the genital to the pregenital, anal-sadistic organization in which the wish to be loved by the father is transformed into a wish to be beaten by him. In Freud's account, beating is both a punishment and the regressive substitute for the desire being punished.

Characteristically, Laplanche locates this confusion between beating-as-punishment and beating-as-a-kind-of-loving in the adult who beats. The equation between beating and loving inhabits the father's message before it structures the child's unconscious fantasy. Behind this traditional rationalization for beating children, Laplanche suggests that an unconscious fantasy sustains it of an anal-sadistic scene involving an assault from the rear. If 'he loves only me' is the child's binding and only tolerable translation of the father's culturally and unconsciously loaded act of beating, it is the obscure, violent aspects of the message in which loving involves such a beating that are excluded, but which form the unconscious scenario. This scenario Laplanche calls

> a fixed and immutable fantasy, not historicized but de-signified, senseless and inaccessible directly—a truly original fantasy, which can only be identified by the perverse derivatives with which we are all familiar. (Laplanche 1991, 159)

The sadomasochistic significance of beating, and of beating a child, is not so much generated spontaneously out of an internal drama of guilt and regression in the unconscious of the child, as always already present and at work in the parental other of the infantile scene with his already constituted unconscious. The unconscious fantasy—'I am being beaten by my father'—marks the insertion of the little voyeur-recipient of the father's message into the scene he or she watches (the unconscious fantasy is common to both sexes). Such a petrified scene acts as a source, not only of a drive to view or imagine such a scene, as in the conscious masturbation fantasy of the third phase—'I am probably looking on'—but of a drive that marks the subject's own body, evident in Freud's further addition to the beating formula—"A child is being beaten on its naked bottom" (1919e, 181). It is the parental targeting of the beaten child's body, in particular the buttocks, rather than any ontogenetic developmental sequence of stages that maps its anal-sadistic significance and provokes the watching child's fantasmatic identification with his rival as the imagined object of the enigmatic love that beats from behind.

Freud's scenographic mapping of the beating fantasies through their three phases (continued through an elaborate cycle of further phases by Anna Freud) has clear affinities with the earlier 1915 essay of the woman's paranoid fantasy, discussed at the beginning of the last chapter. In both cases Freud's aim is to locate the fantasist's position in the fantasy through its shifts and permutations. To Freud's initial questions as to the possible relations between the beaten child, the fantasizing child, and the various beaters (father, mother, authority figures), he receives "only the hesitant reply: 'I know nothing more about it: a child is being beaten'" (ibid.). The fantasy's formula offered by the analysand indicates this. The scene is fixed; its elements are the action of beating and a child, but phrased in the passive mood grammatically, it is not a fantasy of 'beating a child' but a fantasy that 'a child is being beaten' (*"wird Geschlagen"* in Freud's German). While the child fantasist in both the first and third moments of the sequence is on the outside—'I am probably looking on'—the impersonal *passive* construction hints at what is to come. It is as if the subject first internalizes a scene and the action that takes place within it, prior to and as the condition of identifying with any of the subject positions within that scene. Here the position of spectator is part of the scene, while one of the positions—that of the beater (in most, but not all, versions, the father)—despite being the active agent in the scene, is the object of the fantasy-wish rather than a figure available for identification.

It is also notable that Freud's argument enacts a logic characteristic of so many of his theoretical developments. What began as a detailed analysis of a minority pathological formation—trauma, narcissism, and here masochism—ends up discovering in them a general structural condition of the mind.

> The most obvious result of such a discussion is its application to the origin of the perversions . . . but it is seen not to comprise the whole truth. The perversion is no longer an isolated fact in the child's life, but falls into place among the typical, not to say normal processes of development which are familiar to us. It is brought into relation with the child's incestuous love-object, with its Oedipus complex. (Freud 1919e, 192)

The earliest phase of sibling rivalry "shows us the child involved in the agitations of the parental complex" (ibid., 186), while Freud concludes, *"the beating-phantasy has its origin in an incestuous attachment to the father* (ibid., 198), in the case of both male and female children. Whatever the diversity of the later-phase masturbatory fantasies, involving being beaten by the mother (for boys), of boys beaten by teachers and other authority figures (for girls), the unconscious fantasy of the formative second phase is the simultaneous expression and repression of the positive female Oedipus complex and the inverted male Oedipus complex.

This essay allows a glimpse of an alternative causal sequence in which rather than fantasy repeating a single traumatic event from personal or collective prehistory as its literal or disguised memory, various but convergent experiences are translated into an unconscious fantasy scene and fixed by repression, a scene that is never remembered as such but that continues to act as a template that is remodeled and reprocessed in later scenes and dramas. It thus has affinities with the palimpsestic nature of Leonardo's screen memory with its condensation of various scenes and moments rather than with the Wolf Man's reconstruction of a supposed single moment of origins or real event. Rather than a 'primal' fantasy (*Urphantasie*), a set of phylogenetic memory traces that simply replicates an archaic scene (of the *Urvater* and his aggressions), we have an 'original' fantasy (*ursprüngliche Phantasie*), 'originary' in the sense that it is not just at the origins but that it originates, as *Vorbild*, or prototype, successive fantasy sequences. It is an ontogenetic emergence (in response to the signifying actions of the actual adult) of fantasy, the unconscious and the sexual all in the same formation, an original theoretical moment that is bypassed and forgotten (the beating fantasy of 1919 is completely rewritten in 1925,[26] as André has demonstrated at length), to be replaced by the dominance of the primal fantasies and the repetitions of the death instinct.

26. Sigmund Freud, "Some Psychical Consequences of the Anatomical Distinction between the Sexes" (1925j), *SE* 19.

**Part V  Trauma and the Compulsion to Repeat**

## Trauma and the Genealogy of the Death Drive

> "It must be that after the ego-resistance has been removed the power
> of the compulsion to repeat—the attraction exerted by the unconscious
> prototypes upon the repressed instinctual process—has still to be
> overcome."[1]

In the case study of the Wolf Man that we examined in Chapters 9 and 10,
Freud announced a return of "the old trauma theory," devoted an extraordinary effort to a detailed scenographic reconstruction of an unremembered
'primal scene' behind the subject's dream of wolves, sought to bolster this
with an ingenious elaboration of another early scene with the maid, Grusha,
the memory of which did emerge in the course of the analysis, and then
abandoned any definite claim to the actuality of either scene in the face of a
hypothetical alternative account of each of them as retrogressive fantasies.
While leaving these competing claims in this instance as undecidable with a
final judgment of *non liquet*, he exited from his quandary by a recourse to
phylogenesis. Stubbornly attached to a temporal schema of traumatic repetition, to the action of an unresolved and still active ur-event seeking representation in the wolf dream, at the nodal point of its convergent network of

1. S. Freud, *Inhibitions, Symptoms and Anxiety* (1926d), *SE* 20, 159.

associations and recollections, Freud shifted his ground from the prehistory of childhood to the prehistory of the species. Yet within months of his ending the case study, with its exposition of primal fantasies (*Urphantasien*) as collective and unconscious primal memories, and without either disowning the idea of an archaic heritage or invoking it for his analysis, Freud had written up his analysis of childhood beating fantasies as *originary* fantasies (*ursprüngliche Phantasien*). The originary fantasy originates precisely here, as a translation of various jealous and wishful feelings but ungrounded in any one determining event. Formed in a moment of guilt-driven repression, as a punishment fantasy, it simultaneously plays out a genital-phase oedipal desire for the father in an unconscious scenario of beating. Thus, as I have tried to demonstrate in the Coda to Chapter 10, following Jean Laplanche's suggestion, Freud's essay of 1919 opens up briefly the possibility of a multiphase genealogy of a fantasy, which has its own determining power, but without recourse to prehistory and phylogenesis.

The moment does not last and is soon rewritten, whereas the problematic of trauma and its repetition appears again twice in two highly speculative texts, published nearly twenty years apart. The original fantasy model of 1919 is swept away by the radical recasting of the theory of the drives in 1920, where a model of trauma appears both explicitly and, I shall argue, in disguised biological form. Trauma is to make one further and final reappearance in the great anthropological fresco of *Moses and Monotheism* of 1939, the year of Freud's death. Despite the centrality of trauma to both these texts and their shared invocation, not just of repetition but of the *compulsion* to repeat, they bypass each other in silence. Neither the origin of life, with its vesicles and protozoa, nor the death drive appears in *Moses*, nor does any inkling of the beginnings of the species with its primal horde and *Urvater*—already elaborated in *Totem and Taboo* (1912–13)—appear in *Beyond the Pleasure Principle*.

*Topography and Its Contradictions*

The problematic of trauma has always had both a spatial and a temporal dimension, and these find themselves distributed between the two texts, with *Beyond the Pleasure Principle* specializing in a topography of trauma and the

*Moses* in a temporal and historical sequence. The two fundamental topographical figures in Freud's thought are that of the mechanical system open to inputs from its environment and characterized by a reflex action of discharge, and that of a closed homeostatic system that seeks to maintain an optimum energy level for survival and functioning. Both are regulated by opposed logics or principles, and an essential problem at the heart of Freudian thought is how they are to be articulated in a coherent picture of the workings of what Freud calls the psychical apparatus or apparatus of the soul (*psychischer* or *seelischer Apparat*).[2] The former first appears theoretically in the "Project for a Scientific Psychology," sent in draft form to Wilhelm Fliess in 1895 but not published until 1950, after Freud's death. Here it is the principle of neuronic inertia that regulates a network of neurones (the basic units of the nervous system) in which neuronal excitation is conceived as "quantity in a state of flow."[3] Its consequence is "that neurones tend to divest themselves of Q [quanta of energy—JF]," and that "this discharge represents the primary function of the nervous system" (1950a [1895], 296). What is curious about this postulation of a so-called "nervous system" is that it is not a biological model of a living organism at all but a mechanical model governed by the logic of the reflex arc, which in the words of Laplanche and Pontalis is seen as "transmitting the energy it receives in its entirety" (1973, 359). Freud reaffirms it again in the abstract model of perception and the memory systems proposed in Chapter 7 of *The Interpretation of Dreams*: "The psychical apparatus must be constructed like a reflex apparatus. Reflex processes remain the model of every psychical function" (1900a, 538).

It is only in a later moment of theoretical construction that Freud invokes what he calls a "secondary [function] imposed by the exigencies of life." This involves the accumulation of a store of energy that would enable this strange "nervous system" to perform "specific actions" that would meet the satisfaction of "the major needs: hunger, respiration, sexuality" (1950a, 297). In other words, "The nervous system is obliged to abandon its original trend to inertia . . . to zero." The trend persists, however, in modified form as "an endeavour at least to keep the Qn [quantity of intercellular

2. See entry in Jean Laplanche and J.-B. Pontalis, *The Language of Psychoanalysis*, trans. Donald Nicholson-Smith (London: The Hogarth Press, 1973), 358–59.
3. S. Freud, "Project for a Scientific Psychology," Part I (1950a [1895]), *SE* 1, 296.

energy—JF] as low as possible and to guard against any increase of it—that is, to keep it constant" (ibid.). The result is that the principle of constancy that regulates the second topographical figure of the closed homeostatic system and seeks to maintain an optimum level for functioning is subordinated to the first principle. Furthermore, it is described as a reluctant modification of its opposite, the zero principle of discharge, as if they were variant expressions of the same logic.

Jean Laplanche has made a trenchant critique of these founding assumptions of Freud's that initiate his "Project for a Scientific Psychology" and that remain foundational through to his last texts. Pointing to the assignment of a primary function to the model of a free circulation and discharge of energy, Laplanche observes that "at the beginning we are given a description of an organism which would be as yet . . . *non-living*": "Constancy of level and homeostasis, although they characterize the vital function itself, would thus be introduced only *secondarily* into what should have been, supposedly from the beginning, an *organism*."[4] This is part of Laplanche's critique of a model Freud takes from Hughlings Jackson, sometimes called the 'Father of British Neurology,' of a neurological hierarchy of brain functions from the primitive and simplest, integrated under the control of the more complex higher centers, and of a possible entropy or regression down the scale. In particular, he targets the notion of the 'primary,' which for Freud comes to include a coalescence of regressions: the topographical (regression to the unconscious), formal (regression from the conceptual to the sensory and perceptual), and temporal (regression to older, infantile, and primitive psychical structures, ultimately to a time before the organic).[5] Laplanche argues that Freud's description of an abstract 'circulation-and-discharge' model of functioning that would be 'primary' cannot be taken as a biological stage: "It is biologically unthinkable that the living being could pass through a first stage in which it was a mechanical system open to all the winds, seeking nothing but to empty itself completely of its energy" (1992b, 69, n. 33). Its value is as a description of a second-order process that *becomes* topographically and formally 'primary.' "It is rightly interpreted as a model not of the living being, but of the process occurring

---

4. Jean Laplanche (1992b), "The Unfinished Copernican Revolution," in *Essays on Otherness*, ed. John Fletcher (London: Routledge, 1999), 68–69.
5. S. Freud, *The Interpretation of Dreams* (1900a), *SE* 5, 538.

in a preliminary living being *from the moment when an unconscious comes to exist*" (ibid.).

Laplanche's reversal of Freud's so-called primary and secondary functions, in which the 'circulation-and-discharge' model figures instead as a *secondary* formation of the unconscious within an *already* constituted living being, can find some support from Freud's own text. It is certainly true that the "Project's" programmatic opening announces bravely a "natural science" that will "represent psychical processes as quantitatively determinate states of specifiable material particles" in the reductionist rhetoric of the biophysics program of Bruche and Helmholtz.[6] Freud admits, however, that what he calls his "First Principal Theorem" is in fact derived from "pathological clinical observation" of hysteria and obsessions and their "excessively intense ideas." In particular, "processes such as stimulus, substitution, conversion and discharge"—that is, the unconscious *psychical* processes at work in the formation of symptoms—"directly suggested the conception of neuronal excitation as quantity in a state of flow" (1950a, 295–96). What is implicitly at stake here is the question as to whether the unconscious and its specific forms of functioning—the so-called 'primary' processes of condensation and displacement—are there from the beginning and primordial (the id of the second topography of 1923) or are the by-products of the ego's defensive and binding strategies of repression and sublimation (the repressed unconscious system of the "Papers on Metapsychology" of 1915).

## The Pleasure Principle and Its Ambiguities

Freud's decision in the "Project" to subsume the second principle of constancy under the first principle of neuronic inertia, as a special case of the

6. See Frank J. Sulloway, *Freud, Biologist of the Mind* (1979), rev. ed. (Cambridge, Mass.: Harvard University Press, 1992), 14, 65–67. Sulloway argues that the older 'biophysics' program was of less significance for Freud's thought than the later 'psychophysics' of Fechner (which Helmholtz and Freud's director, Theodore Meynert, later embraced), and whose principles of stability and conservation of energy are crucial elements in both the "Project" and *Beyond the Pleasure Principle*. However, the biophysical model of a neurological reflex arc, previously elaborated by Bruche and Meynert, remains central, as we have seen, to Freud's metapsychology. See George Makari, *Revolution in Mind: The Creation of Psychoanalysis* (New York: HarperCollins, 2008), 57–74.

latter, despite their opposing tendencies, is reproduced in the opening section of *Beyond the Pleasure Principle*. In this section Freud sets up a correlation between feelings of pleasure and unpleasure and "the quantity of excitation that is present in the mind but not in any way 'bound' [i.e., freely flowing—JF]." This economic hypothesis proposes that "unpleasure corresponds to an *increase* in the quantity of excitation and pleasure to a *diminution*."[7] Freud then invokes Gustav Fechner's definition of pleasure and unpleasure, which he claims "coincides in all essentials" with his own. He quotes a passage in which Fechner argues that pleasure and unpleasure have "a psycho-physical relation to conditions of stability and instability," such that pleasure results "beyond a certain limit" from a return to stability, while unpleasure results "beyond a certain limit" from a deviation from stability (Freud 1920g, 8). These definitions, however, are *not* identical to Freud's. For Fechner, pleasure might result from either a rise or a drop in the level of excitation, as long as either returns to stability, while, similarly, unpleasure might result from either a rise or a drop in excitation that introduces instability. It is not assumed by Fechner that a rise is always unpleasurable or a diminution pleasurable; it is a question of their relation to and maintenance of stability.

Freud next equates his definition of the pleasure principle with the principle of neuronic inertia, as stated in the "Project": "The dominance of the pleasure principle in mental life finds expression in the hypothesis that the mental apparatus endeavours to keep the quantity of excitation present in it as low as possible or at least to keep it constant" (1920g, 9). This exactly replicates the ambiguity in the "Project" by which a tendency to maintain constancy is subsumed under a tendency to keep a level as low as possible (which would, under certain circumstances, include zero). At this point in his argument, however, Freud claims that "the pleasure principle follows from the principle of constancy," and that the principle that regulates the mental apparatus "is subsumed as a special case of Fechner's principle of 'the tendency towards stability'" (ibid.). Thus an irreducible contradiction is introduced into Freud's definition of the pleasure principle, which is si-

7. S. Freud, *Beyond the Pleasure Principle* (1920g), *SE* 18, 7–8, though he adds a rather undeveloped qualifier that they may be a function of increase or decrease over different periods of time.

multaneously equated with the principle of constancy/stability and with the old principle of neuronic inertia or drive to reduction.

Certainly in Fechner's account a return to stability (whether by reduction or increase of excitation) is accompanied by pleasure and deviation by unpleasure. Consequently, the pleasure–unpleasure series can be said to follow from his principle of stability, and both reduction and increase are in the service of its maintenance. However, as we have seen, this is not so with Freud's definitions, where the regulative aim of the mental apparatus is "to keep the quantity of excitation as low as possible or at least to keep it constant" ibid.), where constancy is a second-best compromise forced on it by what he calls in the "Project" "the exigencies of life" (1950a, 297). It is also clear, from the very passage Freud quotes from Fechner, that his stability principle regulates a homeostatic system that finds its optimum level of excitation for functioning between two limits, within which either increase or diminution is neutral, neither pleasurable nor unpleasureable: "Between the two limits, which may be described as qualitative thresholds of pleasure and unpleasure, there is a certain margin of aesthetic indifference," where, as the *Standard Edition* editor reminds us, " 'Aesthetic' is here used in the old sense of 'relating to sensation or perception' " (1920g, 9).

The difference between the two positions of Fechner and Freud can be illustrated by a diagram (Figure 6) of Laplanche's taken from his lucid exposition of the relation between their respective accounts of the 'Pleasure Principle' and the 'Constancy Principle.'[8]

I have taken the left-hand arrow of Laplanche's diagram as illustrating Fechner's pleasure principle in relation to constancy (or homeostasis) and the arrow on the right as illustrating Freud's. According to Fechner's model, those movements of the arrow toward the constant level of energy, N, that is to be maintained represent Fechner's definition of pleasure (whether it requires decreases or increases in energy level), and those movements away from it (whether increases or decreases) represent unpleasure. By contrast, the right-hand arrow represents Freud's conception of the pleasure principle. The upper section of the arrow heading toward homeostasis at the transverse

8. Jean Laplanche, *Life and Death in Psychoanalysis*, trans. Jeffrey Mehlman (Baltimore: The Johns Hopkins University Press, 1976), 113–14.

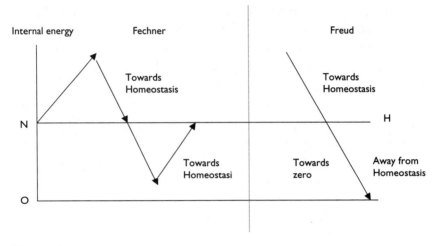

**Figure 6**
The Pleasure Principle: Fechner and Freud
Adapted from Jean Laplanche, *Life and Death in Psychoanalysis*, 114.

line N appears to coincide with the downward section of Fechner's arrow above the line, but its continued progress reveals its essential tendency toward the bottom line of zero. It is only arrested at line N by the intervention of another requirement—the exigencies of life—where it forms a compromise, while constantly seeking opportunities for its further progress to a lower level of excitation. Figure 7 further illustrates the workings of homeostasis in Fechner's models.

A central zone of neutral fluctuation, neither pleasure nor unpleasure, between two thresholds, the upper and lower limits, represents the optimum range of homeostatic functioning. Only increases above or decreases below these thresholds incur unpleasure, just as a return to the central zone in each case would be experienced as pleasurable. With Fechner, discharges and recharges of energy serve the maintenance of the system, whereas with Freud the maintenance of a 'store of energy' is only a moderation of the fundamental and persisting drive to evacuate energy from the system.

Despite Freud's claim that the pleasure principle follows from the principle of constancy and is a special case of Fechner's stability principle, when

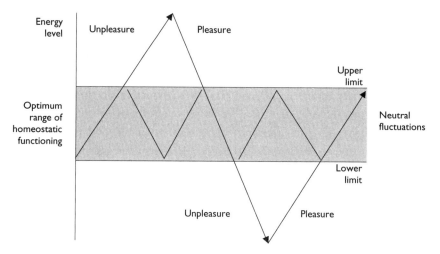

**Figure 7**
Fechner's Principle of Constancy

considering the various countervailing forces that can produce an outcome of unpleasure, he immediately goes on to identify the pleasure principle with the opposite of constancy and stability, the drive toward discharge. This is "proper to a *primary* method of working on the part of the mental apparatus," which is "from the very outset inefficient and even highly dangerous" when viewed by the ego "from the point of view of the self-preservation of the organism." The pleasure principle is then further identified with "the method of working employed by the sexual instincts, which are so hard to 'educate'" (1920g, 10). Cumulatively, by the end of the section, the pleasure principle is repositioned on the side of the primary processes, and the sexual drives pressing for gratification, as against the ego and its self-preservative instincts. The paradoxical outcome is that when the repressed sexual drives achieve a substitutive gratification (as instanced in the anxiety dream or the hysterical conversion symptom), "what would in other cases have been an opportunity for pleasure is felt by the ego as unpleasure." This leads to the general proposition that "all neurotic unpleasure is of that kind—pleasure that cannot be felt as such" (ibid., 11). This neurotic unpleasure is not, however, an increase in excitation but rather the gratification of the drives in *discharge*. This recognition calls into question Freud's opening economic hypothesis that unpleasurable feelings are the result of an increase and pleasurable feelings a result of a decrease of excitation in the nervous system.[9] Furthermore, Freud's definition of the constancy principle, as a modification and special case of the fundamental drive to reduction, acts as a conceptual switch mechanism that allows the pleasure principle to be identified first with one term of a primary opposition and then with the other, with the result that 'beyond the pleasure principle' as constancy, stability, the store of energy necessary for a living system to survive and function, we find—once again the pleasure principle, this time as the reflex drive to reduction, discharge, and ultimately zero.

## Trauma Revisited

Sections II and III of *Beyond the Pleasure Principle* pursue a search for phenomena that might testify to that "beyond" by focusing on forms of repetition that do not appear to conform to the operations of the pleasure principle. In particular, Freud interrogates the repetition of painful or distressing experiences in order to ascertain what forces might be responsible for such behavior. The main objects of consideration are traumatic repetition, children's repetitious play, the analytic transference, and what he calls "fate neurosis."

He begins by revisiting an entity from prepsychoanalytic times, the "traumatic neurosis," the result of violent physical accidents and concussions. We have seen in the first chapter of this book how, with Charcot's account of trauma and its effects, Freud had encountered a model of the

9. It is the case that in introducing the economic hypothesis, Freud had raised the possibility of a more complex relation between feelings of pleasure and unpleasure and simple quantities of excitation: "The factor that determines the feeling is probably the amount of increase or diminution in the quantity of excitation *in a given period of time*" (1920g , 8). In "The Economic Problem of Masochism" (1924c), due to the problems of the original purely quantitative equation—the recognition that "there are pleasurable tensions and unpleasurable relaxations"—Freud returns to this possible refinement that the relation may involve a question of rhythm, of "the temporal sequence of changes, rises and falls in the quantity of stimulus." This remains undeveloped. Consequently, he alters the *equation* of the pleasure principle with what he now calls the Nirvana principle ("the purpose of reducing to nothing . . . the sums of excitation"), making the pleasure principle a "modification" of the latter (Freud 1924c, 159, 160), a distinction without a difference.

ideogenesis of certain bodily symptoms that appeared only after an incubation period, due to the shock of a violent accident producing a mental splitting off of the memory-traces of that forceful bodily impact. The range
of hysterical panic attacks, paralyses, and contractures without apparent
physical damage was explained by the retention of strong affects attached
to the memory-traces of the event, to which the ego no longer had access.
While Charcot's model of *la grande hystérie* and its dramatic symptomology
had been criticized and rejected after his death in 1893, even by his own
students, the First World War, with its shell-shock and battlefield traumas,
had put the anomalies of a fully *psychical* trauma, apparently resulting from
the violent impact of external *physical* events, back on the agenda.

The range
Freud begins with two features that seem to characterize traumatic neuroses: first, the factor of surprise and fright; second, the puzzling feature
that a physical wound or an injury makes the development of a psychical
neurosis less likely. He distinguishes a set of three psychological states often confused with each other, in terms both of their relation to a possible
object and to the state of preparedness of the potential subject of trauma.
*Fear* is apprehension of a definite object; *anxiety* is a state of expectation of
a danger or a preparedness for it, even though the dangerous object is indeterminate; and *fright* is the result of having been overtaken by danger
without expecting or preparing for it, being taken by surprise. Anxiety so
defined cannot lead to a traumatic neurosis, Freud suggests; something
about anxiety protects against "fright neuroses" (1920g, 13). What seems at
stake here in these distinctions (which Freud does not himself always abide
by) is a question of boundaries and defenses.[10]

The repetitive phenomena he first considers briefly here are traumatic
dreams, in which the dreamer is repeatedly put back into the situation of
the bomb blast or the accident and wakes up in a state of fright. The traumatized dreamer, like the hysteric who in Freud's classical formulation
"suffers from reminiscences," is fixated to his trauma (in Freud's Lecture
27, "Fixation to Traumas—The Unconscious," he illustrates it with cases of

10. Strachey notes (Freud 1920g, 13, n. 1) that the fright/anxiety distinction reappears
in Freud's later distinction between automatic anxiety—when overwhelmed by a traumatic situation—and signal anxiety, warning of a danger to come, in *Inhibitions, Symptoms and Anxiety* (1926d).

obsessional neurosis).[11] However, for dreams to enact such distressing repetitions should not be taken simply as a testimony to the strength of the initial trauma. It contradicts the wish-fulfilling nature of dreams as specified by psychoanalysis, which, to be consistent with their function, Freud suggests, should be producing scenes of a healthy past or a future cure. He does little more than point the anomaly here from the point of view of psychoanalytic theory other than to suggest that "the function of dreaming . . . is upset in this condition and diverted from its purpose," or to gesture toward "the mysterious masochistic trends of the ego," before passing on to a more detailed consideration of children's play.

The repetition of distressing experiences in play is pursued through the famous example of the *fort/da* game of Freud's grandson, in which the absences and returns of the child's mother are rehearsed through repeated acts of throwing away a toy and retrieving it, accompanied by these two German words meaning 'gone/here.' Even when Freud focuses on the fact that most often the negative first half of the game—the throwing away of the toy that is made to be 'gone'—is repeated without its joyful return as a compensatory restoration, he points to motives such as punishment of the mother for going away—'Go away then!'—or mastery of an overwhelming experience and toleration of loss, which converts the passive experience into an active one. As a result, the experience becomes 'ego-syntonic,' self-comforting. Freud concludes at the end of section II that the sources of pleasure constituted by these various motives for the repetition of the distressing experiences of maternal absence presuppose the existence of the pleasure principle. Consequently, "they give no evidence of the operation of tendencies *beyond* the pleasure principle, that is, of tendencies more primitive than it and independent of it" (ibid., 17). It is clear that at this point Freud is placing the pleasure principle on the side of the secondary processes, mastery and the ego, rather than with "the *primary* method of working of the mental apparatus" and the sexual drives that pose the danger of "overcoming the reality principle, to the detriment of the organism as a whole" (10), as he had just done in the previous section.

With his turn to the analytic transference as a form of repetition in section III, Freud brings to the fore the idea of "the compulsion to repeat," first

11. Freud, *Introductory Lectures on Psycho-Analysis* (1916–17), *SE* 16.

formulated in one of the key papers on transference, "Remembering, Repeating and Working-Through" (1914g, 112), which we examined in Chapter 8. In the conceptual architecture of the earlier essay, the compulsion to repeat gives rise to two different and alternative processes: remembering and acting out. The analytic aim is to bring to consciousness repressed material, but because the repressed cannot be recalled directly due to the resistances of the ego that had originally repressed it, it makes its appearance in the form of acting out. One of the forms of this acting out is the transference. This term appears earlier on in *The Interpretation of Dreams* to describe the attachment of the repressed infantile material onto the more recent feelings, memories, and unfinished business of the day before the dream, which Freud calls 'the day's residues.' These tend to supply a lot of the material from which the manifest scene of the dream is largely formed, and onto which is transferred the infantile wishes and the memorial and fantasy material in which those wishes are encoded. In the analytic transference the person of the analyst and the analytic situation are the equivalent of the day's residues in the dream. The infantile material that cannot be remembered as such is repeated by being acted out in the current situation of the analysis, and in relation to the analyst who is recruited into the particular scenarios of the transference. Where the analyst seeks to bring the compulsion to repeat onto the side of memory and analysis, the ego seeks to keep it acted out in the transference, so as not to undo its repressions. The transference, once considered an obstacle to analysis, is now seen as providing an essential arena in which the repressed can enact its repetitions in the forms of a special transference-neurosis. The repressed cannot be overcome, Freud says, *in absentia* or *in effigy* but only as it comes alive again and repeats in the analytic situation and is captured in the nets of the transference and its interpretation.

Where a key issue in the 1914 essay is the kind of reality constituted by the transference, in *Beyond the Pleasure Principle* the key issue is the relation of the compulsion to repeat to the pleasure principle, whether it can be explained as motivated by the latter (in the sense of constancy, self-preservation, and the ego's mastery of the drives, or even just actual feelings of pleasure) or whether it provides evidence for a psychical force that is autonomous of and so *beyond* it. Freud argues that the ego "operates under the sway of the pleasure principle: it seeks to avoid the unpleasure which would be produced by the liberation of the repressed" (1920g, 20). While the compulsion to repeat acts to produce this unpleasure from the return of repressed impulses, this does not contradict the pleasure principle, Freud argues, because the two outcomes are topographically distinct: "unpleasure for one system [the ego—JF] and simultaneously pleasure for the other [the drives—JF]" (ibid.). Again, it is important to note that this unpleasure of the ego in reduction and discharge (rather than a taking pleasure in them) is not explicable in terms of the simple economic hypothesis with which Freud had begun in section I. However, Freud's point is that neither does this necessarily consign the compulsion to repeat to the side of the pleasure principle, because what is repeated are also, perhaps predominantly, "past experiences which include no possibility of pleasure, and which can never, even long ago, have brought satisfaction even to instinctual impulses which have since been repressed" (ibid.). As examples, Freud cites in some detail the frustration of the child's oedipal wishes, his failed sexual researches, disappointed hopes of parental intimacy or favoritism, and jealousy of siblings, all of which are so often reenacted in the transference to the analyst. Freud suggests that having not produced pleasure in the past, they would lead to less unhappiness if repeated as memories or dreams rather than as new versions of the old experiences. But no lessons are learned: "In spite of that, they are repeated, under pressure from a compulsion" (ibid., 21). Thus a certain paradox emerges from Freud's account regarding the situation of the ego caught up in the analytic transference. "Clinging as the ego does to the pleasure principle," it avoids the unpleasure of having to relax the resistances of repression and to acknowledge, if not embrace, the existence of the repressed. Consequently, it enlists the compulsion to repeat in order to keep the repressed acted out afresh in the transference, and so unacknowledged with all its historical baggage, but with all its consequences of the repeated disappointment, frustration, and bitterness of childhood revivified. So the pleasure principle here seems to lead to a choice for the ego of either one form of unpleasure or another. It also seems clear that Freud is using the terms pleasure and unpleasure here to refer to actual feelings of pleasure or unpleasure, and not to their supposed economic bases of either an increase or a decrease of excitation (neither of these terms seems to map easily onto the alternatives of remembering or acting out).

"Fate neuroses," Freud's final example of phenomena that might be witness to forces that act beyond the pleasure principle, are the equivalents of transference phenomena, which can be observed in the lives of 'normal' people who are generally asymptomatic. Nevertheless, they exemplify the compulsion to repeat in such a way as to give the impression "of being pursued by a malignant fate or possessed by some 'daemonic' power." Their fate, however, according to psychoanalysis, is "arranged by themselves and determined by early infantile influences" (ibid.). Though the *Standard Edition* translates the German as "fate neurosis," Freud's term for it is *Schicksalzwang*, or 'fate compulsion.' They are indeed characterized by the repetition of painful and distressing experiences. Freud distinguishes them from events where the subject is manifestly active in bringing them about, such that they seem to exemplify certain fixed character traits, however self-thwarting. Fate neurosis refers to events in which the subject is passive, apparently having no influence in bringing them about, but in which the same or similar fatalities occur in a repeating scenario. Freud gives as examples people whose relationships all finally have the same painful outcome: the benefactor whose generosity is met by ingratitude and abandoned by successive beneficiaries; the man whose friendships always end in betrayal by his erstwhile friends; the person who idealizes others, granting them at first authority and then overturning the pedestal on which he has set them; or the woman who marries three husbands in turn, each of whom falls ill and has to be nursed by her on their deathbeds.

The negative therapeutic transference of childhood distresses, the fated life histories, Freud suggests, point to the possibility that "there really does exist in the mind a compulsion to repeat which over-rides the pleasure principle" (ibid., 22), while the traumatic dreams are perhaps the least dubious, as there seems with them no coincidence of drive satisfaction with the compulsion to repeat, as is observable in the other examples. The identification of the ego in the transference with the pleasure principle is at best paradoxical, given the option of either one unpleasurable repetition or another, while both of these unpleasurable options are products of that compulsion. So Freud ends by proposing "the hypothesis of a compulsion to repeat—something more primitive, more elementary, more instinctual than the pleasure principle" (23). However, what must be noted again is the conceptual instability that haunts the pleasure principle as Freud defines it: sometimes identified with the constancy principle, sometimes with the primal drive to reduction, and sometimes an empirical reference to actual states and feelings of pleasure or unpleasure, outside any economic equation at all. In its final form, however, it is clearly an equation of the pleasure principle with something like the constancy principle, on the side of the ego and its attempts at recuperation and mastery, while what overturns it and so functions enigmatically *beyond* it is the instance of traumatic repetition, an instance without any pleasurable supports, reinforcements, or by-products, an instance, apparently, of pure— and purely self-destructive—repetition.

## *The Topography of the Vesicle*

A striking thing about Freud's enunciation of the death instinct (in sections V and VI) as the essence of all instinctuality (thus creating a problem with the possibility of a *life* instinct that would be opposed to it, while still being an 'instinct') is that he needs to tell another story first. This is the story of the vesicle in section IV, with its recapitulation and reworking of the apparatus of the "Project," and of the vicissitudes of pain and trauma that befall it. The vesicle and its trauma are necessary to situate the compulsion to repeat, which was, at the close of section III, the bearer of the possibility of a 'beyond' of the pleasure principle, even if we were to find there a radicalized, antithetical version of what we thought to have left behind.

The abstract model of the vesicle, defined initially as "a living organism in its most simplified possible form" (ibid., 26), hovers as a theoretical fiction ambiguously between being a mythical ur-organism, a prototype from which the human brain and cerebral cortex supposedly evolved, and a model of the psychical apparatus with memory systems, receptive surface, and primitive ego. Rather than the mechanical 'circulation-and-discharge' model that was the starting point for the "Project" of 1895, and to which the conditions for a living organism were only added secondarily, here the vesicle is a boundaried entity designed to model the conditions under which it might remain intact and survive. Freud's exposition begins with the differentiation of a special consciousness system as a reception apparatus, in which excitatory processes leave behind them no permanent traces as a form of material memory of their passage through the system. Instead, their excitation is transmitted to an adjoining system where a memorial trace or deposit is registered. The principle here is that "becoming conscious and leaving behind a memory trace are processes incompatible with each other within one and the same system," which is the case because permanent traces in the receptive system itself "would very soon set limits to the system's aptitude for receiving fresh excitations" (25).

The sensitive, exposed surface of the vesicle, by virtue of its liminal position, functions as "an organ to receive stimuli." At this point its biological character is emphasized by Freud, who refers to the origins of the nervous system in the ectoderm of the embryo: "The grey matter of the cortex remains a derivative of the primitive superficial layer of the organism and may have inherited some of its essential properties" (26). However, in the following description of the formation of the receptive apparatus by virtue of its exposed position, something like the "Project's" neuronic network is evoked with its contact barriers and facilitations. Perhaps because of the elementary or primitive nature of the model, what it receives from the outside are not described as perceptions but as quantities of energy. The vesicle is an economic model, described in terms of an energetics, not a hermeneutics. The receptive layer is said to be formed "as a result of the ceaseless impact of external stimuli," so that "its substance to a certain depth may have become permanently modified." Freud describes this modification in terms of a metaphor: "A crust would thus be formed which would at last be so thoroughly 'baked through' by stimulation that it would . . . become incapable of any further modification" (ibid.). This would constitute, Freud claims, "the most favourable possible conditions for the reception of stimuli." To picture this, Freud invokes his early model of the network of neurones, in which "in passing from one element to another, an excitation has to overcome a resistance, and that diminution of resistance is what lays down a permanent trace of the excitation, that is, a facilitation." While this indicates how memory-traces are left in the adjoining systems, in contrast, "in the system *Cs.*, then, resistance to this kind of passage from one element to another would no longer exist" (ibid.). He then maps this picture, of a network of elements without resistance to the free passage of excitations, onto what he takes to be Breuer's distinction between quiescent and mobile energy: "The elements of the system *Cs.*, would carry no bound energy but only energy capable of discharge" (ibid., 27). In fact, Breuer's distinction is between a 'quiescent energy' that is an optimal condition or base level that ensures the mobility of energy within a closed system rather than, as with

Freud, 'bound' and 'free' states of energy that are alternatives to each other.[12] Here the resistance of the contact barriers between elements or neurones either creates 'bound' energy stases at such points, equivalent to 'memory-traces,' or it is worn down to create facilitated pathways. Such a 'baked' system without resistances would be a system without memories. The assumption seems to be that such a completely receptive system, open to "energy capable of free discharge," would "have become capable of giving rise to consciousness" (ibid., 26). The model is in fact a mechanical one (but derived, Freud admits, from the observation of the primary processes in dreams and symptoms). Here, however, it is intended to represent the emergence of consciousness within a primitive organism, a consciousness that would be little more than a registering surface for external excitations that "expire, as it were, in the process of becoming conscious" (15),[13] while passing on to permanent registration in the adjoining memory systems.

If the system of consciousness without resistances and without memory-traces is completely receptive to what comes from without, then, as a "little fragment of living substance suspended in the middle of an external world charged with the most powerful energies," it needs a protective barrier to safeguard it, else "it would be killed by the stimulation emanating from these" (27). This deduction of a function necessary for the survival of the vesicle is pursued via a somewhat surprising dialectic of the dead and the living. Freud posits a death of "the outermost surface" that ceases to have "the structure proper to living matter," which becomes inorganic and functions as "a special envelope or membrane resistant to stimuli" (ibid.). By virtue of this death, the outer layer constitutes a filter that diminishes and attenuates the force of the incoming stimuli, such that the still-living layers are able to continue their receptive activity. Freud proposes that "*Protection against* stimuli is an almost more important function for the living organism than *reception of* stimuli" (ibid.). Curiously, Freud's previous metaphor, of a crust that has been baked through by intense stimuli, applies more fittingly to the idea of dead skin that forms a protective carapace (compare the function of shells among

12. For a clarification of the differences between Freud and both Breuer and Helmholtz, see Laplanche, *Life and Death in Psychoanalysis*, 17–20.
13. In a later discussion of these issues, Freud refers to "the flickering up and passing-away of consciousness in the process of perception," in "A Note upon the 'Mystic Writing-Pad'" (1925a), *SE* 19, 231.

the lower life-forms) than to a still-sensitive receptive surface that can function only beneath the crust. Paradoxically, both the protective layer, with its resistant filters, and the protected layer, without resistances, in Freud's metaphorical account, are the effect of the same high-intensity impact (being "baked through") of the surrounding powerful energies that assail them. A further paradox is that the dead crust, with its retained coefficient of resistance necessary for its filtering function—the crust of a crust—turns out to have some of the properties of a 'living' homeostatic system. The protective shield, we are told, has "its own store of energy," which it must preserve, along with "the special modes of transformation of energy operating in it" (ibid.), against the destructive effects of a leveling out should the surrounding forces overwhelm it. So we have a "dead" and "inorganic" outermost layer that protects a still-living inner layer; while the latter has lost the specific density of its resistances, the dead layer retains both its resistance, at least in part, and its own 'store of energy' (the same phrase Freud had used in the "Project" to describe what meets the exigencies of life) necessary to enable its own homeostatic functioning. This subordination of death to the survival of the vital principle (and a 'death' with some lifelike attributes) in an unpromising, hostile environment does not lead the reader to expect the celebration of the death instinct that is to come in sections V and VI.

So important is the protective shield that it enables a process of sampling of the excitations from without in manageably diminished quantities, which Freud compares to "feelers that are all the time making tentative advances towards the external world and then withdrawing from it" (ibid., 28). It is to this rhythm that he attributes an awareness of time, a temporal consciousness that arises, he suggests, from "the method of working of the system *Pcpt.-Cs.* [Perception-Consciousness—JF]" and that corresponds to "a perception on its own part of that method of working" (ibid.). It is another way of providing a filtering and protective process for the still-sensitive receptive second layer.

## Trauma and the Compulsion to Repeat

Having set out the model of the vesicle as a doubly boundaried homeostatic entity, armed with defenses that protect both its internal energy level and containing form against excessive incursions of stimuli from without, Freud addresses the question of trauma. The common traumatic neurosis involving a traumatizing external event, which he had invoked briefly in sections II and III in relation to its repetitive dreams, is now situated in terms of a specific topographic model. The idea of an "extensive breach" in the protective shield might look like a return to the root meaning of the word 'trauma' (from the Greek for a wound), and to the "old naïve theory of shock," with its postulation of physical damage to the tissues at the micro-anatomical level of the nervous system. This was the model associated with the Berlin neurologists Thomsen and Oppenheim, which in Chapter 1 we saw Charcot challenging with his subsuming of traumatic cases under the rubric of hysteria. Freud makes clear that it is not, after all, a biological organism subject to histological damage and lesions with which he is concerned, and that the vesicle has become at this stage of his exposition a model of the psychical apparatus: "What *we* seek to understand are the effects produced on the organ of the mind by the breach in the shield against stimuli and the problems that follow in its train" (ibid., 31).

With the breaking through of the protective shield by excessive amounts of excitation that overwhelm its filtering function, the system of the psychical vesicle is thrown into crisis. Freud tells us that the pleasure principle that would normally act to reduce the intolerable levels of stimuli is put out of action. Instead, more urgently there is "the problem of mastering the amounts of stimuli that have broken in and binding them, in the psychical sense, so that they can be disposed of" (30). The relations between mastery, binding, and disposal are not spelled out here, while Freud passes on to consider the related but different question of pain. Pain also involves a breach of the protective shield, but one that is restricted to a limited area. In response to invasion by a stream of excitations from the periphery, the mind reacts by rallying large amounts of psychic energy to block the inflow and bind it "in the environs of the breach": "An 'anticathexis' on a grand scale is set up, for whose benefit all the other psychical systems are impoverished, so that the remaining psychical functions are paralyzed or reduced" (ibid.). The greater the store of internal energy, the more capacity it has to take up and bind whatever has breached the protective shield. The example of pain as a localized breakthrough of the shield, however, indicates an emergency counterinvestment of psychical energy—

"anticathexis on a grand scale"—that is not available to the "extensive breach" of trauma.

In considering trauma, Freud returns to the psychological idea of "fright" and the subject's unpreparedness for a sudden danger to life that takes it by surprise, which he had distinguished in section II from fear of a particular danger or a generalized anxious expectation without a specified object. He translates fright into the energetics of his topographical model, such that trauma "is caused by unpreparedness for anxiety, including lack of hypercathexis of the systems that would be the first to receive the stimulus" (ibid., 31). Where the protective shield, equipped with its own store of bound energy, would normally be "in a good position for binding the inflowing amounts of excitation," as in the example of pain, with the extensive breach of the shield, this "last line of defence of the protective shield" is lost (ibid.).

Here Freud turns again to the question of the repetitive dreams that cast the dreamer back into the original situation of the trauma, the moment when the shell hit the trench and killed the dreamer's friend but let him survive (or the car crashed, or the train came off the rails). These dreams, in which the dreamer wakes up in a state of renewed fright, are clearly not regulated by the principle of disguised wish fulfillment of unconscious impulses that would otherwise disturb sleep. That would assume the dominance of the pleasure principle, acting to reduce tension and any disturbance of the state of sleep. Freud states that "dreams are here helping to carry out another task, which must be accomplished before the dominance of the pleasure principle can even begin" (ibid., 32). He offers two distinct formulations as to what these dreams of traumatic repetition are doing. The first is the proposition that "these dreams are endeavouring to master the stimulus retrospectively, by developing the anxiety whose omission was the cause of the traumatic neurosis" (ibid.). This is, at first—and even second—glance, a puzzling claim. How would belated anxiety (*nachträglich* anxiety?) master the excessive flood of excitations that had in an earlier moment paralyzed the ego's defenses (for the psychical vesicle is clearly the beleaguered ego)? How would *retrospective* mastery work? How would it be compatible with the renewed state of fright in which the dreamer awakes—yet again?

Without elaborating the terms of the first proposition, Freud goes on to distinguish between anxiety dreams and punishment dreams, both of which have negative and distressing affects, on the one hand, and traumatic dreams, on the other. The former do not contradict the principle of wish fulfillment, as it is precisely the forbidden wish fulfillment in the dream that provokes the anxiety or the punishment that characterizes them. Traumatic dreams, however, cannot be considered as driven by wish fulfillment but "arise in obedience to the compulsion to repeat" (ibid.), although Freud concedes that in analysis they may be supported by the conscious wish to uncover forgotten and repressed material. This revision of dream theory leads him to speculate that the protection of the state of sleep, "by fulfilling the wishes of the disturbing impulses" (ibid., 33), may not be the original function of dreams, as it implies the already established dominance of the pleasure principle, so dreams that are driven by the compulsion to repeat are performing a more primal or foundational task, located not so much *beyond* the pleasure principle as *before* it. Freud describes this primitive dream function in the same terms as the crisis measures required by the destructive effects of trauma, that of mastering and binding the excessive stimuli that have invaded the psychical apparatus: these dreams "obey the compulsion to repeat" but "with a view to the psychical binding of traumatic impressions" (ibid.). Freud's earlier description of the system's crisis measures adds, "binding them, in the psychical sense, so that they can then be disposed of" (ibid., 30).

## *Trauma and the Function of Binding*

Freud is speaking a kind of Freudian shorthand in the previous quotation in his use of the opposition between binding and unbinding, which he gives no theoretical explication of, either in itself or its relations to adjacent concepts. We have binding and mastery, which might seem virtually synonyms; mastery achieved retrospectively, presumably by going back over the memory of something that was overwhelming and even isolating as an experience; the achievement of the latter through developing a belated anxiety, understood as a free-floating expectation of danger, that would have allowed the traumatized subject to prepare its defenses and not be taken by surprise; and a binding that is a necessary prerequisite for the establishment of the pleasure principle, and for the disposal of the excitations that have flooded and paralyzed the ego in its defensive operations. There is the further suggestion that binding is involved in the very establishment of the psychical apparatus as a coherent system in the first place, with its own external boundaries and defenses and its own internal energy levels and exchanges that need protecting from the destructive leveling out potentially inflicted by a high-energy environment and its intensities. We are back then with the two topographies with their opposed logics that we saw in the opening moves of the "Project" of 1895, only now it is the principle of binding (the principle of constancy) that is foundational rather than discharge.

More problematical is the claim that the rescue operations of binding are achieved by the compulsion to repeat. While there is an intuitive plausibility in assuming that an active mastery of distressing experience was the aim of little Ernst's *fort/da* game, it is not at all clear that mastery and binding would be either the aim or the effect of the traumatic repetition in dreams of an original moment of trauma, especially when that is a scene with various perceptual elements—sight, sound, surprise timing, violent force—of an event that threatened life. This would be even more the case when the repetition resulted in a repeated state of fright. The idea of aiming to produce the warning or signal anxiety that had been missing the first time around seems contradicted by the end result of repeated fright, unless one were to posit a different kind of repetition that took anxious expectation as its starting point, such that fright and violent surprise were preempted. The latter, however, sounds more like a kind of training or dressage than a *compulsion*. Freud, in fact, talks of "*endeavouring* to master the stimulus, by developing the anxiety" (ibid., 32, emphasis added) but does not consider its success or its likelihood. It seems more like a fantasy, of the kind Freud describes when he talks of the use of the outer-oriented protective shield against internal drive impulses that have been disavowed and projected outward, which is of course the formula for the production of anxiety phobias, as compulsive as they are notoriously unsuccessful in protecting the phobic subject from the *internal* source of his fear.

Then there is the repeated formula of binding as a prerequisite for disposal or discharge of the invading excitations. It might seem puzzling that Freud introduces his standard distinction between "a freely flowing cathexis that presses towards discharge and a quiescent cathexis" (ibid., 31), the latter being identified with bound energy, into a text that argues for binding as a *condition* for discharge. Are binding and discharge alternatives, or is the former a condition for the latter? Freud does not describe the processes he includes under the heading of binding. So why is binding necessary, and what is it? The entry under the term in the great psychoanalytic dictionary of Laplanche and Pontalis distinguishes three related conceptions of binding. One is that of "a relation between several terms which are linked up, for example, as by an associative chain," and along which energy might flow; another is virtually its opposite, "the idea of a fixation in one place of a certain quantity of energy which can no longer flow freely"; and a third is "the idea of a whole in which a certain cohesion is maintained, a form demarcated by specific limits or *bound*aries."[14] The first and the third, however, are compatible, in the maintenance of a homeostatic system with a stable core and capacities for receiving inputs of stimuli and excitations, and differentiated pathways allowing for regulated discharge of tensions, rather than the unmanageable surplus of excitations pressing by the shortest route to a massive, unregulated, and exhausting discharge. It is not clear, however, just how the repeated production of a belated anxiety missing from the original breaching event *could* achieve the binding and mastery that Freud seeks.

Section IV ends with another description of a possible form of binding that would be simultaneous with the—in this case literal—breach. Freud takes up again the puzzling instance of a violent event in which a physical wound or an injury is sustained without an accompanying psychical trauma. He suggests indeed that the former may be the condition of the latter. He argues that the violence and sheer mechanical agitation of the event, coming unexpectedly and without any defensive preparation, would release a quantity of sexual excitation that would be unregulated and overwhelming. However, the simultaneous breach in the body's boundary and physical integrity, by commandeering "a narcissistic hypercathexis of the injured organ, would bind the excess of excitation" (ibid., 33). What emerges overall from Freud's argument is an emphasis on binding as "a function of the mental apparatus which . . . is nevertheless independent of and seems to be more primitive than the purpose of gaining pleasure and avoiding unplea-

14. Laplanche and Pontalis, *The Language of Psychoanalysis*, 52.

sure" (32). A function both beyond and before the pleasure principle, binding manifests itself in response to trauma as an attempt at restoring the conditions for the functioning of the pleasure principle, and in traumatic dreams, Freud argues, binding manifests itself precisely in the compulsion to repeat.

## From Compulsion to Repeat to the Death Instinct

Freud's proposal of a 'death instinct' begins two and a half pages into section V, after a summary of already discussed phenomena and the connections between them, but without adducing any new evidence or analyses. Having considered trauma a consequence of external events and their impact on the psychical apparatus, Freud begins with a consideration of "economic disturbances comparable with traumatic neuroses" initiated by "the organism's instincts" (ibid., 34).[15] He equates these *Triebe*—"the representatives of all the forces originating in the interior of the body and transmitted to the mental apparatus"—with unbound "*freely mobile* processes which press towards discharge" and obey the laws of the primary process, of condensation and displacement, knowledge of which "is derived from our study of the dream-work" (ibid.). In the model of the dream and the dream-work, as we know, a central place is given to the dream censorship and the function of repression, with the dream formation being driven by the disguised fulfillment of *repressed* infantile wishes. The primary process characteristics of the unconscious as a system are the product of the processes of both primary and secondary repression that have formed it, as set out in the Papers on Metapsychology of 1915 ("Repression" [1915d] and "The Unconscious" [1915e]). It is all the more surprising, therefore, to find Freud's opening statement claiming that "the cortical layer which receives stimuli

---

15. Freud continues to use the term *Trieb* and not *Instinkt* when talking of the death instinct (*Todestrieb*). Where the terminological problem in English has been the *Standard Edition*'s translation of *Trieb* as 'instinct,' at this point we are faced with Freud's continuing use of the term *Trieb* for the life and death instincts, when he is engaged in *what looks like* a wholesale biologizing of the *Trieb*/drive, by postulating forces that are inherent not just in human biology but in all living, organic matter, and that seek to return to the inorganic, although the issue has further complications, as we shall see.

is without any protective shield against excitations from within" (ibid.), when previously he had spent some effort in elaborating boundaries between the unconscious system, the preconscious system, and the perception-consciousness system, and the censorship/repression of impulses from within that operates at those boundaries.

What seems to be taking place already in Freud's thinking is a shift from the repressed unconscious to something like the primordial id of the second topography (*The Ego and the Id* [1923b]), which is said to open directly onto the body and its instincts. This is a correlative of the collapse of the previous distinction between the sexual drives, on the one hand, and those inherited but weak self-preservative functions that are essentially *instincts*, that is, inherited, species-specific, with pregiven objects and preformed aims serving the survival of the organism, on the other. These are now to be assimilated and regrouped together as the new 'life instinct.' Freud had acknowledged in 1915 that it was only of the sexual drives and not the self-preservative instincts that psychoanalysis had any systematic knowledge, and that it was only to them that applied the characteristics of precisely a *deviation* from the instinctual function, a contingency and substitutability of the object, a capacity to act vicariously for each other, the aim of immediate 'organ-pleasure,' their susceptibility to the famous "vicissitudes" of repression, sublimation, reversal into its opposite, turning round on the subject's self ("Instincts and Their Vicissitudes" [1915c], 125–26). If there is an obvious affinity between the sexual drives so conceived and the characteristics of the repressed unconscious system, with its atemporality, its absence of coordination and negation or the law of noncontradiction, its primary process functioning, then it is also obvious that there is a radical *incompatibility* between such an unconscious and the self-preservative functioning of any living organism, governed by homeostasis and the law of constancy. The forgetting or marginalization of repression as both the genesis of the unconscious system and its characteristics, and a protective shield against the sexual drives (it scarcely makes sense to conceive of an organism having a protective shield against its own self-preservative instincts), is clearly the sign of Freud's reshuffling of his conceptual cards.

Before turning to the compulsion to repeat, once again Freud rehearses the need for binding the potentially traumatic "instinctual excitation reaching the primary process" (1920g, 34–35), but without specifying either the nature of the 'instincts' (sexual or self-preservative) involved or the process of binding and its agents. It is all the more surprising, then, that Freud immediately proceeds to locate the compulsion to repeat on the side of the 'instincts' and the primary process, not on the side of the foundational principle of binding, which is where he had just previously located its purest manifestation in traumatic dream repetition and its struggle for mastery of overwhelming excitations: "The manifestations of a compulsion to repeat . . . exhibit to a high degree an instinctual character and, when they act in opposition to the pleasure principle, give the appearance of some 'daemonic' force at work" (ibid., 35). He runs through his standard examples of repetition: children's play, the clinical transference, and, oddly enough, *nontraumatic* dreams, because they are formed by unbound wishful fantasies based on the repetition of repressed 'primaeval' memory-traces (such dreams are thereby claimed to be manifestations of hitherto incompatible terms: repetition, but, instead of binding, its opposite unbinding, *and* wish fulfilment, hence contradictorily the pleasure principle). However, puzzlingly, neither traumatic neuroses and their repetitive dreams nor fate neuroses are mentioned. The whole paragraph has the air of seizing examples of repetition at will—repetition on the side of the pleasure principle (nontraumatic dreams and children's play), and also opposed to the pleasure principle (children's play again and painful transferences). Instead of the compulsion to repeat being an agent of the foundational principle of binding, endeavoring to achieve retrospective mastery through belated anxiety, it is now, without explanation, placed on the side of unbinding, and the drive-pressure toward discharge. It is as if silently a conceptual switch had been thrown and the compulsion to repeat was now proceeding along a quite different track in the opposite direction. The effect is one of rhetorical amplification overriding conceptual instability and radical incoherence rather than theoretically consistent analysis and argument.

Posing once again his previous identification of the compulsion to repeat and the instinctual as an apparent question, Freud asks: "How is the predicate of being 'instinctual' related to the compulsion to repeat?" Here as on the previous occasion of combining the two terms, Strachey footnotes 'instinctual' as '*Triebhaft*,' to bring out its sense of urgency as compared to his chosen English translation "instinct," and certainly Freud's twice-repeated adjective, 'daemonic,' conveys that sense. Freud's response to his own question, however, is instead the reverse move of attaching the predicate of being a repetition to the notion of instinct, instead of attaching the predicate of being instinctual to repetition. Repetition (Does it still make sense to call it a 'compulsion'?) is now "a universal attribute of instincts and perhaps of organic life in general" (ibid., 36). The psychical disappears into "organic life in general," and we are offered a redefinition of the very term 'instinct'/*Trieb*: "*It seems, then, that an instinct is an urge inherent in organic life to restore an earlier state of things*" (ibid.). Despite Strachey's insistence on the term *Trieb*, with its functional deviance, its vicissitudes and its "daemonic" urgency, Freud's sudden transplantation of this theoretical entity from the specific level of human *psychical* life to "organic life in general" indicates rather that, at first and even second glance, what is really at stake is a biological concept of instinct/*Instinkt* (human, animal, vegetable?). That this is Freud's intention—or at least one of Freud's intentions—is testified to by his later recourse in section VI to the laboratory experiments of Weismann, Woodruff, Maupas, Calkins, and others to establish whether death is a property of single-cell protozoa and thus natural and intrinsic, or whether the protozoa, with no differentiation as yet between germ cell and soma, are immortal, and death is instead acquired at the level of complex, multicellular organisms. If protozoa are subject to senescence, however prolonged, then the "earlier state of things" that all organic life instinctively seeks to restore is the inorganic state of inert matter before the appearance of life. "If . . . everything living dies for *internal* reasons—becomes inorganic once again—then . . . '*the aim of all life is death*' and . . . '*inanimate things existed before living ones*'" (ibid., 38).

Freud acknowledges that "this view of instincts strikes us as strange because we have become used to see in them a factor impelling towards change and development, whereas we are now asked to recognize in them the precise contrary." This contrary he calls "the *conservative* nature of living substance" (36). However, rather than an alternative *biological* proposition, and despite the invocation of the migratory flights of birds, and the spawning patterns of fish species, what Freud offers in response to the question of the relation between the compulsion to repeat and the instinctual is a direct transfer of the formulation of the *psychical* process across to the instinct (more *Instinkt* than *Trieb*, despite Freud's retention of the latter term), and not just as a predicate but as its very definition. Hence, in the very next paragraph he talks of "the organic compulsion to repeat" (37), as if the phrase needed no explaining and organic repetition would be much the same thing as psychical repetition. What sense can a psychical term such as 'compulsion' have, with its reference to a return of repressed unconscious processes, when attributed to spawning fish and migrating birds? Freud attempts to give some conceptual substance to this transfer of a verbal formula from one domain to another by alluding to Lamarckian recapitulation theory, often summed up by Freud in Haeckel's biogenetic law that "ontogeny repeats phylogeny": the development of the individual recapitulates the stages of development of the species (strictly speaking of the *phylum* or subgroup of the species). He locates in passing this supposed "organic compulsion to repeat" in "the phenomena of heredity and the facts of embryology" (ibid.). However, both the Lamarckian thesis that acquired characteristics in one generation could be transmitted to successive generations, and the claim that the embryo's stages of development recapitulated the earlier developmental stages of its phylum, had been substantially discredited within biology and zoology by the time Freud was writing, though he refused to abandon them right up to his final text, *Moses and Monotheism* (1939a). Discredited or not, it is hard to see that the conceptual content of Lamarckianism is really the substance of Freud's "organic compulsion to repeat," or its extreme development in the death instinct that supposedly leads organic life back to a preorganic state. This notion of the regression of individual life-forms to the inorganic is not the same thing as the transmission of acquired characteristics, nor as individual developmental stages recapitulating earlier ones. The direction of these 'Lamarckian' processes is from the past into the future, and Lamarck posited inherent progressive tendencies toward greater complexity. Despite the claims of Sulloway, that Freud's 'psycho-Lamarckianism' and his invocation of 'the biogenetic law' solved a number of his metapsychological problems, including our problem of the enigmatic nature of traumatic fixation-repetition, Freud's deployment of Lamarckian terminology at this point seems little more than a self-legitimating *façon de parler.*[16]

16. Sulloway, *Freud: Biologist of the Mind*, 393–415.

*Freud's Bio-traumatology*

In fact, Freud's attempt to subsume the psychical process of the compulsion to repeat into a biological redefinition of 'instinct' that would ground and explain such a repetition has a paradoxical reverse effect. The specificity of the biological concept of instinct as an inherited adaptational and survival mechanism, with its specific behavioral sequences and triggers, is abandoned for an ambiguous, simplified "organic compulsion to repeat," in which the specificity of the psychical process is also abandoned. In the psychical phenomenon of the repetition-compulsion, what is repeated is a highly specific, perceptual, and memorial configuration or gestalt, in which is invested the original affect of fright and a range of painful and distressing emotions that have not been worked through. The power of the fixation is puzzling and the function of its repetition is ambiguous, being described by Freud as either implementing or assisting the ego's mastery of the excess of affect and excitation, or, alternatively, repeating the original attack of excessive and negative affects on the ego's composure and resources, leading to enfeeblement, demoralization, and even, in extreme instances, suicide. What is being repeated in trauma is a highly specific formation, the product of a particular subjective history with its own preexisting fault lines and residues (despite its adjacent memory systems, the model of the vesicle does not allow for the reactivation of earlier scenes and their inscriptions).[17] The logic of *Nachträglichkeit*, or afterwardsness, with its associated themes of retranscription and translation, and thus the specific *temporality* of trauma, which has been a central thread of this book, is noticeably absent.

The compulsion to repeat was first formulated in 1914 in relation to both the clinical transference and to the resistance that manifests itself in the analytic situation. The epigraph for the current chapter, taken from Freud's revision of the theory of resistance in 1926, reverses his previous position to allow a resistance distinct from that of the ego and the super-

17. In a brief introductory note to a volume on war trauma, Freud raises the question of the traumatic neuroses of war being made possible or promoted by "a conflict in the ego," between a self-preservative "peace ego" and what he calls "its newly formed, parasitic double," the "war ego." See Freud, "Introduction to *Psycho-Analysis and the War Neuroses*" (1919d), *SE* 17, 209. However, the conflict is contemporary and not located in the subject's history.

ego, and specific to the unconscious. This takes the form precisely of the compulsion to repeat, which is attributed to "the attraction exerted by the unconscious prototypes upon the repressed instinctual process" (1926d, 159). We have already seen the notion of a prototype (*Vorbild*) or template invoked by Freud in relation to both the clinical transference, as well as the erotic transference, that produces adult 'object-choice.' In this late reformulation, we have a form of binding to an unconscious traumatic scene, whose affective burden has the power to replicate itself to the discomposure and even undoing of the ego. A form of binding in the second sense of the term defined earlier by Laplanche and Pontalis, it is a fixation in one site of a charge of affect, in which the ego is trapped and over whose repetitions it has no control. We have caught a glimpse of such an unconscious prototype in Freud's detailed and multilayered analysis of the childhood 'beating fantasies,' especially the unconscious, never remembered second phase, in which the fixated punishment scene of beating, with its masturbatory *jouissance*, exercises a compulsion in the repetitive production of fantasies from childhood into adulthood, and in which the perverse, masochistic underside of the oedipal structuring of sexuality can also be glimpsed.

In contrast, the so-called 'organic' repetition repeats nothing from the subject's history, and even the supposed 'death' or inorganic state it results in can only by a slight of hand be considered a repetition: the living subject has never been dead before, nor 'inorganic,' simply not yet born. The 'repetition' can only be conceived at the level of evolutionary history as a myth of origins, not even that of the phylum or species but that of "life"—all organic life—itself. Hence the Freudian 'Just So' fable:

> The attributes of life were at some time evoked in inanimate matter by the action of a force of whose nature we can form no conception. . . . The tension which then arose in what had hitherto been inanimate substance endeavoured to cancel itself out. In this way the first instinct came into being: the instinct to return to the inanimate state. (1920g, 38)

We have here a 'proto-vesicle' for whom life itself is a traumatic intrusion from the outside to be canceled out by a reflex discharge of its constitutive tension. As the smallest possible distance between input and discharge, it is less a vital phenomenon than a mechanical reflex arc, a nonvital anti-instinct, for which the vital order in its most minimal manifestation is itself a trauma to be abreacted. Freud's fable is a mythical restatement of the principle of neuronic inertia from the opening paragraphs of the "Project" of 1895, a simplified 'traumatology' in thin disguise, passing itself off as biology.

What looks like a wholesale recourse to biology turns out in fact to be a ruse by which biology is itself canceled out. So the biological experiments and consequent arguments rehearsed in section VI, as to whether protozoa that die from their inability to void sufficiently their own waste products can be taken as dying from internal causes or not, are abruptly dismissed by Freud with an affirmation that is little more than a restatement of the hypothesis to be confirmed or disproved:

> The instinctual forces that seek to conduct life into death may be operating in protozoa from the first. . . . But even if protista [a synonym for protozoa—JF] turn out to be immortal in Weismann's sense, his assertion that death is a late acquisition would apply only to *manifest* phenomena and would not make impossible the assumption or processes *tending* towards it. (1920g, 49)

It is clear that for Freud nothing biological, experiments or arguments, would make impossible that assumption, which does not depend on them.[18] Similarly, his speculations on the life instinct, apparently 'biological' in character, take up the formation of multicellular organisms as a life-promoting synthesis of single cells, at which point another metaphorical transfer from the psychical register takes place:

> Accordingly, we might attempt to apply the libido theory which has been arrived at in psychoanalysis to the mutual relationship of cells . . . the life instincts which are active in each cell take the other cells as their object, they partly neutralize the death instincts . . . in those cells and thus preserve their life; while the other cells do the same for them. . . . The germ-cells themselves would behave in a completely "narcissistic" fashion. (1920g, 50)

Beneath the stalking horse of biological speculation, libido theory, especially the theory of the libidinal synthesis of the self-preservative instinctual functions and the narcissistically constituted ego, is exported into the place of a general theory of Eros as a universal life principle. The overall

18. "To begin with it was only tentatively that I put forward the views I have developed here, but in the course of time they have gained a hold on me that I can no longer think in any other way." See Freud, *Civilization and Its Discontents* (1930a), *SE* 21, 119.

result is a kind of 'meta-biology' whose logic is really that of a transferred psychical dualism. This dualism obtains between a colonizing tendency on the part of "His Majesty the Ego" toward a narcissistic synthesis and subsumption of pragmatic life functions, and a countertendency, for which all living systems, forms of homeostasis and binding, are a blockage, an obstacle to be broken open and abreacted, whether the subject's first centered and totalized object, the ego, as in masochism, or as in sadism, the other, who receives the gift of the ego's narcissistic love.

## Freud's "Strange Chiasmus"

In the reorganization of his instinct/drive theory, Freud appears to move from one dualism to another:

self-preservative/ego-instincts　sexual drives/
death instincts　　　　　　　　　Eros/life instinct

Assuming that sexuality remains the same in each dualism, when Freud redefines instinct/*Trieb* as an 'organic compulsion to repeat,' the ego instincts are what he attempts, rather counterintuitively, to redefine as death instincts: "The ego-instincts arise from the coming to life of inanimate matter and seek to restore the inanimate state" (1020g, 44). Their self-preservative function is redefined as a preservation of the organism's own circuitous path to death via forcibly acquired detours imposed on it by external circumstances over time, as opposed to any abrupt termination of life. In the second dualism, the sexual drives are redefined essentially in terms of the reproductive "coalescence of two germ cells" (ibid.), and the whole question of nonreproductive infantile sexuality, of the pregenital component *Trieb*, is left aside.

However, Freud is compelled to change the equation of ego and death instincts in midtext by the consideration of the narcissistic libido that invests the ego, and with which he then identifies the self-preservative functions. The narcissistic self-preservative instincts have to be recognized as also libidinal, at which point Freud is in danger, as he himself acknowledges, of having his dualistic theory collapse back into a Jungian monism of a generalized libido that he had for so long been opposing. If the self-preservative instincts are then moved over to the side of the life instincts because of their shared libidinal basis, Freud is only left with a mysterious x, an as-yet undiscovered 'ego-instinct' to act as a placeholder for the death instincts for which it would be a concrete agent, opposed to the life instincts. Later, sadism and masochism suggest themselves as candidates, except that they are also libidinal and lead to the proposition that the death instincts can only manifest themselves in combination with the life instincts. Yet Freud wants, and in late texts will go on to affirm, a nonlibidinal instinct of pure destructiveness.

Jean Laplanche has mapped out a certain paradoxical pattern in the relocation of sexuality within each of Freud's dualisms, together with an underlying conceptual consistency, which enables an interpretation of the conceptual equilibrium of the Freudian theoretical field and of the anomalies of this late affirmation within it of the death instinct, with its failed arguments, internal contradictions, abandoned experimental evidence, and opposite values given to the same term.

Laplanche points to what he calls "a strange chiasmus" that structures the Freudian field can be seen in Figure 8. The diagram dramatizes both the apparent *anomaly* by which sexuality moves from the pole of the primary process, free energy in the first theory to the pole of the secondary process, bound energy and the ego in the second theory, and the underlying *consistency* of the opposition of unbinding and binding that organizes these pairs of opposites. To these one can add further Freudian opposites, such as the pressure toward absolute discharge versus homeostasis or the principle of constancy. I have argued elsewhere[19] that the crossover point of Freud's strange chiasmus, where the sexual drive crosses over into its opposite, Eros, although unnamed on Laplanche's diagram, is in fact primary narcissism in its earliest form, as given in Freud's 1914 paper "On Narcissism: An Introduction" (1914c). The sexuality of the first dualism is the component drive with its part-objects, aiming at organ pleasure and pressing by the shortest available route toward discharge, subject to all the vicissitudes of the drive, a potential danger in its intractability to the ego and its guardianship of the reality principle, and brought under the dominance of

19. John Fletcher, "'His Majesty the Ego': From Freud to Laplanche," *Sitegeist: A Journal of Psychoanalysis and Philosophy* 4 (Spring 2010): 67–69.

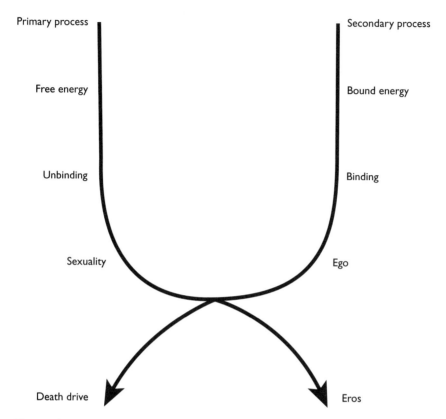

**Figure 8**
Freud's 'strange chiasmus'
Jean Laplanche, *Life and Death in Psychoanalysis*, 124

the reproductive function through the processes of repression, reaction formation, and sublimation, and then only with difficulty. The Eros of the
second dualism is the agent of libidinal synthesis, in alliance with the ego
and its self-preservative functions that it supplements and encloses. It is the
bound and binding form of sexuality, with its investment of the total object, both in the form of the narcissistically constituted ego and its narcissistically invested others.

Laplanche argues:

> In the face of the risk that a victorious, narcissistic Eros might take over
> completely, there arises . . . an imperious need to re-affirm the drive in its most

radical form: as something 'daemonic,' obeying nothing but the primary process and the compulsions of unconscious fantasy."[20]

With the death instinct unprovided with its own energy source—a 'destrudo' to match the libido—Laplanche proposes, in a later refinement of his critique of Freud's formulation of the second dualism (Laplanche 1999a), that the opposition between life and death principles is one between different regimes of the sexual, between "sexual life drives" and "sexual death drives." Faced with the predominance of Eros in alliance with the ego, of narcissistic ego libido and its transfers to narcissistically loved objects (from "His Majesty the Ego" to "His Majesty the Baby"), the unbound, destabilizing, and self-shattering aspect of the drive—"Lucifer-Amor"[21] —is affirmed, albeit in the displaced form of a supposedly nonlibidinal pure aggressiveness.

## *Coda: Moses and Repetition*

To give an account of the place of the repetition-compulsion within the argument of Freud's final text, as well as in the proliferating repetitions of its formation *as* a text, would require virtually a book in its own right, and a number of such have indeed been written.[22] For the purposes of the current argument, it is perhaps only necessary to reiterate the point made at the beginning of the present chapter with regard to the apparent nonrelation between *Beyond the Pleasure Principle* of 1920 and *Moses and Monotheism* of 1939: despite the centrality to both texts of trauma and the compulsion

20. Jean Laplanche, "The So-Called 'Death Drive': A Sexual Drive," in *The Death Drive: New Life for a Dead Subject*, ed. Rob Weatherill (London: Rebus Press, 1999), 44. A revised version appeared in *The British Journal of Psychotherapy* 20, no. 4 (2004).

21. "Everything is in flux and dawning, an intellectual hell, with layer upon layer; in the darkest core, glimpses of the contours of Lucifer-Amor," Letter to Fliess, July 10, 1900. See Jeffrey Moussaiff Masson, trans. and ed. (1985a), *The Complete Letters of Sigmund Freud to Wilhelm Fliess 1887–1904.* (Cambridge, Mass.: Harvard University Press, 1985), 421.

22. See Yosef Hayim Yerushalmi, *Freud's Moses: Judaism Terminable and Interminable* (New Haven, Conn.: Yale University Press, 1991); Richard J. Bernstein, *Freud and the Legacy of Moses* (Cambridge: Cambridge University Press, 1998).

to repeat, what is striking is their silent mutual exclusion. Freud does not acknowledge, let alone build on, his previous transposition of their shared concern with traumatic repetition into the field of the biological, and the supposed regrounding of the repetition-compulsion in the death instinct. Instead, the *Moses*, in contrast, rehearses in elaborate detail the previous model of traumatic repetition, to the extent that it virtually subsumes the later drive theory of neurosis under the meticulously reconstructed trauma model. In particular, deploying a two-stage temporal schema, it addresses the first moment of the reception of traumatic experience, distinguishing its three defining characteristics—its early receptivity, its later availability only in the form of screen memories, and its content of sexual-aggressive acts and narcissistic mortifications—and a second moment in which the later effects of trauma are specified in carefully distinguished forms of positive and negative repetitions: positive repetitions in attempts at conscious remembering, in literal repetitions, and in transferential repetitions with other persons, and negative repetitions in the form of defensive reactions such as avoidances, inhibitions, and phobias. All of these repetitions are said to be forms of fixation to the trauma and exercise a compulsive power that accumulates intensity and dominance in the subject's psychic life.[23] What is striking here is the reconstruction of an entire conceptual problematic, in which various mechanisms and processes are specified that articulate trauma and the compulsion to repeat in a systematic, intelligible manner. There is no need to invoke biology or the vital order, and the questions of the topographic and economic dimensions of trauma, the pleasure and constancy principles, the function of binding, and protective shields and their breaches are all notable by their absence. Rather than psychic space, the question of the psychic temporality of trauma is what is central. *Moses and Monotheism*, in what it excludes as much as in what it meticulously assembles, silently and systematically undoes its predecessor text, even as it redeploys anew their shared conceptual matrix. Never have the organizing antitheses and contrary tendencies that constitute the Freudian field been so pointedly, even geometrically, exhibited.

23. S. Freud, *Moses and Monotheism* (1939a), *SE* 23, 72–80.

## Uncanny Repetitions: Freud, Hoffmann, and the Death-Work

Freud's essay "The Uncanny" was written in 1919, during the same months in which he was working on his new theory of the life and death instincts to appear the following year (1920) as *Beyond the Pleasure Principle*; this was the same period in which the other major transformation of Freud's metapsychology was incubating—that is, the second topography of id, ego, and superego, which was to appear in 1923 as *The Ego and the Id*. During this incubation period Freud turned to what might seem something completely unrelated: the aesthetic phenomenon of the uncanny, which brought in its train an engagement with the work of the early nineteenth-century Romantic writer, E. T. A. Hoffmann, and in particular with his novella *The Sandman*. There is a certain parallel here with Freud's turn in his letter to Fliess of October 15, 1897, barely three weeks after his temporary repudiation of his seduction theory, in a moment of theoretical impasse, to the tragedies of Sophocles and Shakespeare, with the incubating seeds of the Oedipus complex developing through a reading of the two tragedies. In 1919 the frisson of the uncanny in both life and literature invited Freud to think through the question of repetition as a form of thought-experiment in the alternative context of the aesthetic. His speculations in *Beyond the Pleasure Principle* were taking him to what he regarded as a salutary regrounding of the psychical—in particular, the anomaly of trauma and its outcomes in the compulsion to repeat—in the order of the instinctual and the biological. Once again, however, his chosen writer and text elaborate a vision of the repetition-compulsion that reinstates the very 'traumatology,' with its originary scenes and prototypes, its daemonic figures of the other, which he was in the process of replacing with the epic struggle of the life and death instincts.

One of the things this chapter will be concerned with is what one might call Hoffmann's theory of the death drive. In fact, as a writer of fantastic narratives, Hoffmann does not present a 'theory' as such, although the characters in his tales are quite capable of entering into sustained disquisitions on those 'phantoms of the ego,' of which Clara in *The Sandman* warns the fated protagonist, Nathaniel, in an idiom that uncannily anticipates Freud's own: Clara warns of dark, uncanny psychic powers that can lead us into madness and death, if we believe in them and so allow them to triumph. Like so many Anglophone readers of Hoffmann, I read him because Freud in his classic essay "The Uncanny" had introduced us to him through his commentary on Hoffmann's novella *The Sandman*. However, reading Hoffmann's tales, unavoidably in a Freudian framework, one might wonder not so much whether Hoffmann is a Freudian precursor who anticipated in his intuitive–poetic way what Freud one hundred years later came to theorize systematically, but whether Freud should be read as a belated Hoffmannesque theorist, and nowhere more so than in the matter of the compulsion to repeat and its relation to the so-called death instinct.[1] Hoffmann, of course, was not just a naive genius; apart from being a successful writer, he

---

1. Strachey's translation in the *Standard Edition* notoriously elides the distinction between the psychical *Trieb* (drive) and the biological *Instinkt* (instinct) by translating them both as 'instinct.' With the *Todestrieb*, however, for which he ultimately evokes a biological explanation, Freud continues to use the term *Trieb*. I will use the phrase 'death instinct' when citing Strachey's translation but otherwise will use the phrase 'death drive.' See the entries under 'Instinct,' 'Death Instincts,' and 'Anaclisis,' in Jean Laplanche and J.-B. Pontalis, *The Language of Psychoanalysis*, trans. Donald Nicholson-Smith (London: The Hogarth Press, 1973).

was also a composer of music and opera, a conductor and a dramaturge, and these careers alternated with a successful career in the Prussian civil service as a magistrate and judge. He was conversant with the psychiatric literature of his day and particularly concerned with the psychopathology of the criminal cases he dealt with in his court.

My point, however, is not really to adjudicate priority between Hoffmann and Freud on the question of the death drive but to bring out a distinctive, original understanding in Hoffmann's narratives of the same psychic phenomena that led Freud one hundred years later to embark on his final metapsychological speculations: the theory of the life and death 'instincts' as well as the theory of the superego function from the second topography. This is to say that Hoffmann's tales seem to present a particular framing of compulsive repetitions, of inner persecutory voices, and what also, after Freud, we might call sublimation. Embedded in Hoffmann's dramatization of these phenomena, at least in the two tales with which I am concerned, is also an implicit 'theory' of literary production as a compulsion-to-imitate, a seductive but deadly mimesis that unleashes a daemonic transmission between writer and reader in *The Sandman*, while an opposite association prevails in *Mademoiselle de Scudery*, an association of literary production with a sublimatory function that lays to rest the murderous repetitions of the death drive.

The relationship between Hoffmann and Freud, then, is far from being a straightforward one of reflection in which metapsychology explains theoretically what literature presents in narrative form. The relationship between the two bodies of work is somewhat paradoxical. It is true that certain psychoanalytic concepts enable us to recognize and begin to analyze the inner logic of the fantastical features of Hoffmann's tales that had seemed to early critics, such as Sir Walter Scott and Thomas Carlyle, merely self-indulgent, morbid, or willfully eccentric, that is, that psychoanalysis can perform something of the function of a so-called master discourse. Nevertheless, the tales' presentation of what psychoanalysis understands as repetition phenomena, superego functions, and self-destructive drives are distinctively different from Freud's account of them. Hoffmann could even be said to make his own intervention retrospectively in the debates that Freud's controversial postulation of the death instinct has provoked and to reconfigure some of the key terms in the debate. In other words, Hoffmann's tales both resist and reorganize the psychoanalytic propositions whose application they appear to solicit or invite.

## Repetition and the Uncanny

In those passages of "The Uncanny" that deal with the motifs of the double and repetition as sources of the feeling of the uncanny, Freud in effect sketches out the postulate of a compulsion-to-repeat that proceeds, he claims, from the very nature of the drives, a compulsion that is powerful enough to overrule the pleasure principle and that is responsible for what Freud calls the 'daemonic' character of certain aspects of mental life. He then concludes "that whatever reminds us of this inner 'compulsion-to-repeat' is perceived as uncanny."[2] The essay's reigning proposition that the uncanny is that species of the frightening and alien that leads back to what was once known of old and long familiar but has been alienated by repression, implies that the uncanny is characterized by the return of the repressed. Despite this Freud's conclusion in the section of the essay on repetition shifts the emphasis away from the *content* that is being repeated, with its combination of the alien and the *déjà vu*, to the sheer fact of repetition itself. The uncanny feeling proceeds not from the return of the once familiar but no longer recognized *in itself* but from what that repetition testifies to: the activity of an autonomous— daemonic—inner compulsion-to-repeat independent of the content of what is repeated.[3] However, the term 'death instinct' appears nowhere in the essay and the whole train of metabiological speculation that goes with it in *Beyond the Pleasure Principle* is also absent.

Similarly, with the motif of the double, Freud outlines the production of the double as a narcissistic formation designed to safeguard the ego, and as an "energetic denial of the power of death" in order to guarantee the ego immortality; but the double then goes on to reverse its significance, Freud claims, and from "an assurance of immortality, it becomes an uncanny harbinger of

2. Sigmund Freud, "The Uncanny" (1919h), *SE* 17, 238.
3. Neil Hertz makes this point forcefully in "Freud and the Sandman," in *Textual Strategies*, ed. Josue V. Harari (Ithaca, N.Y.: Cornell University Press, 1979), reprinted in Neil Hertz, *The End of the Line* (New York: Columbia University Press, 1985).

death" (1919h, 235). With his references to the immortal soul as the first double of the body as well as to Egyptian death masks, Freud here seems to be
talking primarily about social practices and belief systems, especially religious
and funeral rites, rather than psychic structures as such; presumably the
reversal Freud refers to is that of the reassuring immortal soul turning into
the threatening ghost or *revenant*, in popular beliefs and superstitions.

Freud goes on to outline a transformation in the double after the phase
of primary narcissism. This comes with the development of the ego and the
agency that is "able to stand over against the rest of the ego, which has the
function of observing and criticizing the self and of exercising a censorship
within the mind, and which we become aware of as our 'conscience'" (ibid.).
Clearly the conceptual profile of what Freud is soon to call the 'superego' is
being sketched in here, but without the concept being named as such. The
term 'superego' does not appear in the essay any more than the term 'death
instinct.' In extreme pathological conditions, such as paranoia, with its
characteristic delusions of being watched, Freud writes, "this mental agency
becomes isolated, dissociated from the ego, and discernible to the physician's eye" (ibid.), hence a persecutory double that haunts the ego, as found
in the tales of doubles by Hoffmann, James Hogg and Poe, among others.
Freud suggests that in such literary doublings, "when poets complain that
two souls dwell in the human breast . . . what they are thinking of is this
division (in the sphere of ego-psychology) between the critical agency and
the rest of the ego, and not the antithesis . . . between the ego and what is
unconscious and repressed" (ibid., 235, n2). However, this identification of
the double–as-superego is radically qualified by Freud's simultaneous claim
that the fact of an agency devoted to self-criticism makes it possible to
ascribe to the double "those things which seem to self-criticism to belong
to the old surmounted narcissism of earliest times"(235). Between the
self-reproachful critic of narcissism and the narcissistic object of that self-
criticism, who is the double: the double-as-superego, the double-as-primary
narcissism, the double-as-return of the repressed ? Indeed Freud goes on to
ascribe various contents to the figure of the double – "all the unfulfilled but
possible futures to which we still like to cling in phantasy" and all our "suppressed acts of volition"(236).

It is clear, however, that Freud wants to explain the feeling of uncanniness through the motif of a return of an earlier surmounted narcissistic

stage in a later psychic formation, perhaps in the very one self-critical of that narcissism. This recapitulates, somewhat cryptically, the transformation of the narcissistically loved 'ideal ego' in Freud's 1914 paper "On Narcissism" into the 'ego ideal,' an agency that might be described as a forerunner, both theoretically and psychically, of the superego itself. Here the narcissistic content of the repetition does seem to matter more than the mere tendency to return. Consequently, it is not at all clear how the theme of the double relates to the autonomous compulsion-to-repeat, except that both of them are held to be sources of the uncanny. Equally, it is not clear how their later avatars—the superego and the death instinct—are to be articulated together.

## Oedipal Readings

All these themes are in solution in Freud's essay—the double, the compulsion-to-repeat, narcissism, the inner voice or self-critical agency, the fear of death or the dead—all are cited as sources for the feeling of the un- canny under the general rubric of the return of past stages in unfamiliar form in the present. However, the essay is content to list them rather than to articulate them as a theoretical system. What is more puzzling is that when Freud explores Hoffmann's novella *The Sandman* as his most extended ex- ample of the uncanny, the interpretation he elaborates virtually ignores all these themes as sources for the uncanny in the story. He argues instead for the story's uncanniness being a function of the return of the infantile castration complex embodied in the figure of the titular Sandman with his threat to tear out children's eyes. Freud's oedipal reading is all the more curious when we realize that his uncanny themes, explored at length in the rest of his essay but more or less excluded from his reading of *The Sandman*, are in fact to be found insistently all over Hoffmann's text. Freud could not be more concerned than Hoffmann is with the double, the persecutory in- ner voice, the death-dealing repetition-compulsion. Paradoxically, Freud seems to scotomize almost entirely the presence in Hoffmann's tale of those very themes he is most concerned with in the bulk of his essay.

It is standard practice at this point for commentators on Freud's essay on the uncanny to criticize at length or even to dismiss out of hand his oedipal reading of *The Sandman* as the imposition of a psychoanalytic shibboleth on a literary text whose concerns are otherwise. Critics accuse Freud of being insensitive to the text's literary values and construction, and of structuring a reading of the text around an attempt to discredit the German psychologist Ernst Jentsch, who had published an essay on the uncanny thirteen years before Freud, in 1906. Jentsch had attributed the feeling of the uncanny to intellectual uncertainty and had cited as a privileged example "doubt as to whether an apparently living being is animated and, conversely, doubt as to whether a lifeless object may not in fact be animate."[4] Jentsch had also cited Hoffmann in general as a master of the uncanny, but with no specific references to particular tales.

Now Hoffmann's story, discussed by Freud but not by Jentsch, turns not only on the Sandman of the title and his successive embodiments in a series of father figures, including briefly the protagonist Nathaniel's actual father, but also on the figure of Olympia, the daughter of Professor Spalanzani, with whom Nathaniel falls besottedly in love and who suddenly replaces his fiancée, Clara, in his affections. Nathaniel's courtship of Olympia is a bizarre stage-by-stage process in which he pours out his heart to her, claiming that "only you understand me completely" and directing at her a positive torrent of literary production: "From the profoundest depths of his writing desk Nathaniel fetched up everything he had ever written: poems, fantasies, visions, novels, tales, daily augmented by random sonnets, stanzas, *canzoni* and he read them all to Olympia for hours on end. And he had never before had so marvellous an auditor."[5] Olympia, the perfect listener, has one repeated response to Nathaniel's passionate utterances: "ah! ah!" His courtship climaxes in the traumatizing discovery that Olympia is in fact a mechanical doll, constructed by a conspiratorial collaboration of her supposed 'father,' Spalanzani, and the itinerant Italian eyeglass seller, Giuseppe Coppola. Coppola had earlier sold Nathaniel a telescope, spying through which he had first fallen in love with the vision of the heavenly Olympia, who previously had failed to interest him at all. He later stumbles

4. Ernst Jentsch, "On the Psychology of the Uncanny" (1906), trans. Roy Sellars, *Angelaki* 2, no. 1 (1995): 11.
5. E. T. A. Hoffmann, *The Sandman*, in *Tales of Hoffmann*, trans. and ed. R. J. Hollingdale (Harmondsworth: Penguin, 1982), 117.

upon Spalanzani and Coppola quarreling over the lifeless and eyeless figure of the doll, which Coppola seizes and runs away with, leaving behind "a
pair of blood-flecked eyes . . . lying on the floor and staring up at him,"
while Spalanzani boasts enigmatically "my finest automaton. . . . The clock-
work, speech, walk—all mine! The eyes, the eyes purloined from you!"
(Hoffmann 1982, 120). Freud is concerned to argue polemically against the
location of the story's uncanny effect in the figure of 'the living doll,'
Olympia, and in the reader's consequent intellectual uncertainty as to
whether she is a living being or a dead machine, which was the motif privileged by Jentsch as the source of the uncanny (although with no specific
reference to Olympia). Freud's alternative reading privileges instead the
Sandman (who, as Freud points out, gives his name to the story) over
Olympia the doll-woman, as the source of the feeling of the uncanny. This
folkloric figure, who threatens children with the loss of their eyes, is interpreted by Freud as "the dreaded father at whose hands castration is expected" (1919h, 232). Freud offers two grounds for this reading: one is the
symbolism of the eyes and their loss; the other is a repeated pattern of triangular relations that structure the narrative. Although my larger argument is that Freud's reading is organized around a blind spot that scotomizes
in Hoffmann's texts the presence of his own most disturbing concerns, I
want briefly to defend Freud's oedipal reading in order to indicate both its
strengths and limitations so as to glimpse Hoffmann's own different configuration of their shared concerns.

Freud posits a "substitutive relation between the eye and the male organ
which is seen to exist in dreams and myths and fantasies" (ibid., 231). In particular, he references the self-blinding of the mythical criminal Oedipus as
a self-punishment for his incest with his mother, Jocasta. Freud argues that
Oedipus's blinding is a mitigated form of castration, the latter to be understood as the ancient *lex talionis* (the law of retaliation) by which the offending organ responsible for the crime is punished, the thief's hand cut off and
the incestuous parricidal son subjected to blinding as a displaced symbolic
castration.[6] Freud's argument can be supported by evidence internal to the

6. Thomas Gould, the Classics scholar and translator of Sophocles's *Oedipus Tyrannus*,
argues at length in his commentary on the play that blinding is "a kind of voyeur's castration" for transgressive looking at a forbidden sexual sight. See Sophocles, *Oedipus the*

tale as Hoffmann makes extensive use of the traditional imagery of the courtly love tradition, whereby the eyes are the organs of desire and shoot burning and flaming glances into the heart of the recipient. Hence, when Coppola lays out his eyeglasses, which will lead to Nathaniel's fatal love for the vision of Olympia shown him by Coppola's telescope, he initially appals Nathaniel by offering him "lovely *occe*, lovely *occe*" (Italian: eyes), and as he spread out his optical wares "a thousand eyes gazed and blinked and stared up at Nathaniel . . . and flaming glances leaped more and more wildly together and directed their blood-red beams into Nathaniel's breast" (Hoffmann 1982, 109). This violent and dangerous penetration and implantation of erotic energy from eye to heart is both a long-standing motif in the European love tradition and part of a series of similar transmissions of energy in the tale that are intimately related to the figuration of the repetition-compulsion that drives both Nathaniel and the tale's action into death. The eyes, with their flaming glances, are presented by Hoffmann as organs of desire, and so plausibly they are appropriate objects of punishment by the castratory oedipal father figure.

Freud locates the castration motif of the loss of the eyes within a shrewdly observed triangular pattern of relations—first, the splitting of the imago of the father into good and bad fathers, whereby Nathaniel's own beloved actual father is paired with the evil old lawyer, Coppelius, with whom he engages in uncanny nighttime activities, which lead to the death of Nathaniel's father in a mysterious nocturnal explosion from which Coppelius escapes unharmed; this first pair is then doubled by Professor Spalanzani, Olympia's supposed father, who appears to favor Nathaniel's courtship of Olympia, and the disturbing Coppola (from the Italian *coppo* = eye socket), who steals the eyeless figure of Olympia. This proliferating father series is bound together by the fantasm of the legendary Sandman, with his threat to the eyes of naughty children who refuse to close their eyes and go to sleep. Freud asks pertinently:

> Why does Hoffmann bring anxiety about eyes into such intimate connection
> with the father's death? And why does the Sandman always appear as a
> disturber of love? He separates the unfortunate Nathaniel from his betrothed

---

*King: A Translation and Commentary*, trans. and ed. Thomas Gould (Englewood Cliffs, N.J.: Prentice Hall, 1970), 50, 145.

> Clara . . . and he destroys the second object of his love, Olympia, the lovely
> doll; and he drives him into suicide at the moment when he has won back his
> Clara and is about to be happily united to her. (1919h, 231)

In other words, Freud points to a repeated triangular scenario of a distinctly oedipal cast in which the male lover is violently separated from the beloved woman by the intervention of the father figure, whose threat involves the loss of the beloved's eyes. This narrative pattern, Freud claims, is the refiguration in fantasy of the universal male oedipal situation of childhood and its accompanying castration complex, whose return in adulthood generates the tale's feeling of the uncanny, and not any intellectual uncertainty about the doll being alive or dead. Freud goes on to interpret Olympia, instead, not in relation to castration and the uncanny but as a dissociated narcissistic complex of Nathaniel's that confronts him as a person.

At this point we reach the limit of Freud's oedipal reading, which insulates the oedipal dynamics he identifies from the larger pattern of uncanny repetitions in Hoffmann's tale. For the term 'uncanny' is used eight times in Hoffmann's tale, three of them in relation to the Sandman, equally balanced against three citations in relation to Olympia. More significantly, rather than *counterposing* the Sandman and his avatars to the doll, as Freud does, thereby reducing her to secondary status, Hoffmann goes out of his way to weave the father figures and the doll together, implicating the two motifs of the doll and the Sandman *together*. It is, after all, the second pair of father figures, Spalanzani and Coppola, who construct the doll in the first place and metaphorically 'purloin' Nathaniel's own eyes in order to bring the doll to life (cf. Spalanzani's boast: "the eyes, the eyes purloined from you" [Hoffmann 1982 , 120]). The doll is, as Freud recognized, a satiric representation of a particular male fantasy of the woman who exists as the perfect listener, returning an admiring echo to the male lover's own narcissism: "ah! ah!," just as Olympia's eyes, which at first "seemed to him strangely fixed and dead," as he gazes at her "were at that moment acquiring the power of sight," and "Olympia's hand was icy cold," but "at that instant it seemed as though a pulse began to beat in the cold hand and a stream of life blood began to glow" (ibid., 110, 114). Nathaniel finds again his own gaze and his own warmth of feeling projected onto the unliving doll Olympia and is captured narcissistically by it (whereas Clara we are told is impatient of flattering male fantasists and is a critical even protesting listener to Nathaniel's paranoid literary fantasies). However, reducing Olympia to being merely a complex of Nathaniel's, as Freud does, excludes the question of the place of the woman in the narrative structure, in particular, the idealizing male fantasy of the woman, for in Hoffmann's narrative, the figure of the doll-woman is bound up with both the loss of the eyes, the castration trauma, and the compulsion-to-repeat leading to death. When Nathaniel buys the telescope from Coppola and falls for its seductive but delusional vision of Olympia, which will replace Clara, the real woman in his life, we are told he seems to hear a death sigh in the room and fears that he has paid too high a price for the telescope. This price, we learn only later, is the loss of "the eyes purloined from you" (ibid., 120), revealed in the traumatic moment of the discovery of Olympia's eyeless, mechanical form, which leads to Nathaniel's first attack of madness. The fantasy of the doll, the delusional gift of the fathers, binds Nathaniel into a particular narcissistic structure of desire, while the traumatic undoing of the fantasy of Olympia seems to unleash both psychosis and the death drive. The loved woman as fantasy and simulacrum, one might infer, functions to keep castration at bay and to tame the death drive.

Hoffmann shows us these interconnections between the fantasy of the woman and the compulsion-to-repeat, which locate the death drive at the very heart of the oedipal drama. In contrast, in Freudian metapsychology the successive theorizations of the Oedipus complex, from *The Ego and the Id* in 1923 through the run of papers in the 1920s centering on the castration complex, take place contemporaneously with the introduction of Freud's death instinct but without any systematic articulation with it. The partial exception to this is Freud's attempt in *The Ego and the Id* to connect the death instinct to the sadistic pathologies of obsessional neurosis and melancholia, and his haunting remark, which has considerable resonance for any reading of Hoffmann's tales, that in melancholia "what holds sway in the superego is, at it were, a pure culture of the death instinct, and in fact it often enough succeeds in driving the ego into death" (1923b, 53). In *The Sandman*, however, the oedipal configurations that Freud persuasively identifies are brought about not at Nathaniel's initiative, as the expression of *his* desire, but by the dogged persecutory attentions of the succession of father figures—Coppelius the lawyer, Coppola the eyeglass seller, and Professor Spalanzani. Coppelius and Coppola, as their names suggest, are direct transformations of each other, and they exist independently of Nathaniel, their existence vouched for by the narrator. As Freud points out, the effect of their interventions is to break up the love pairings that Nathaniel enters into, first with Clara, next with Olympia, and finally with Clara, again. They also set off fits of madness that in their final occurrence drive Nathaniel to suicide, a suicide that is predicted mockingly by Coppelius the lawyer, who reappears in person from Nathaniel's childhood after a twenty-year absence to witness the tale's deathly climax.

> Some wanted to enter the tower and overpower the madman, but Coppelius laughed and said: 'Don't bother: he will soon come down by himself,' and gazed upward with the rest. Nathaniel suddenly stopped as if frozen; then he stooped, recognized Coppelius, and with the piercing cry: 'Ha! Love-ly *occe!* Love-ly *occe!*' he jumped over the parapet.
>
> As Nathaniel was lying on the pavement, with his head shattered, Coppelius disappeared into the crowd. (Hoffmann 1982, 124)

The figure of Coppelius-as-Sandman predicts, provokes and presides over Nathaniel's final act of self-shattering.

### Hoffmann and the 'Pure Culture' of the Death-work

The tale's image for this madness that descends on Nathaniel, identified by Neil Hertz in a brilliant discussion of the tale and of Freud's reading of it, is the 'circle of fire,' or *Feuerkreis*. This is associated with the figure of the puppet who is seized and carried away by forces over which he has no control. In both moments of madness, when he discovers that Olympia is a mechanical doll and later when he tries to kill Clara, thinking she is Olympia, and then ends by killing himself, Nathaniel's delirium invokes this image. He bellows, "Circle of fire, circle of fire! Spin, spin, circle of fire, lovely puppet, spin, spin!," and attacks Spalanzani, attempting to strangle him (Hoffman 1982, 120); in the final scene, bellowing "spin, puppet, spin," he first attacks Clara and attempts to hurl her off the tower on which they are standing. Spying Coppelius in the crowd below, he screams, "spin, spin, circle of fire," and finally jumps over the parapet, his last words being Coppola's grim play on words, "lovely *occe*, lovely *occe*" (ibid., 124).

These moments look like the enactment of the classical description of the death-work. I take the term from a very suggestive essay by J.-B. Pontalis, who coins the term by analogy with Freud's concepts of the dream-work and the joke-work which, through the primary processes of condensation and displacement, produce the dream and the joke as wishful or wish-driven compromise-formations. By contrast with these productions, the death-work *undoes* complex formations, breaking up complex unities, unraveling the synthesizing and binding work of the life instincts in alliance with the ego. He argues that the death drive is a "fundamental process of *unbinding*, of fragmentation, of breaking up, of bursting . . . that mimics death in the very kernel of being."[7] What is at stake here are psychic processes that disorganize the living being from within. Hoffmann's *Feuerkreis* and the jerking, bellowing maddened puppet that it reduces Nathaniel to, certainly seem compelling representations of the deathly unbinding that is unleashed by the repetition-compulsion. Disintegration and death seem to be its defining terms. Pontalis shares this emphasis with his former collaborator and cothinker, Jean Laplanche, whose work on the death drive argues that the death drive with no energy of its own apart from that of libido—Freud declined to posit a *destrudo* that would be the parallel but alternative energy source to the *libido*—is in fact but a modality or regime of the sexual drive itself: "The death drive does not possess its own energy. Its energy is libido. Or, better put, the death drive is the very soul, the constitutive principle, of libidinal circulation."[8] The distinction between life and death drives is not a question of instincts or tendencies inherent in all living matter, as Freud speculates, but of drives that operate in 'the human, all too human' field of sexuality. This is what Laplanche calls a 'sexual death drive', not bound to totalized objects or people but passing through part-objects, zones, and organs—*occe*, lovely *occe*—pressing repetitively to-

7. J-B. Pontalis, "On Deathwork in Freud, in the Self, in Culture," in *Psychoanalysis, Creativity and Literature*, ed. Alan Roland (New York: Columbia University Press, 1978), 92.
8. Jean Laplanche, *Life and Death in Psychoanalysis*, trans. Jeffrey Mehlman (Baltimore: The Johns Hopkins University Press, 1976), 124.

ward absolute discharge and so shattering the ego and its constructions in its wake.

While the end result of the repetition-compulsion in *The Sandman* bears this out, what seems to me so striking in Hoffmann's tale is the way the motifs of the circle-of-fire and the puppet-out-of-control bear witness to a complex structure of repetition that, rather than itself breaking down or disintegrating, appears to proliferate in complex sequences of scenes in which the component elements of one scene are reconfigured and augmented in later scenes. One can trace back both the circle-of-fire and puppet motifs from scene to scene, to what I will call the 'primal scene' of both Hoffmann's narrative and of Nathaniel's biography, using the phrase in the sense of an originary scene as—so I have argued in Chapter 9—Freud used it. By invoking this term 'primal scene,' I am revisiting the officially abandoned seduction theory from the period 1895–97 at the start of Freud's psychoanalytic development. Here he uses it to indicate a moment of originary trauma in which the subject's defenses are breached by sexual excitations that cannot be integrated or bound within the ego but that are split off in a psychic quarantine that is reactivated and reworked through associational processes in later moments (Freud's *Nachträglichkeit* or 'afterwardsness,'[9] as discussed in Chapters 2–4).

Hoffmann's narrative not only embeds the deathly processes of repetition in the oedipal-familial configuration but sees this configuration as itself but a repetitive refiguring of a primal scene of trauma in which Nathaniel spies from a closet on the uncanny nighttime activities of his father and the lawyer, Coppelius. The two adults appear to be making something in his father's chamber with the aid of a secret forge or hearth—a 'circle of fire'—but which appears to involve the use of 'eyes' as raw materials. In this primal scene of the narrative, Coppelius's call for eyes precipitates the screaming child, Nathaniel, out of his hiding place in the closet, and he is dragged to the hearth to supply what Coppelius calls "a lovely pair of children's eyes" (Hoffmann 1982, 91), or "lov-ely *occe*" as later in Coppola's salesman's pitch (ibid., 124), and Nathaniel's last words as he is precipitated to his death in the final scene. Spared his eyes by the pleadings of

---

9. See Jean Laplanche, "Notes on Afterwardsness," in *Essays on Otherness*, ed. John Fletcher (London: Routledge, 1999).

his father, his arms and legs are then violently twisted and screwed in and out in different ways by Coppelius, who works him over like a puppet or mechanical doll, which is what one infers the two men are secretly making. This all-male scene has affinities with the primal scene in a narrower, later psychoanalytic usage—that of a scene of violent sexual encounter between the mother and the father, either overheard or overseen by the childish voyeur. This later parental configuration of the primal scene is in fact reproduced in a second scene, of the father's death. Here a loud explosion and a violent exit of someone from the house (presumably Coppelius) awakens Nathaniel to confront, not his father and Coppelius at work before the secret hearth in his study, but the parental couple: "Before the billowing hearth, his face blackened with smoke and hideously distorted, my father lay dead on the floor, my sisters lamenting and wailing all around him, my mother unconscious beside him" (92). Although a realist explanation is implied and later stated by Clara (the two men working together, the mother's belated arrival on the scene and fainting), what the scene presents *visually* is a familial configuration with the parental couple lying side by side at its center. This second scene resumes the earlier one but substitutes the mother for Coppelius as the father's partner, at least at the level of its scenic (if not narrative) form. Both are transgressive and dangerous scenes of making.

The scene's symbolic components—the threat to the eyes, the implied making of the doll, the treatment of Nathaniel as a mechanism or puppet, the hearth with its flickering flame and the "brightly gleaming substances" drawn out of its smoke and fire, and, finally, the alliance between the much-loved father and Coppelius-as-Sandman—recur throughout the tale in such a way as to determine Nathaniel's fate. In commenting selectively on Hoffmann's tale, I have, by a process of theoretical bricolage, drawn on elements of Freud's conceptual arsenal, from both the early and officially abandoned theories of seduction and trauma and the later theories of the Oedipus and castration complexes. I have done so in order to try to trace the ways in which Hoffmann embeds the most extreme forms of the compulsion-to-repeat leading to death, not in a grand struggle of biological forces—the life and death instincts as postulated in *Beyond the Pleasure Principle*—but in a proliferating and baroquely complex symbolic machine or series. This series is unleashed by an originary moment whose traumatic elements are encoded in a *mise-en-scène*, a governing fantasy that has a seemingly autonomous power to increase and multiply unto death.

Hoffmann's vision of the death-work is not simply that of a work of un-binding, fragmentation, and entropy, although all of these result spectacu-larly from its operations. Rather, the death-work in Hoffmann's texts appears to operate through and as a kind of symbolic or cultural machine. It involves more than the psychodynamics of one subject, Nathaniel, the fated protagonist, even though Nathaniel himself offers up his life story in the tale's opening exchange of letters, as if it were an exemplary proto-psychoanalytic case study. The death-work also involves a process of trans-mission between people that circulates throughout an ever-widening circuit. The figure of the Sandman is not just a paranoid oedipal projection of one disturbed young man but a generative representation that circulates from generation to generation. As I have argued elsewhere,[10] Nathaniel inherits the idea of the Sandman initially from his mother and his nurse. The Sand-man who sprinkles sand in children's eyes is a fanciful personification of the red, sore eyes of the child refusing to go to bed, first invoked by his middle-class mother, who does not believe in his actual existence but ex-plains him as a figure of speech. It is Nathaniel's old nurse who next elabo-rates the Sandman as the cruel and punitive figure of peasant folklore, who steals naughty children's eyes and carries them in a sack up to the moon to feed his own children. So Nathaniel acquires the fantasy of the Sandman from the older generation and the cultural traditions they transmit.

It is the mystery of the relation between the Sandman and his beloved father—"what it could be that he had to do with my father" (Hoffman 1982, 88)—that drives him to spy on them in the first place. This is the formative moment from which, as from the traumatic power of the scene, Nathaniel dates his "possession" by the Sandman, tracing it back to this primal scene and asserting that "Coppelius was in reality an evil force which had taken possession of him as he was hiding and listening behind the curtain" (ibid., 103). As he spies on the two men, he is distressed to see his father's "gentle honest features" distorted "into a repulsive devil-mask. He looked like

---

10. John Fletcher, "The Sins of the Fathers: The Persistence of Gothic," in *Romanticism and Postmodernism*, ed. Edward Larrissy (Cambridge: Cambridge University Press, 1999), 129.

Coppelius" (91). After his father's death, he is relieved to note that "his features had again grown mild and gentle, as in life," and he is consoled by the thought that "his bond with the diabolical Coppelius had in any event not plunged him into eternal damnation" (94). The father's relation to Coppelius, however, remains enigmatic, and it is as if, in this scene, Nathaniel inherits this figure from his father as a persecutory paternal legacy.

The Sandman is also the "dreadful voice" who speaks Nathaniel's literary production, and hence he is the very figure of a daemonic possession by the power of transmitted representation. The phrase comes from the narrator's description of Nathaniel's composition of a poem, given only in paraphrase, which combines both the oedipal triangle Freud points to— Nathaniel and Clara standing before the marriage altar, where the ceremony is disrupted by the appearance of Coppelius, who touches Clara's eyes "which sprang out like blood-red sparks, singeing and burning, on to Nathaniel's breast" and the unleashing of the death drive in the form of the "circle of fire": "While Nathaniel was composing this poem he was very quiet and self-possessed. . . . Yet when he had finished the poem and read it aloud to himself, he was seized with horror and exclaimed: 'Whose dreadful voice is this?'" (Hoffmann 1982, 105). In Hoffmann's text, the Sandman, as both the agent and fantasmatic embodiment of the death drive, is the very figure of transgenerational transmission, of cultural inheritance and reproduction as the persecutory relay of a deathly, mortifying enigma, and of a past that contains an untranslatable reserve. Paradoxically, the repetition-compulsion here powers cultural apparatuses, and while it may unbind or shatter its hapless or fated bearers such as Nathaniel, it constitutes a cumulative, ramifying form of binding that is both deathly and libidinal.

## *The Dead Seizes the Living: Tradition as a Psychotic Enclave*

In his work on the psychopathology of inheritance and its relation to the work of mourning, Éric Toubiana, in commenting on the French Code Civil, isolates behind the legitimate heir's active seizure, in the modern sense, of his inheritance, an archaic moment of 'seisin' (Old French, *la saisine)* in which, as a precondition for his entering into possession, he is 'seized of' his property. The passive grammatical form and the archaic legal usage testify to an earlier feudal property form in which property comes *from the other*, whether feudal suzerain or deceased benefactor. In the case of inheritance, as distinct from investiture, agency is located in the dead. This is summed up in the legal maxim *'le mort saisit le vif.'* Toubiana comments:

> The law substitutes here a passive and paradoxical form: *the living is seized by the dead*. It is the dead who is in the active position and in order to insist on this paradox, the jurist specifies that the dead seizes the living without the latter doing anything or without his knowledge. Seisin [*la saisine*] places the successor in the possessive situation of the deceased . . . we are faced with a perpetuation of the person of the deceased by the successor.[11]

This legal decentering of the modern possessive individual and the attribution of agency to the dead testator-as-other is related by Toubiana to the metapsychology of mourning. In parallel to the legal maxim—the dead seizes the living—he places Freud's famous formulation from "Mourning and Melancholia"—"the shadow of the object fell upon the ego" (1917e, 249)—where the bereaved subject internalizes and identifies with his lost object, the deceased. Despite the suggestiveness of much of Toubiana's argument, the homology fails here because the implicit attribution of agency to the deceased in Freud's famous metaphor is purely rhetorical, that is, his argument actually attributes the psychical processes of identification to the mourning *subject*—the "shadow" of the dead is the effect of the *survivor's* psychical action of internalizing the lost object, not of any seizure by the deceased. More suitable as a structural rhyme, at the level of the psychical, to the legal structure of inheritance described by Toubiana, is Laplanche's concept of the psychotic enclave, especially the superego as psychotic enclave.

Laplanche attributes a special mode of agency to the adult other in the normal formation of subjectivity, the implantation of enigmatic messages, enigmatic because compromised by the adult's unconscious, and which would normally stimulate the recipient's capacity both to translate and as-

---

11. Éric Toubiana, *L'héritage et sa psychopathologie* (Paris: Presses Universitaires de France, 1988), 97, my translation.

similate what he receives, and to defend himself against what cannot be assimilated. However, he also posits a "violent variant"[12] of this implantation, which he calls "intromission" that paralyzes the child's capacity to translate and metabolize the parental discourse, to produce his own substitutions, variations, and refusals of what comes from the adult.

> While implantation allows the individual to take things up actively, at once translating and repressing, one must try to conceive of a process which blocks this . . . and puts into puts into the interior an element resistant to all metabolisation. (Laplanche 1990, 136)

Provocatively Laplanche also gives to intromission a role in the formation of the superego whose injunctions and imperatives constitute "a foreign body that cannot be metabolized":

> This means that they cannot be diluted, and cannot be replaced by anything else. They exist and they are immutable . . . they resist the schema for the substitution of signifiers . . . should we not see them as psychotic enclaves inside the human personality as such?[13]

Inscribed in the subject but untranslatable into anything other than themselves, what is to distinguish the categorical imperatives of the superego from these violently intromitted messages that persecute the psychotic subject? Laplanche poses this question: Is the superego a psychotic enclave in the normal/neurotic subject? The analogy here would be with the power of the taboo in tribal cultures, which Freud associates with the Kantian categorical imperative whose nonnegotiable injunctions ("Do this!") contrast with Kant's hypothetical imperative ("Do this, if you wish to be saved . . . if you wish to be happy, etc"), and whose compulsion and transgenerational reproduction cannot be explained pragmatically as a form of practical reason.[14]

---

12. Jean Laplanche, "Implantation and Intromission," in *Essays on Otherness*, ed. John Fletcher (London: Routledge, 1999), 136.
13. Jean Laplanche, *New Foundations for Psychoanalysis* (Oxford: Basil Blackwell, 1989), 139.
14. Sigmund Freud, *Totem and Taboo* (1912), *SE* 13. Laplanche's reflections on the relations between intromission, the superego and psychosis are fruitfully developed by Dominique Scarfone, 1994.

The Sandman as paternal legacy and psychotic enclave (the dead seizes the living), with his relish in contaminating and spoiling the oral pleasures— the cakes and sweetmeats—of Nathaniel's childhood and his sadistic anticipation of Nathaniel's suicide in the final scene, certainly seems, in Lacan's words, "the obscene, ferocious figure in which the true signification of the superego must be seen,"[15] and which presides over the paranoid transactions between the oedipal male subject and a patriarchal culture. He is the emanation of the symbolic order of a whole culture and its system of formative myths and fantasies, the patriarchal unconscious and its collective symbolic reality. For while Coppelius is no aristocrat, and the narrative is located in a distinctively bourgeois milieu, he is nevertheless presented as both an advocate and a representative of the Law: an aged and curiously outdated figure, dressed in old-fashioned court dress with black stockings, shoes with jeweled buckles, a wig, hair bag, and cravat. He seems a figure of the *ancien régime*, which marks the historically archaic quality of the punitive legacy he represents. In his persecutory extremity he has affinities with Freud's formulation, that in melancholia "what holds sway in the superego is, as it were, a pure culture of the death instinct, and in fact it often enough succeeds in driving the ego into death" (1923a, 53). While Freud's German term *Reinkultur* has the artificially purified laboratory culture of microorganisms in mind rather than the culture of Mathew Arnold or Raymond Williams, it is precisely a cultural work of the death drive, the investment of the repetition-compulsion in cultural apparatuses (rather than in the fundamental germ cells of living matter, as in Freud's metabiological fantasy) that Hoffmann's narratives dramatize.

## A Social Ecology of the Death-work

In Hoffmann's other long novella, "Mademoiselle de Scudery" of 1818, which is also a narrative of the death drive, the repetition-compulsion is situated in the story of the obsessed master goldsmith, René Cardillac, who is the first literary representation in modern European literature, of which

---

15. Jacques Lacan, "The Freudian Thing," in *Écrits*, trans. Bruce Fink (New York: Norton & Co., 2002 ), 361.

I am aware, of the stalker and serial killer. He is condemned to live out the repetitious replaying of an originary moment that functions as both the primal scene of the narrative and of his own biography, which he tells as a narrative within the narrative. However, this inner autobiographical narrative of Cardillac the goldsmith is framed and contextualized by Hoffman's panoptic vision of the city of Paris in 1680 as "a scene of horrific atrocities" (Hoffmann 1982, 22), and one that constitutes a virtual social ecology of the death drive. A series of social networks, both opposed yet parallel to each other, is laid out by the narrative, around which circulates, first, an epidemic of poisoning and, second, a moral panic of accusation and execution that actually prolongs the fatalities of the former, while seeking to extirpate them.

The epidemic of poisoning is presented by Hoffmann in the form of a genealogy of transmission of the chemical knowledge of poisons obtained through a kind of pupilage or apprenticeship. It begins with "Herr Glaser, a German apothecary and the finest chemist of his time," then his Italian apprentice, Exili, who under a pretext of learning alchemy sought after his real objective "the mixing, boiling and sublimation of poisons," thus perfecting "a fine potion, odourless and tasteless, quickly fatal or killing slowly, and leaving behind no trace in the human body" (ibid.). Such a dematerialized process might seem more like a malevolent wish fulfillment that works simply through the omnipotence of thoughts. Despite these discreet proceedings, Exili falls under suspicion and ends up in the Bastille, where he shares a cell with and transmits his knowledge to Captain Godin de Sainte Croix, who becomes his pupil, surpasses his master, and goes on to work independently on his release. Sainte Croix, in turn, transmits his knowledge to his mistress, the Marquise de Brinvilliers, a notorious female libertine. In the figure of the Marquise, who poisons her father for revenge and her two brothers and her sister for their inheritance, the motif of inheritance passes from the transmission of poisonous knowledge itself to the familial scene, where the activity of poisoning itself seems to become virtually a form of family relation, following the pathways of consanguinity and inheritance that link its victims: "Death stole into even the closest circles of family, love, friendship . . . mistrust infected the most sacred relationships: husband feared his wife, father his son, sister her brother; meals remained untouched, wine undrunk" (ibid., 24). The sobriquet bestowed on the poison by the Parisians—*la poudre de succession*—sums up this parallel distribution of lineages between the poisoners and the poisoned.

It is also with the Marquise that the activity of poisoning takes the form of a repetition-compulsion:

> This kind of crime can become an irresistible passion: such poisoners have then killed people whose life or death must have been a matter of complete indifference to them . . . the sudden death of several paupers at the Hotel Dieu . . . the pigeon pies which she set before her guests . . . the Chevalier de Guet and several others. (Hoffman 1982, 23)

This proliferation of poisonings, over and above the gains from inheritance or other material benefits, is partly explained as a regime of generalized envy: "[r]iches, a lucrative office, a beautiful, perhaps too youthful wife: these sufficed for a man to be pursued to his death" (ibid, 24). Its contagious or epidemic-like quality soon infects a third social network or apparatus, that of the law, whose activities of prosecution and punishment are described in terms that are curiously parallel to the murderous circulation of the poisons. Hoffmann introduces the law into the successive transmissions of the powder through the motif of inheritance that has regulated its previous circulation. Sainte Croix, through a slipping of his glass mask as he prepares the almost immaterially fine powder, breathes it in and drops instantly dead, in effect self-poisoned. Being without heirs, Sainte Croix's estate is seized by the court which comes into possession of the *poudre de succession*: "there, locked in a case, they found his whole fiendish arsenal of poisons" (ibid., 23). The evidence incriminates both his assistant, La Chaussée, and the Marquise, who are both beheaded, but instead of closure and a bringing of the poisoning compulsion to rest, the execution ends with an image of dispersal: "After the execution her body was burnt and the ashes thrown to the winds" (24). It is not too surprising to learn that the execution leads but to a further round of poisonings and suspected poisoners, as if the dispersal of the Marquise's ashes—another fine powder—had but spread the deathly compulsion even more widely.

Close on the heels of the second wave of poisonings are the judicial and police activities instigated by the court's possession (or inheritance by default) of the *poudre de succession*. The special judicial institution or tribunal appointed by the king "to control the mounting disorder" (ibid.) is given its own punning or metaphorically resonant sobriquet, that of the *Chambre ardente*. So two further name sequences are set in parallel with each other, that of the members or officers of the *Chambre ardente*, Argenson, the Minister for Public Order, La Regnie, the president of the *Chambre*, and "the cunning Desgrais," a law officer and one of the earliest literary detectives (predating Poe's Inspector Dupin by twenty-three years), ranged against the new poisoner, La Voisin, who with her accomplices, Le Sage and Le Vigoureux, is positioned within the genealogy of previous poisoners: "[L]ike Sainte Croix, a pupil of Exili's, she knew how to prepare Exili's untraceable poison and so help sons to early inheritances and wives to younger husbands" (ibid., 25). Discovered by Desgrais, she is burned in the Place de Grève, but not before a list among her papers initiates yet a further sequence of names "of all those who had availed themselves of her assistance, and after that execution followed upon execution" (ibid.). A new sequence of naming further proliferates a network of either suspected poisoners or judicial victims: Cardinal Bonzy, the Archbishop of Narbonne, the Duchesse de Bouillon, the Countess de Soissons, and even the Duke of Luxembourg, the Marshall of the Realm, imprisoned in the Bastille before his innocent consultation of Le Sage for a horoscope is established. These successive listings and 'genealogies' of names concentrated into four pages give the reader a bewildering sense of social density and the networks, either private and secretive or public and institutional, that traverse the social body and open it up to the epidemics and compulsions of the death-work.

The coincidence of social and psychic economies that frames the novella's central story of Cardillac the murderous goldsmith is strikingly figured in the title I remarked on earlier of the judicial institution that seeks to track down and punish the poisoners. This is explicated by its president, La Regnie, who tells Mademoiselle de Scudery, "Evil-doers shall tremble before the *Chambre ardente*, which knows of no punishment other than blood and fire" (ibid., 46). This references the *Chambre* in terms of the exhibition of exemplary bodily punishment, the spectacle of the scaffold in Foucault's phrase,[16] characteristic of the judicial regimes of

16. Michel Foucault, *Discipline and Punish: The Birth of the Prison*, trans. Alan Sheridan (Harmondsworth: Penguin, 1979), 32.

late feudal absolutism in which Hoffmann's narrative is set (the court of Louis XIV). However, the *Chambre ardente* also reads like an allegorical figure, from a traditional book of emblems, for the heart as seat or organ of passion, in this context precisely that "irresistible passion" for which the Marquise de Brinvilliers was publicly beheaded and burned. We are told that La Regnie, in "the blindness of his enthusiasm . . . soon inspired the hatred of those whose avenger or protector he was supposed to be . . . [t]he blood of the guilty and the innocent flowed at the Place de Grève" (25), thus enacting a reversal of the instruments of law and punishment into an expression of the very murderous compulsion they were meant to eradicate. The *Chambre ardente*, with its double reference to both the institutional seat of law, judgment and punishment, and the traditional bodily seat of the passions, fitly designates the investment of the cultural apparatus of the law by the "irresistible passion" of the death drive, and its proliferation through the succession of epidemics and moral panics that Hoffmann invokes as his narrative frame.

## The Goldsmith's Primal Scene

There are, however, no direct causal links between this frame narrative and the events of the story of Cardillac the goldsmith. His enactment of a murderous repetition-compulsion on the streets of Paris by night is presented as merely the latest in the series of "outrages" by which the social space of the city is marked by the work of the death drive. Like Nathaniel's opening letters in *The Sandman*, the goldsmith's inner narrative traces to an earlier infantile scene his murderous adult compulsion to stalk his clients at night and stab them through the heart, in order to retrieve the jewelry he has just completed and supplied to them. This originary scene involves his mother, then pregnant with him, and a male seducer sporting a chain of sparkling diamonds that were, we are told, the object of "her longing, fiery glances"; "[h]er whole being lusted after the sparkling stones" (ibid., 64). As the cavalier embraces Cardillac's mother, her seizure in turn of the cavalier's diamond chain provokes in him a heart attack and immediate death:

> My mother's efforts to free herself from the stiffened arms of the corpse were in vain. His hollow eyes, their sight extinguished, fixed upon her, the dead man

rolled on the ground with her. Her cries for help at last reached some distant passers-by, who hurried to her and rescued her from the arms of her gruesome lover. (Hoffmann 1982, 64)

This grotesque primal scene brings together the desire of the mother and the death of the male object in a complex scenario that is transmitted to the son: "The fear of that terrible moment had got into me. My evil star had risen and sent down fires which kindled in me one of the strangest and most pernicious of passions" (ibid., 64). The "pernicious passion" in question entails the compulsion to steal back the jewelry he has fashioned for his clients. The satisfaction afforded by the thefts is only temporary, for increasingly this is accompanied by a sinister inner voice that urges him, "It is yours really, it is yours really; take it, then—what do diamonds mean to a dead man? . . . Ha, ha, a dead man is wearing your jewels!" (ibid., 65). Cardillac's resultant compulsion entails both the stealing of the jewels and the desire to murder their bearer with a blow to the heart (a form of cardiac arrest, as Hoffmann puns suggestively on the protagonist's name). What is being subject to such deadly arrest is the circulation of the jewels in the narrative as a signifier of desire, which had given them something of a phallic signification in the classic Lacanian sense, as the contextualization of the murderous thefts suggests:

> In the voluptuous court of Louis XIV there were many who, entangled in some amorous intrigue, crept to their mistress in the night, often bearing a rich gift; but often, too, the lover failed to reach the house where he antici- pated enjoyment; sometimes he fell on the threshold, sometimes even before his mistress's door, who, horror-stricken, found his body in the morning. (Hoffmann 1982, 26)

The "rich gift" of the jewels is a signifier of male desire and so a potential object of female desire and thus a bearer of the phallic function as Lacan defines it.[17] Cardillac's primal scene involves the transmission of the desire for the jewels-as-phallus from the mother to the son who is born into that desire of the mother:

17. Jacques Lacan, "The Signification of the Phallus" (1966 [1956]), in *Écrits* trans. Fink: 575–84.

Even when I was very young, sparkling diamonds, golden jewellery, meant more to me than anything else . . . as a boy I stole gold and jewels wherever I could lay hands on them. . . . This inborn urge had to be suppressed in the face of the cruellest punishments by my father. (Hoffmann 1982, 65)

If this positions him by identification with the mother as the bearer of her desire, it must be noted that hostility to the male figure is explicitly not attributed to the mother, even though a previous attempt at seduction without the desirable accoutrements had been rebuffed: "My mother recognised him, but this time he seemed to her, in the gleam of the sparkling diamonds, a being of a higher kind, the embodiment of everything beautiful" (ibid., 64). If the inheritance of the desire of the mother explains Cardillac's adult vocation as a master goldsmith and jeweler, it leaves enigmatic the question as to the origin of the murderous compulsion aimed at the male bearer of the jewels as signifier of desire. The alignment of the dead cavalier, from the primal scene with the mother, with the subsequent clients who commission the jewelry from Cardillac, is clear; the commissioned jewels are repeatedly spoken of as male love-gifts to the woman, and the process of commissioning them, and in particular of delivering them once finished, is invested with an obsessional drama in which, agitated, Cardillac feels "robbed . . . of my sleep, my health—of all my vital energies" (ibid., 65). However, the compulsion is not just to retrieve the jewels, to regain their possession, so repeating the desire of the mother, but to repeat the death of the male subjects of desire, as if the whole scenario of the primal scene must be repeated, not just one of its component elements.

In light of the father's cruel punishments for his childhood thefts, this might be glossed as a classic oedipal desire to appropriate the phallus, eliminate the father as rival, and succeed to his place as the bearer of the object of the mother's desire. It is striking, however, that Cardillac does not enter into any sexual exchanges through a recirculation of the jewels as love-gifts to a wife or mistress; instead, he withdraws them from circulation, hoarding them in his jewel cabinet in a secret vault: "On every piece of jewellery was hung a ticket marked with the name of the person for whom it was made and when it had been taken by theft or robbery or murder" (67). This compulsion seems not about the wish to perpetuate or to participate in the circulation of desire but, rather, to eliminate desire and its male bearer and to memorialize that elimination. As J. M. Ellis argues, based on "a confusion of diamonds and sex" (or, one might rather propose, the symbolization by the former of the latter, that is at once a cultural convention and a compulsive unconscious association): "Cardillac, then, spends his nights punishing his mother's lover, and protecting her from temptation by taking back the diamonds."[18]

Cardillac's revelation of his hoard to his prospective son-in-law, Olivier Brusson, is made in terms of the thematics of inheritance that mark the narrative's frame. Cardillac makes a curious double or contradictory gesture:

> "On your wedding day Olivier," said Cardillac gloomy and solemn, "you shall swear to me a sacred oath, with your hand on the image of Christ on the cross, that as soon as I am dead you will reduce all these riches to dust by a means which I will make known to you. I do not want any human being, least of all Madelon and you, to come into possession of a hoard which has been purchased with blood." (Hoffmann 1982, 67)

Cardillac has already agreed to the marriage of his apprentice, Olivier, to his daughter, Madelon, in return for Olivier's silence about his secret crimes. As a result, Olivier feels that his love for Madelon is "a passion that binds him to the crime" (ibid., 67). The invocation of the wedding day and the oath seems like an attempt on Cardillac's part to reverse the logic of transmission and inheritance that has regulated the circulation of the repetition-compulsion in its various forms. As well as his silence, Olivier must now pledge, in return for Madelon, to destroy Cardillac's inheritance that would normally pass on to him on Cardillac's death. This is one of Cardillac's two attempts to reverse or abort the transmission and reactivation of the original primal scene. Liquidating the "hoard which had been purchased with blood" is an attempt to prevent the repetition of the "irresistible passion" in the next generation.

18. J. M. Ellis, "E. T. A. Hoffmann's 'Das Fraulein von Scuderi," *Modern Language Review* 64 (1969): 344, 345.

*Old Maids and Virgin Mothers:*
*Is There a Sublimation of the Death Drive?*

Cardillac's other attempt to reverse the operation of his compulsion occurs in relation to Mademoiselle de Scudery, the famous *précieuse* and writer who is both virginal and elderly, "an old maid who sometimes went to court," in her own words. She is drawn into the circuit of Cardillac's compulsion by a witty pair of verses she produces at court in opposition to another poem importuning the king "on behalf of all the imperilled lovers," and which presented a picture of "the lover, creeping on his secret way to his beloved, . . . filled with such fear and distress that his anxiety killed all joy in love." Speaking against the creation of another court with even wider powers than the *Chambre ardente*, she replies: "*Un amant qui craint les voleurs/n'est point digne d'amour*" (A lover who fears thieves/is not worthy of love) (Hoffmann 1982, 29). The jewel-bearing lovers under threat are clearly aligned with the Spanish cavalier in the primal scene, and Mademoiselle de Scudery appears to be speaking enigmatically here in defense of the necessary risks attached to desire. A further ironic complication is added by the location of the scene in question in the apartments of Madame de Maintenon, the king's mistress. As if taking Mlle. de Scudery's epigram as a defense of his own activities, Cardillac praises Mlle. de Scudery's virtue to Olivier, his apprentice, and as the latter reports to her, declared that "gifted as you were with such virtue . . . his evil star faded and was powerless before it; even if you were wearing the most beautiful jewellery ever made by him it would never raise any evil spirit or murderous thought within him" (ibid., 68). He consequently decides to send a set of jewelry to her as "a humble sacrifice to virtue and piety itself" and claims that "a deep inward voice—quite different from the one which demands bloody acts like a ravenous beast of prey—has commanded me to do this" (69). However, neither the promised destruction of the secret hoard of jewels nor their decathexis or libidinal disinvestment as a gift to the virginal mother (she turns out to have adopted Olivier as a child and acted the role of a substitute mother to him) is sufficient to lay the compulsion to rest. Indeed, the jewelry reasserts its role as signifier of desire, even in relation to Mademoiselle de Scudery and despite her refusal of the gift and her presentation of herself as desexualized and outside the circuit of desire: "What will such splendour do for these wrinkled arms, what will this sparkling finery do for this scrawny neck?" Cardillac's response is that of a traditional tongue-tied lover; overwhelmed with an excess of feeling, he "dropped to his knees, kissed the hem of Mademoiselle's skirt, kissed her hands, moaned, sighed, wept, sobbed, and ran out upsetting the armchair and table" (39). Although offered as a tribute to her "virtue," the gift of jewels positions her within the circuits of desire and its deadly nemesis, so much so that she becomes the butt of court raillery, with Madame de Maintenon prophesying "the unexampled spectacle of a seventy-three-years-old lady of irreproachable aristocracy becoming the bride of a goldsmith" (ibid.). Unsurprisingly, Cardillac's old compulsions resurface, regretting his gift and brooding ill-humoredly over it, in preparation, so Olivier fears, for a possible murderous reclaiming of the jewels.

Cardillac's sudden death by stabbing in an attempt on the life of another client preempts the danger to Mademoiselle de Scudery, but it leads to Olivier's arrest for his master's murder, and he is seized by La Regnie as the chief suspect for the wave of murderous jewel thefts. The narrative interest of the novella's final section turns largely on the intrigues and manipulations at court on the part of Mademoiselle de Scudery, necessary to free Olivier, her long-lost foster child, from the clutches of the *Chambre ardente*. The question of the possible *decathexis* of the jewels and the quelling of the repetition-compulsion appears to be forgotten as Cardillac's plans to outflank his "evil star" are forestalled by his own death.

However, the question of the *aftereffects* of the narrative's primal scene reappears in a strange moment that is in excess of its function in the intrigue-plot, and which operates outside any case-study narrative centered on Cardillac and his murderous psychopathology. Seeking to approach the king to persuade him to initiate an investigation of Cardillac's crimes independent of La Regnie and the *Chambre ardente*, Mademoiselle de Scudery is faced with the king's horror of the crimes and his refusal to discuss them. Her stratagem to catch the king's attention and divert it onto the forbidden topic involves the staging of a *scene* at court that turns on the wearing of the jewels given to her by Cardillac. "She clad herself in a black dress of heavy silk, adorned herself with Cardillac's jewels, draped a long black veil over her shoulders," and appears before the astonished king:

The diamonds of the necklace and bracelets flashed before his eyes, and he cried: "By Heaven, that is Cardillac's jewellery!" Then, turning to Madame de Maintenon with a smile, he added: "Look, Madame Marquise, how our beautiful bride grieves for her bridegroom." (Hoffmann 1982, 78)

She seems here to be acting out the previous jest of the Marquise in which she was portrayed as the goldsmith's bride and object of desire. Dressed in what appears to be both bridal and mourning dress and wearing the jewelry as signifier of Cardillac's desire, she appears both to accept and to mourn the meanings they carry. The moment resonates with the original primal scene itself, aligning her with Cardillac's lustful and entranced mother and the goldsmith with the long-dead Spanish cavalier (not to mention the host of murdered male bearers of the jewelry). However, having positioned herself outside the circuit of desire, she also rewrites that scene (of which she is unaware) in a moment of renunciation and mourning. Her reply to the king, which we are told she speaks "as if continuing the joke," is enigmatic. She repudiates the role of "grief-stricken bride" desiring her lost husband:

No, I have severed all connection with that goldsmith and would think no more of him, did not the horrible sight of his body borne past me appear from time to time before my eyes. (Hoffmann 1982, 78)

While this allows her to segue cunningly into a narrative of her involvement in the affair (she enacts perfectly Freud's description of the joke-work, bypassing the king's resistance to take him by surprise), it also positions her not as moved by desire but as haunted by the dead. The effect of the scene is not accountable for merely in terms of Cardillac's personal psychopathology. The significance of the jewels in terms of their role in the primal scene seems to persist or repeat outside of his personal associations. Mademoiselle de Scudery herself had commented on Cardillac's giving them to her: "I shudder at the blood that seems to cling to these gems. And now even Cardillac's behavior has, I must confess, for me something peculiarly unnerving and uncanny about it. . . . I shall never dare to wear these jewels." To which Madame de Maintenon replies, "Sooner throw the jewels into the Seine than ever wear them" (ibid., 40). In fact, the particular jewels in question have not involved the death of anyone, but especially in light of Cardillac's excessive investment of them, they carry the phallic signification of all the jewels in the narrative, which Hoffmann persistently connects to the compulsion to appropriate and to kill their bearer.

Mademoiselle de Scudery's assumption of Cardillac's jewels in this *tableau* of the mourning virginal bride seems not so much an unwitting or compulsive repetition of the lost scene that gives them their uncanny power, as a resignification or sublimation of it in relation to her withdrawal from the circuits of desire. It is as if she acts out a mourning for both Cardillac and all the dead men who have borne the jewels and even for the death of desire itself. In this she is associated with religious sublimation. Cardillac had previously attempted to withdraw the jewelry from libidinal circulation, but failed: "I resolved to make a diamond crown for the Holy Virgin in the Church of St. Eustace. But then that incomprehensible fear overcame me whenever I wanted to start the work, so that I left it altogether" (ibid., 69). His gift to Mademoiselle de Scudery was another such attempt. Neither the Holy Virgin of St. Eustace nor Mademoiselle de Scudery is able to function alone as a sublimatory substitute object for the desires signified by the jewels. It is only the death of Cardillac, and the mediating role of Mademoiselle de Scudery in bringing the young lovers together (rather than Cardillac "giving away" his daughter in exchange for Olivier's complicity—"a passion that binds him to the crime" (67)—and his inheritance of the hoard of stolen jewels), that lays to rest the repetitions of the death-work and ends its transmission. The narrative concludes with the disposal of Cardillac's secret jewel hoard. A discreet advertisement appeals to the rightful owners of jewels stolen before the end of the year 1680. Those who survived reclaim them. Of the jewels whose owners perished and are unable to reclaim them (i.e., the jewels that played their role in the murderous repetition of the primal scene), the novella's final sentence tells us: "What was left fell to the treasury of the church of St. Eustace." They remain outside of libidinal circulation and are assigned by implication to the *mortmain* of the virginal mother without desire.

Cardillac himself is unable to lay to rest the murderous repetition-compulsion, of which he is the possessed subject and agent. Even when the recipient is a figure of the virgin mother who stands outside the circuit of desire, the very act of fashioning the jewels is invested with a passion and an unconscious fantasy which entails that giving or parting from them leaves him "robbed . . . of all my vital energies" (65) which they carry and

embody. Even as a gesture intended as a tribute to the virgin mother's virtue, it capsizes into its opposite, a transgressive, ineradicably erotic act, as
his kneeling, kissing, weeping and comical exit from her presence makes
clear. His repeated acts of killing desire in the person of the successive avatars of the Spanish cavalier are driven by the very desire for the jewels they
seek to extinguish. It is only when he too joins the long line of murdered
jewel–bearers that finally he punishes the right person, the one who makes
the jewels, kills for them, and hoards them, over and over again. Nevertheless it is the figure of Mademoiselle de Scudery who presides over the
narrative's conclusion and by her act of mourning, as bride and widow, acknowledges Cardillac's contradictory position as both avenging son and
murdered lover, presides also over the liquidation of his hoard, cheats the
*Chambre ardente* of its latest victim, and enables the Cardillac's daughter to
marry her young jeweler, while as a maternal figure she provides her son
with an alternative object of desire.

In Freud's encounter with Hoffmann's novella and the aesthetic phenomenon of the uncanny at the moment of theoretical crisis and revision in 1919,
we have, appropriately enough, a replication of his encounter with the tragedies of Sophocles and Shakespeare in the earlier crisis of 1897. The instability and oscillations that plagued his reformulation of the seduction
theory in the letters and drafts to Wilhelm Fliess in the late 1890s are virtually identical with the oscillations that beset his 1914 draft of the Wolf
Man case in the additions of 1918. The crisis of 1897 was partly resolved by
the official abandonment of the model of traumatic seduction as an explanation of the psychoneuroses. This was replaced with a model of infantile
sexuality and the sexual *Trieb* with its vicissitudes, as an explanation of human sexuality in general. The latter was increasingly framed within a conception of sexual development as determined by a pregiven program of
stages, modeled on and determined by biological development. However,
the conceptual arsenal of the theory of traumatic seduction, as Jean Laplanche
has suggested and this book seeks to demonstrate at length, makes a number of returns under different names, and in simplified or fragmented
forms, to challenge or temporarily displace its antagonist theoretical twin,
the homeostatic living organism, with its biological model of development.
Indeed, in what looks like the final triumph in 1920 of the biological and
the instinctual, which appears to subsume the traumatic into the death instinct and the libido into the life instinct, in fact, by a certain *legerdemain*,
the reverse happens. The instinctual is redefined by the export of the
psychical compulsion to repeat into the field of the organic and the vital
order. Instead of the living homeostatic organism, with its boundaries and

protective defenses, being the victim and possible survivor of the incursions of the traumatic, rather life itself, with its intolerable raising of tensions and energy levels, is declared to be the primal trauma that afflicts inanimate matter. The trauma of life must be abreacted and extinguished by that blindest and most mechanical of principles, the discharge to zero, itself modeled, as Freud acknowledged at the beginning of the "Project for a Scientific Psychology" in 1895, on the observation of the primary processes of the dream-work and the repressed unconscious.

I have tried to trace the complexities of the formation of the traumatic in Freud's thought, especially in his writings of the 1890s and his relation to and break from 'the great Charcot' and in the theoretical crisis revealed in his correspondence with Fliess. I have also sought to trace the returns of the model of traumatic repetition, of seduction with its temporal schemas and relation to the other, and their persistent manifestations in the form of a scenography of trauma, in the decades that followed their so-called abandonment. These are most obvious in either the clinical case studies, from *Studies on Hysteria*, or in the great set pieces such as the Wolf Man case (the Rat Man case would have provided equally rich material), or in Freud's engagement with the narrative and scenic forms of literature, drama, and painting. These engagements with the arts at critical turning points seem to be driven by Freud's unresolved alternation between the antithetical problematics of trauma and bio-development, the pathological and the normative, the progressive and the retrogressive—the exogenous-'Copernican' and the endogenous-'Ptolemaic'—that structure the Freudian conceptual field with its contrary gravitational pulls. As I have argued in Chapters 5 and 12, Freud is drawn to, even magnetized by, literary and dramatic works that stage elaborate scenic sequences driven by the forces of traumatic repetition, embodied in persecutory figures of a daemonic or spectral other (Apollo, old Hamlet's ghost, the Sandman and his avatars, Cardillac and his voices) and bound to originary, traumatic—'primal'—scenes and fantasmatic prototypes. In other words, these are works that stage the very 'traumatology' that Freud is in the process of apparently marginalizing or repudiating theoretically, and which he subjects to an endogenous, normalizing—'oedipal'—interpretation. The case of Leonardo represents a fascinating reverse instance here, where the strange, even uncanny, serenity of his Madonnas and St. Johns, religiously and culturally orthodox icons as they are, receives a compelling interpretation that traces back their deviant sublimations and 'secrets of love' to the seductive traumas inscribed within the frozen, perverse moment of the baby Leonardo and his *nibio*, both scene and screen. An interpretation even more fascinating for its casual reversal of the oedipal prototype: for where with Sophocles, Shakespeare and Hoffmann, the traumatic was rendered oedipal by Freud's interpretation, with Leonardo for a brief moment the Oedipus appears as itself both seduction and trauma.

ABBREVIATIONS

*SE: The Standard Edition of the Complete Psychological Works of Sigmund Freud.* Edited by James Strachey and translated by James Strachey, Alix Strachey and Alan Tyson. Vols. 1–24. London: The Hogarth Press, 1953–74. The references to Freud's works carry a lower-case letter after each date, which follows the listing of works for each year as given in the *Standard Edition.*

NOTE ON DATES

Where more than one date appears within a given entry, the date immediately after the author's name is the date of the first publication, followed by the date of composition/delivery in square brackets where this is significantly different. References are to the English translations where they exist; otherwise, the original foreign language edition is cited. The date of publication of the English translation is given at the end of the reference, for example:
Laplanche, Jean. 1981 [1977–79]. *The Unconscious and the Id.* Translated by Luke Thurston. London: Rebus Press, 1999.

Aeschylus. *Agamemnon.* Translated by Hugh Lloyd-Jones. Englewood Cliffs, N. J.: Prentice Hall, 1970.
André, Jacques. "Feminine Sexuality: A Return to Sources." Translated by Julia Borossa. *New Formations* 48 (Winter 2002–3): 77–112.
Anzieu, Didier. *Freud's Self-analysis.* Translated by Peter Graham. London: The Hogarth Press, 1986.
Bates, Catherine. "Castrating the Castration Complex." *Textual Practice* 12, no. 1 (1998): 101–19.
Bourneville, D. M., and P. Regnard. *Iconographie Photographique de la Salpêtrière.* 3 vols. Paris: Aux Bureaux du Progrès Médicale, DelaHaye & Cie., 1876–80.
Carter, K. Codell. "Germ Theory, Hysteria, and Freud's Early Work in Psycho-pathology." *Medical History* 24 (1980): 259–74.

Charcot, Jean-Martin. 1887–8. *Charcot the Clinician: The Tuesday Lessons: Excerpts from Nine Case Presentations on General Neurology Delivered at the Salpêtrière Hospital in 1887–8.* Translated and edited by Christopher Goetz. New York: Raven Press, 1987.

———. 1889. *Clinical Lectures on Diseases of the Nervous System.* Vol. III. Translated by Thomas Savill. London: The New Sydenham Society, 1889; reprinted and intro. Ruth Harris. London: Routledge, 1991.

———. "Concerning Six Cases of Hysteria in the Male," Lecture XVIII. In *Clinical Lectures on Diseases of the Nervous System.* Vol. III. 1889.

———. "On Two Cases of Hysterical Brachial Monoplegia in the Male (continued)," Lecture XXII. In *Clinical Lectures on Diseases of the Nervous System.* Vol. III. 1889.

———. Appendix I: "Two Additional Cases of Hystero-Traumatic Paralysis in Men." In *Clinical Lectures on Diseases of the Nervous System.* Vol. III. 1889.

———, and Pierre Marie. 1892. "HYSTERIA mainly HYSTERO-EPILEPSY." In *A Dictionary of Psychological Medicine*, ed. D. Hack Tuke. London: J. & A. Churchill, 1892: 627–641.

Chase, Cynthia. "Oedipal Textuality: Reading Freud's Reading of *Oedipus.*" In *Psychoanalytic Literary Criticism*, ed. Maud Ellmann. London: Longman, 1994: 56–75.

Critchley, E. M. R., and H. E. Cantor. "Charcot's Hysteria Renaissant." *British Medical Journal* 289, (July-December 1984): 1785–88.

da Vinci, Leonardo. *The Notebooks of Leonardo da Vinci.* vol. 2. Edited by E. MacCurdy. London: Jonathan Cape, 1938.

de Marneffe, Daphne. "Looking and Listening: The Construction of Clinical Knowledge in Charcot and Freud." *Signs* 17, no. 1 (1991): 71–111.

Eissler, Kurt. *Leonardo da Vinci: Psychoanalytic Notes on the Enigma.* New York: International Universities Press, 1961.

———. *Freud and the Seduction Theory: A Brief Love Affair.* New York: International Universities Press, 2001.

Ellis, J. M. "E. T. A. Hoffmann's 'Das Fraulein von Scuderi.'" *Modern Language Review* 64 (1969): 340–50.

Fletcher, John. "The Sins of the Fathers: The Persistence of Gothic." In *Romanticism and Postmodernism*, ed. Edward Larrissy. Cambridge: Cambridge University Press, 1999: 113–40.

———. "Gender, Sexuality and the Theory of Seduction." In *Women: A Cultural Review* 11, nos. 1 and 2 (2000): 95–108. Reprinted and enlarged, in *The Academic Face of Psychoanalysis*, ed. L. Braddock and M. Lacewing. London: Routledge, 2007: 224–40.

———. "'His Majesty the Ego': From Freud to Laplanche." *Sitegeist: A Journal of Psychoanalysis and Philosophy* 4 (Spring 2010): 47–71.

Foucault, Michel. *Discipline and Punish: The Birth of the Prison*, trans. Alan Sheridan. Harmondsworth: Penguin Books, 1979.

Freud, Anna. 1922. "Beating Fantasies and Daydreams." In *The Writings of Anna Freud*, vol. 1. New York: International Universities Press, 1974.

Freud, Sigmund. 1888b. "Hysteria" *SE* 1.

———. 1892–94. "Preface and Footnotes to Charcot's *Tuesday Lectures*" *SE* 1.

———, with Josef Breuer. 1893a. "On the Psychical Mechanism of Hysterical Phenomena: Preliminary Communication" *SE* 2.

———. 1893. "Quelques Considérations pour une Étude Comparative des Paralysies Motrices Organiques et Hystériques." *Archives de Neurologie* 26 (July 1893): 29–43.

———. 1893c. Translated as "Some Points for a Comparative Study of Organic and Hysterical Motor Paralyses" *SE* 1.

———. 1893f. "Charcot" *SE* 3.

———. 1893h. "On the Psychical Mechanism of Hysterical Phenomena: A Lecture" *SE* 3.

———. 1894a. "The Neuro-Psychoses of Defence" *SE* 3.

———, with J. Breuer. 1895d. *Studies on Hysteria SE* 2.

———. 1896a. "Heredity and the Aetiology of the Neuroses" *SE* 3.

———. 1896b. "Further Remarks on the Neuro-Psychoses of Defence" *SE* 3.

———. 1896c. "The Aetiology of Hysteria" *SE* 3.

———. 1898a. "Sexuality in the Aetiology of the Neuroses" *SE* 3.

———. 1899a. "Screen Memories" *SE* 3.

———. 1900a. *The Interpretation of Dreams SE* 4–5.

———. 1901b. *The Psychopathology of Everyday Life SE* 6.

———. 1905d. *Three Essays on the Theory of Sexuality SE* 7.

———. 1905e. "Fragment of Analysis of a Case of Hysteria" *SE* 7.

———. 1906a. "My Views on the Part Played by Sexuality in the Aetiology of the Neurosis." *SE* 7.

———. 1908c. "On the Sexual Theories of Children" *SE* 9.

———. 1908e. "Creative Writers and Day-Dreaming" *SE* 9.

———. 1909b. "Analysis of a Phobia in a Five-Year-Old Boy" ['Little Hans'] *SE* 10.

———. 1909d. "Notes upon a Case of Obsessional Neurosis" ['The Rat Man'] *SE* 10.

———. 1910c. *Leonardo da Vinci and a Memory of His Childhood SE* 11.

———. 1910h. "A Special Type of Choice of Object Made by Men" *SE* 11.

———. 1912b. "The Dynamics of Transference" *SE* 12.

———. 1913d. 'The Occurrence in Dreams of Material from Fairy Tales" *SE* 12.

———. 1912–13. *Totem and Taboo SE* 13.

———. 1914c. "On Narcissism: An Introduction" *SE* 14.

———. 1914d. "On the History of the Psycho-Analytic Movement" *SE* 14.

———. 1914g. "Remembering, Repeating and Working-Through" *SE* 12.

———. 1915a. "Observations on Transference-Love" *SE* 12.

———. 1915c. "Instincts and Their Vicissitudes" *SE* 14.

———. 1915d. "Repression" *SE* 14.

———. 1915e. "The Unconscious" *SE* 14.

———. 1915f. "A Case of Paranoia Running Counter to the Psychoanalytic Theory of the Disease" *SE* 14.

———. 1916–17. Lecture 23: "The Paths to the Formation of Symptoms". In *Introductory Lectures on Psycho-Analysis SE* 16.

———. Lecture 27, "Fixation to Traumas—The Unconscious." In *Introductory Lectures on Psycho-Analysis SE* 16.

———. 1917a. "A Difficulty in the Path of Psycho-Analysis" *SE* 17.

———. 1917b. "A Childhood Recollection from *Dichtung und Warheit*" *SE* 17.

———. 1917e. "Mourning and Melancholia" *SE* 14.

———. 1918 [1914]. *Aus der Geschichte einer infantilen Neurose. Gesammelte Werke: Werke aus den Jahren 1917–1920*, (Frankfurt am Main: Fischer Taschenbuch Verlag, 1999) Band 12.

———. 1918b [1914]. "From the History of an Infantile Neurosis" ['The Wolf Man'] *SE* 17.

———. 1919d. "Introduction to *Psycho-Analysis and the War Neuroses*" *SE* 17.

———. 1919e. "'A Child Is being Beaten': A Contribution to the Study of the Origin of Sexual Perversions" *SE* 17.

———. 1919h. "The Uncanny" *SE* 17.

———. 1920g. *Beyond the Pleasure Principle.SE* 18.

———. 1923b. *The Ego and the Id SE* 19.

———. 1923e. "The Infantile Genital Organization" *SE* 19.

———. 1924c. "The Economic Problem of Masochism" *SE* 19.

———. 1925a. "A Note upon the 'Mystic Writing-Pad'" *SE* 19.

———. 1925d. *An Autobiographical Study SE* 20.

———. 1925j. "Some Psychical Consequences of the Anatomical Distinction between the Sexes" *SE* 19.

———. 1926d. *Inhibitions, Symptoms and Anxiety SE* 20.

———. 1930a. *Civilization and Its Discontents SE* 21.

———. 1937d. "Constructions in Analysis" *SE* 23.

———. 1939a. *Moses and Monotheism SE* 23.

———. 1940a. *An Outline of Psycho-Analysis SE* 23.

———. 1950a [1895]. "Project for a Scientific Psychology" *SE* 1.

———. 1956 [1886]. "Report on My Studies in Paris and Berlin" *SE* 1.

Gelfand, Toby. 1988. "'Mon Cher Docteur Freud': Charcot's Unpublished Correspondence to Freud, 1888–1893." Translation with annotation and commentary. In *Bulletin of the History of Medicine* 62 (1988): 563–88.

————. 1989. "Charcot's Response to Freud's Rebellion." *Journal of the History of Ideas* 50, no. 1(1989): 293–307.

Goetz, Christopher, Michel Bonduelle and Toby Gelfand. *Charcot: Constructing Neurology*. Oxford: Oxford University Press, 1995.

Goux, Jean-Joseph. *Oedipus Philosopher*, trans. Catherine Porter. Stanford, Calif.: Stanford University Press, 1993.

Grove, Robin. "The *Oresteia* and the Furies," *The Critical Review* (Melbourne) 13 (1970): 2–33.

Hertz, Neil. "Freud and the Sandman." In *Textual Strategies*, ed. Josue V. Harari. Ithaca, N.Y.: Cornell University Press, 1979: 296–321. Reprinted in Neil Hertz, *The End of the Line*. New York: Columbia University Press, 1985.

Hoffmann, E. T. A. *The Sandman*. 1816. Translated by R. J. Hollingdale. In *Tales of Hoffmann* ed. R. J. Hollingdale, Harmondsworth: Penguin Books, 1982.

————. *Mademoiselle de Scudery*. 1818. Translated by Sally Hayward and R. J. Hollingdale. In *Tales of Hoffmann* ed. R. J. Hollingdale, Harmondsworth: Penguin Books, 1982.

Jensen, Wilhelm. *Gradiva: A Pompeiian Fantasy*. 1904. Translated by Helen M. Downey. Los Angeles: Sun and Moon Press, 1993.

Jentsch, Ernst. "On the Psychology of the Uncanny" (1906). Translated by Roy Sellars. *Angelaki* 2, no. 1 (1995): 7–16.

Jung, C. G. "Psychoanalysis and Neurosis." 1913. In *Freud and Psychoanalysis: The Collected Works of C. G. Jung*, vol. 4, ed. Herbert Read, Michael Fordham, and Gerhard Adler. London: Routledge and Kegan Paul, 1961.

————. "The Theory of Psychoanalysis: 7. The Aetiology of Neurosis." 1915. In *Freud and Psychoanalysis: The Collected Works of C. G. Jung*, vol. 4, ed. Herbert Read, Michael Fordham, and Gerhard Adler. London: Routledge and Kegan Paul, 1961.

Kemp, Martin. *Leonardo da Vinci: The Marvellous Works of Nature and Man*. Oxford: Oxford University Press, 2006.

Lacan, Jacques. "The Freudian Thing." 1966[1955]. In *Écrits*. Translated by Bruce Fink, with Héloïse Fink and Russell Grigg. New York: Norton & Co., 2002.

Lanouzière, Jacqueline. 1994. "Breast-feeding as Original Seduction and Primal Scene of Seduction." Translated by John Fletcher. *New Formations* 48 (Winter 2002–3): 52–68.

Laplanche, Jean. 1970. *Life and Death in Psychoanalysis*. Translated by Jeffrey Mehlman. Baltimore: The Johns Hopkins University Press, 1976.

————. 1980. *Problématiques III: La sublimation*. Paris: Presses Universitaires de France.

————. 1981. *The Unconscious and the Id*. Translated by Luke Thurston. London: Rebus Press, 1999.

————. 1987. *New Foundations for Psychoanalysis*. Translated by David Macey. Oxford: Basil Blackwell, 1989.

————. 1990. "Implantation and Intromission." In *Essays on Otherness*, ed. John Fletcher. London: Routledge, 1999.

————. 1991. "Interpretation between Determinism and Hermeneutics: A Restatement of the Problem." In *Essays on Otherness*, ed. John Fletcher. London: Routledge, 1999.

————1992a. "The Drive and Its Source-Object." in *Essays on Otherness*, ed. John Fletcher. London: Routledge, 1999.

————. 1992b. "The Unfinished Copernican Revolution." In *Essays on Otherness*, ed. John Fletcher. London: Routledge, 1999.

————. 1992c. "Transference: Its Provocation by the Analyst." In *Essays on Otherness*, ed. John Fletcher. London: Routledge, 1999.

————. 1993. "A Short Treatise on the Unconscious." In *Essays on Otherness*, ed. John Fletcher. London: Routledge, 1999.

————. 1999a. "The So-Called 'Death Drive': A Sexual Drive." In *The Death Drive: New Life for a Dead Subject?*, ed. Rob Weatherill. Translated by Luke Thurston. London: Rebus Press, 1999: 40–59. Revised translation by John Fletcher. In *The British Journal of Psychotherapy* 20, no. 4 (2004): 455–71.

————. 1999b. "Notes on Afterwardsness." In *Essays on Otherness*, ed. John Fletcher. London: Routledge, 1999.

————. 1999c. "Sublimation and/or Inspiration." Translated by John Fletcher and Luke Thurston. *New Formations* 48 (Winter 2002–3): 30–50.

————. 1999d. *Essays on Otherness*, ed. John Fletcher. Translated by Luke Thurston, revised by John Fletcher, Leslie Hill and Jean Laplanche. London: Routledge, 1999.

————. 2000a. "Drive and Instinct: Distinctions, Oppositions, Supports and Intertwinings." In *Freud and the Sexual*, ed. John Fletcher. New York: International Psychoanalytic Books, 2011.

————. 2000b. "Sexuality and Attachment in Metapsychology." In *Freud and the Sexual*, ed. John Fletcher. New York: International Psychoanalytic Books, 2011.

————. 2006. *Problématiques VI: L'après-coup*. Paris: Presses Universitaires de France, 2006.

————. 2007. *Freud and the Sexual*, translated by John Fletcher, Jonathan House, Nicholas Ray, ed. John Fletcher. New York: International Psychoanalytic Books, 2011.

Laplanche, Jean, and J-B. Pontalis. "Fantasy and the Origins of Sexuality." 1964. Translated in *International Journal of Psychoanalysis* 49 (1968): 1–18, reprinted in Victor Burgin et al., eds., *Formations of Fantasy*. London: Methuen, 1986, and in Riccardo Steiner, ed., *Unconscious Phantasy*. London: Karnac Books, 2003.

———. 1967. *The Language of Psycho-Analysis*. Translated by Donald Nicholson-Smith. London: The Hogarth Press, 1973.

Leys, Ruth. *Trauma: A Genealogy*. Chicago: University of Chicago Press, 2000.

Lukacher, Ned. *Primal Scenes: Literature, Philosophy, Psychoanalysis*. Ithaca, N.Y.: Cornell University Press, 1986.

Lyotard, Jean-François. "Emma: Between Philosophy and Psychoanalysis." In *Lyotard: Philosophy, Politics and the Sublime*, ed. Hugh J. Silverman. London: Routledge, 2002: 23–45.

Mahony, Patrick. *Cries of the Wolf Man*. New York: International University Press, 1984.

Maïdani-Gerard, Jean-Pierre. *Léonard de Vinci: Mythologie ou Théologie*. Paris: Presses Universitaires de France, 1994.

Makari, George. *Revolution in Mind: The Creation of Psychoanalysis*. New York: HarperCollins, 2008.

Masson, Jeffrey Moussaieff, trans. and ed. 1985a. *The Complete Letters of Sigmund Freud to Wilhelm Fliess 1887–1904*. Cambridge, Mass.: Harvard University Press, 1985.

———. 1985b. *The Assault on Truth: Freud's Suppression of the Seduction Theory*. Harmondsworth: Penguin Books, 1985.

Micale, Mark S. "Hysteria Male/Hysteria Female: Reflections on Comparative Gender Construction in 19th Century France and Britain." In *Science and Sensibility: Gender and Scientific Inquiry, 1780–1945*, ed. Marina Benjamin. Oxford: Basil Blackwell, 1991: 200–39.

———. "On the 'Disappearance' of Hysteria: A Study in the Clinical Deconstruction of a Diagnosis." *Isis* 84 (1993): 496–526.

———. "Charcot and *les névroses traumatiques*: Scientific and Historical Reflections." *Journal of the History of the Neurosciences* 4 (1995): 101–19.

Obholzer, Karin. *The Wolf-Man: Sixty Years Later*. Translated by Michael Shaw. London: Routledge and Kegan Paul, 1982.

Paget, James. "Nervous Mimicry." In *Clinical Lectures and Essays by Sir James Paget, Bart.*, ed. Howard Marsh. London: Longmans, Green and Co., 1875.

Pallanti, Giuseppi. *Mona Lisa: The True Identity of Leonardo's Model*. Translated by Tim Stroud. Milan: Skira Editore, 2006.

Pankejev, Sergei. 1926. "Letters Pertaining to Freud's 'History of an Infantile Neurosis'" *Psychoanalytic Quarterly* 26 (1957): 449–60.

———. 1970. *The Memoirs of the Wolf-Man*. Translated by Muriel Gardiner. In *The Wolf-Man and Sigmund Freud*, ed. Muriel Gardiner. Harmondsworth: Penguin Books, 1973: 15–149.

Pontalis, J-B. "On Deathwork in Freud, in the Self, in Culture." In *Psychoanalysis, Creativity and Literature*, ed. Alan Roland (New York: Columbia University Press, 1978: 85–95.

Rand, Nicholas, and Maria Torok. "The Concept of Psychical Reality and Its Traps." In *Questions for Freud: the Secret History of Psychoanalysis*. Cambridge, Mass.: Harvard University Press, 1997.

Ray, Nicholas. *Tragedy and Otherness: Sophocles, Shakespeare and Psychoanalysis*. Bern: Peter Lang, 2009.

Reynolds, J. Russell. "Remarks on Paralysis, and Other Disorders of Motion and Sensation, Dependent on Idea." *The British Medical Journal* 6 (November 1869): 483–85.

Scarfone, Dominique. 1994. " 'It was *not* my mother': From Seduction to Negation." Translated by John Fletcher. *New Formations* 48 (Winter 2002–3): 69–76..

Schapiro, Meyer. "Freud and Leonardo: An Art Historical Study." *Journal of the History of Ideas* 17, no. 2 (1956): 147–78. Reprinted in Meyer Schapiro. *Theory and Philosophy of Art: Style, Artist and Society*. New York: George Braziller, 1994.

Schimek, Jean G. "Fact and Fantasy in the Seduction Theory: A Historical Review." *Journal of the American Psychoanalytic Association* 35 (1987): 935–67.

Shakespeare, William. 1600. *The Tragedy of Hamlet, Prince of Denmark*. ed. T. J. B. Spencer. London: Penguin Books, 2005.

Sophocles. *Oedipus the King: A Translation with Commentary*. Translated and edited by Thomas Gould. Englewood Cliffs, N.J.: Prentice Hall, 1970.

Starobinski, Jean. "*Hamlet and Oedipus,*" in *The Living Eye*, trans. Arthur Goldhammer. Cambridge, Mass.: Harvard University Press, 1989.

Sulloway, Frank J. *Freud, Biologist of the Mind* (1979), rev. ed. Cambridge, Mass.: Harvard University Press, 1992.

Toubiana, Éric. *L'héritage et sa psychopathologie*. Paris: Presses Universitaires de France, 1988.

Tuke, D. Hack, ed. *A Dictionary of Psychological Medicine*. London: J. & A. Churchill, 1892.

Vernant, Jean–Pierre. "Oedipus without the Complex." In *Myth and Tragedy in Ancient Greece*, ed. J.-P. Vernant and P. Vidal-Nacquet, trans. Janet Lloyd. Cambridge, Mass.: M.I.T. Press, 1988.

Viderman, Serge. *Le Céleste et le Sublunaire*. Paris: Presses Universitaires de France, 1977.

Wilde, Oscar. *The Importance of Being Earnest*. In *The Importance of Being Earnest and Other Plays*, Harmondsworth: Penguin Books, 1954

Wohl, R. Richard, and Harry Trosman. "A Retrospect of Freud's *Leonardo*." *Psychiatry* 18 (1955): 27–39.